Emerging Cancer Therapeutics

Jame Abraham, MD, FACP

Editor-in-Chief

Bonnie Wells Wilson Distinguished Professor and Eminent Scholar
Chief, Section of Hematology-Oncology
Medical Director, Mary Babb Randolph Cancer Center
West Virginia University
Morgantown, West Virginia

Editorial Board

Forthcoming Volumes

Multiple Myeloma
Shaji Kumar, MD, Guest Editor
Mayo Clinic, Rochester, Minnesota

Breast Cancer
Antoinette R. Tan, MD, Guest Editor
The Cancer Institute of New Jersey, New Brunswick, New Jersey

Emerging Cancer Therapeutics

VOLUME 1, ISSUE 1

Gastrointestinal Malignancies

M. Wasif Saif, MD, MBBS
Guest Editor

Associate Professor of Medicine, Medical Oncology
Director, GI Cancers Program
Yale Cancer Center
Yale University School of Medicine
New Haven, Connecticut

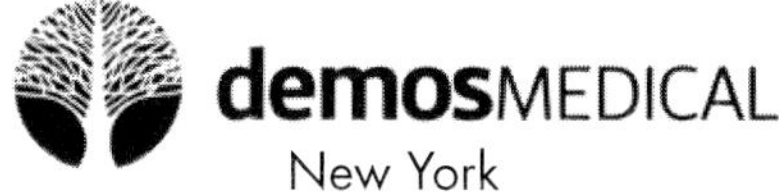

demosMEDICAL
New York

Acquisitions Editor: Richard Winters
Cover Design: Joe Tenerelli
Compositor: NewGen North America
Printer: Hamilton

Visit our website at www.demosmedpub.com

Emerging Cancer Therapeutics is published three times a year by Demos Medical Publishing.

Business Office. All business correspondence including subscriptions, renewals, and address changes should be sent to Demos Medical Publishing, 11 West 42nd Street, 15th Floor, New York, NY, 10036.

Subscription Rates. Volume 1, 2010. For Institutions: $275, For Individuals $225, Single Copy Price: $85. Outside the United States: For Institutions $315, For Individuals $255. Individuals residing outside the United States wishing to purchase individual issues of *Emerging Cancer Therapeutics* should contact their local reseller/agents for pricing and shipping details. Payment must be made in advance by check (in U.S. Dollars drawn on a U.S. bank) or international money order made payable to Demos Medical Publishing, or MasterCard, Visa, or America Express.

The ideas and opinions expressed in *Emerging Cancer Therapeutics* do not necessarily reflect those of the Publisher. The Publisher does not assume any responsibility for any injury and/or damage to persons or property arising out of or related to any use of the material contained in this periodical. The reader is advised to check the appropriate medical literature and the product information currently provided by the manufacturer of each drug to be administered to verify the dosage, the method and duration of administration, or contraindications. It is the responsibility of the treating physician or other health care professional relying on independent experience and knowledge of the patient, to determine drug dosages and the best treatment for the patient. Mention of any product in this issue should not be construed as endorsement by the contributors, editors, or the Publisher of the product or manufacturer's claims.

ISSN: 2151-4194
ISBN: 978-1-933864-90-7

Library of Congress Cataloging-in-Publication Data

Gastrointestinal malignancies / M. Wasif Saif, guest editor.
    p. ; cm. — (Emerging cancer therapeutics ; v. 1, issue 1)
  Includes bibliographical references and index.
  ISBN 978-1-933864-90-7
  1. Digestive organs—Cancer. I. Saif, M. Wasif. II. Series: Emerging cancer therapeutics ; v. 1, issue 1.
  [DNLM: 1. Gastrointestinal Neoplasms. WI 149 G2571 2010]

RC280.D5G3775 2010
616.99'43—dc22

2010002375

Reprints. For copies of 100 or more of articles in this publication, please contact Reina Santana, Special Sales Manager.

Special discounts on bulk quantities of Demos Medical Publishing books are available to corporations, professional associations, pharmaceutical companies, health care organizations, and other qualifying groups. For details, please contact:

Reina Santana, Special Sales Manager
Demos Medical Publishing
11 W. 42nd Street
New York, NY 10036
Phone: 800–532–8663 or 212–683–0072
Fax: 212–941–7842
E-mail: rsantana@demosmedpub.com

Made in the United States of America
10 11 12 13 14   5 4 3 2 1

Contents

Foreword   vii

Preface   ix

Contributors   xi

Screening of Colorectal Cancer   1
M. Wasif Saif

Assessment of KRAS and BRAF Mutations in Metastatic Colorectal Cancer:
A Step Toward Personalized Medicine   9
Richard Kim, Brooke Phillips, and M. Wasif Saif

Esophageal Cancer

    Advances in Surgical Therapy for Esophageal Cancer   19
    Heather Yeo, Amir Shariff, and Charles Cha

    New Developments in Combined-Modality Therapy   37
    Bryan Chang

    New Developments in Radiation Therapy Planning   61
    Bryan Chang

    Chemotherapy and Targeted Agents for Stage IV Cancer   71
    M. Wasif Saif

Gastric Cancer   79
Sobha Kurian, Susan Alsamarai, and M. Wasif Saif

Hepatocellular Cancer   93
Yun Yen, Chiun Hsu, Ann-Lii Cheng, Antonio Arvelakis, M. Wasif Saif, and Sukru Emre

Colorectal Cancer   117
Robert Diasio and M. Wasif Saif

Pancreatic Cancer   139
M. Wasif Saif and Jonathan Knisely

Gastrointestinal Stromal Tumors   151
Bilal Ahmed and Tanios Bekaii-Saab

Current Management of Anal Cancer   165
David Grew, Bryan Chang, and M. Wasif Saif

Small Bowel Adenocarcinoma   173
Jia Li and M. Wasif Saif

Novel and Targeted Agents for Gastrointestinal Tumors   179
Mohammed Almubarak and Michael Newton

Index   189

Foreword

Cancer treatment is one of the fastest growing specialties in modern medicine, with better understanding of the disease, improved diagnostic tools, better prognostic information, and ever-changing management options. The most important tool a clinician can have in the fight against cancer is access to current information.

The Emerging Cancer Therapeutics (ECAT) periodicals provide a thorough analysis of key clinical research related to cancer therapeutics, including a discussion and assessment of current evidence, current clinical best practice, and likely near future developments. The content is in the form of review articles, but the volume format will allow for much more in-depth discussion than the typical journal review article. As a periodical, the content can be dynamic and updated more frequently and regularly than the typical static textbook discussion. The goal is to provide for the practicing clinician a source of thorough ongoing analysis and translational assessment of "hot topics" and areas of rapidly emerging new data in cancer therapeutics with significant implications for clinical care.

Each ECAT issue is a valuable tool for practicing cancer specialists of all disciplines. It provides the most comprehensive evidence-based review of pathology, radiology, pharmacology, surgical oncology, radiation oncology, and medical oncology of the topic.

Gastrointestinal Malignancies provides a comprehensive approach in the pathophysiology, epidemiology, clinical features, diagnostic modalities, and current and future treatment options. Experts from Yale Cancer Center and around the country contributed to this issue. This will be a valuable tool for any clinician, researcher, or student of oncology, and especially gastrointestinal malignancies.

JAME ABRAHAM, MD, FACP
Editor-in-Chief

Bonnie Wells Wilson Distinguished Professor and Eminent Scholar
Chief, Section of Hematology-Oncology
Medical Director, Mary Babb Randolph Cancer Center
West Virginia University
Morgantown, West Virginia

Preface

Gastrointestinal (GI) cancers (i.e., malignancies of the esophagus, stomach, liver, pancreas, colon, and anal canal, and GIST) as a group are common diseases worldwide. About 400,000 patients are diagnosed with esophageal cancer worldwide each year, and nearly 330,000 die from this disease. Approximately 870,000 patients are diagnosed with gastric cancer worldwide; and over 640,000 die from this disease. An additional 940,000 new cases of colorectal cancer are diagnosed yearly and 490,000 patients die from this disease. Although the incidence of cancer of the organs making up the GI tract varies between regions, overall they share some similar promises and problems.

Management options for patients with GI cancers have undergone dramatic changes over the past decade. In addition to newer cytotoxic agents, novel targeted agents have revolutionized the management of few cancers, such as bevacizumab and cetuximab in colon cancer and sorafenib in hepatocellular carcinoma (HCC). Likewise, surgical and ablative options, as well as an array of supportive medications, have shown substantial progress and undergone a dramatic proliferation over the past decade. With the increased number of therapeutic options from which to choose, the clinician is better able to offer effective therapy to the patient with GI cancers. The clinician is challenged, however, to keep up with the rapidly changing landscape and the rapidly emerging data that shape the options for treatment today and tomorrow. In this publication, leaders in the management of colorectal cancer review the current literature that has led us to where we are today. Critical evaluations of the data are offered, and evidence-based recommendations are made.

Gastrointestinal Malignancies provides a comprehensive and in-depth review of this important group of malignancies. The editors and authors are leaders in their fields who have contributed to develop current standards of care. The chapters update the current screening tools for colon cancers, assessment of predictive markers such as K-RAS and BRAF in the management of colon cancer as well as the state-of-the-art for use of both cytotoxic chemotherapy and the incorporation of the newer biological therapies. Last but not the least, multimodality management is emphasized as only this approach can offer the best chance for a favorable outcome to patients with GI cancers.

This book is directed toward all physicians, including medical, radiation, and surgical oncologists, gastroenterologists, internists, and general surgeons, APRNS, nurses, and scientists involved in the management and improvement of outcomes for patients with GI malignancies. The field of GI oncology is advancing rapidly and within these pages we have attempted to provide a state-of-the-art treatment of these cancers and describe the possible pathways that need to be followed to further improve understanding and outcome for patients with GI cancers.

M. Wasif Saif, MD, MBBS

Contributors

Bilal Ahmed, MD
Hematology/Oncology Fellow
Arthur G. James Comprehensive Cancer Center
The Ohio State University
Columbus, Ohio

Mohammed Almubarak, MD
Assistant Professor of Medicine
Section of Hematology/Oncology
Mary Babb Randolph Cancer Center
West Virginia University Hospital
Morgantown, West Virginia

Susan Alsamarai, MD
Fellow
Department of Medical Oncology
Yale Cancer Center
New Haven, Connecticut

Antonios Arvelakis, MD, PhD
Yale New Haven Transplantation Center
New Haven, Connecticut

Tanios Bekaii-Saab, MD
Medical Director, Gastrointestinal Oncology
Assistant Professor of Medicine and
    Pharmacology
The Ohio State University—Arthur James Cancer
    Hospital
Columbus, Ohio

Charles Cha, MD
Surgical Oncology and Gastrointestinal Surgery
Yale Cancer Center
Yale University School of Medicine
New Haven, Connecticut

Bryan Chang, MD
Assistant Professor
Department of Radiation Oncology
Yale Cancer Center
Yale University School of Medicine
New Haven, Connecticut

Ann-Lii Cheng, MD
Department of Oncology
National Taiwan University Hospital
Taipei, Taiwan

Robert Diasio, MD
William J. and Charles H. Mayo Professor
Director, Mayo Clinic Cancer Center
Professor of Molecular Pharmacology and
    Experimental Therapeutics and Oncology
Mayo Clinic
Rochester, Minnesota

Sukru Emre, MD, FACS
Professor of Surgery and Pediatrics
Department of Surgery
Yale New Haven Transplantation Center
Yale University School of Medicine
New Haven, Connecticut

David Grew, MSPH
Tulane University School of Medicine
New Orleans, Louisiana

Chiun Hsu, MD
National Taiwan University Hospital
Taipei, Taiwan

Richard Kim, MD
Clinical Assistant Professor
Department of Solid Tumors
Taussig Cancer Center
Cleveland Clinic
Cleveland, Ohio

Jonathan Knisely, MD
Medical Oncology and Radiation Oncology
Yale Cancer Center
Yale University School of Medicine
New Haven, Connecticut

Sobha Kurian, MD
Associate Professor
Department of Medicine
Section of Hematology/Oncology
Mary Babb Randolph Cancer Center
West Virginia University
Morgantown, West Virginia

Jia Li, MD
Department of Oncology
Yale Cancer Center
Yale University School of Medicine
New Haven, Connecticut

Michael Newton, Pharm D
Assistant Professor, Clinical Pharmacy
West Virginia University School of Pharmacy
Morgantown, West Virginia

Brooke Phillips, MD
Taussig Cancer Center
Cleveland Clinic
Cleveland, Ohio

M. Wasif Saif, MD, MBBS
Associate Professor of Medicine, Medical Oncology
Director, GI Cancers Program
Yale Cancer Center
Yale University School of Medicine
New Haven, Connecticut

Amir Shariff, MD
Resident, Department of Surgery
Yale Cancer Center
Yale University School of Medicine
New Haven, Connecticut

Heather Yeo, MD
Resident, Department of Surgery
Yale Cancer Center
Yale University School of Medicine
New Haven, Connecticut

Yun Yen, MD, PhD, FACP
Allen and Lee Chao Endowed Chair in
    Developmental Cancer Therapeutics
Attending Physician of Medical Oncology
Professor and Director of Clinical and Molecular
    Pharmacology
Associate Director for Translational Research,
    Comprehensive Cancer Center
City of Hope
Duarte, California

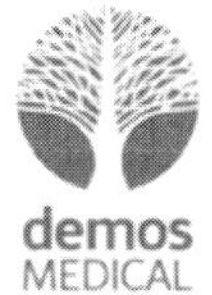

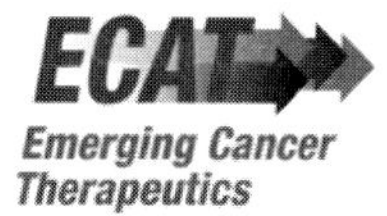

Screening of Colorectal Cancer

M. Wasif Saif*

Yale University School of Medicine, New Haven, CT

■ ABSTRACT

Colorectal cancer (CRC) is the second most common cancer in the United States. The average person's lifetime risk of developing it is about 6–7%. The risk is increased if there is a family history of colorectal polyps or cancer, and is still higher if there is a personal history of breast, uterine or ovarian cancer. Risk is also higher for people with a history of extensive inflammatory bowel disease, such as ulcerative or Crohn's colitis. CRC is commonly known as a "silent" disease, because many people do not develop symptoms, such as bleeding or abdominal pain until the cancer is at an advanced stage. On the other hand, if colorectal cancer is found at an early stage, treatment can lead to cure arte of over 80%. Simple screening is available and should be done in all people staring at an age based on the risk factors or those having symptoms and/or a family history of colorectal cancer. For people who have none of the known risks, digital rectal examination and testing of the stool for hidden blood are recommended annually beginning at age 40. Flexible sigmoidoscopy is recommended every 5 years at age 50 or older. A double contrast barium enema every 5 to 10 years, and colonoscopy every 10 years are acceptable alternatives. This article will focus on the current guidelines of the screening of colorectal cancer and discusses development of newer methods, including stool DNA.

■ INTRODUCTION

Colorectal cancer (CRC) is a major public problem, accounting for approximately 150,000 new cases annually in the United States. More than one-third of these cases will end in death, making CRC the third most common cancer in men and women and accounting for 10% of all cancer deaths in the country (1).

CRC is not biased by gender and affects nearly as many women as men (75,000 and 79,000 cases annually, respectively) (1). The incidence of CRC is likely to increase over time owing to the growing geriatric segment of the population. By 2010, more than 40% of the population will be older than age 50 (2), further confounding the screening challenge associated with this cancer.

■ RISK FACTORS

Approximately 10% to 30% of cases have a family history of CRC, 5% to 8% of cases are associated with hereditary nonpolyposis CRC, 1% of cases have familial adenomatous polyposis, and 65% to 70%

*Corresponding author, Associate Professor of Medicine, Medical Oncology Director, GI Cancers Program, Yale University Center, Yale University School of Medicine, New Haven, CT
E-mail address: Wasif.saif@yale.edu

Emerging Cancer Therapeutics 1 (2010) 01–08.

DOI: 10.5003/2151–4194.1.1.1

of cases result sporadically (Fig. 1) (3). If detected early, however, the survival rate could be as high as 95% (1). The National Polyp Study determined conclusively that relatives of patients with adenomatous polyps have the highest risk of developing CRC (4).

- Annual fecal occult blood testing (FOBT)
- Flexible sigmoidoscopy (FS) every 5 years
- Annual FOBT plus FS every 5 years
- Double-contrast barium enema (DCBE) every 5 years
- Colonoscopy every 10 years

■ EARLY SCREENING INCREASES SURVIVAL

Screening is essential to permit prevention (via polyp removal) and early detection of this cancer. Winawer et al. concluded that the first screening colonoscopy and polypectomy is most effective at reducing the incidence of CRC in patients with adenomatous polyps (4). CRC is most deadly when discovered at an advanced stage. Studies in the United States, United Kingdom, Denmark, and Sweden have shown that the incidence of patients developing stage IV disease could be greatly decreased by implementing screening methods for CRC. Earlier detection and better management of disease improved survival in CRC patients in Denmark between 1977 and 1999 (5). In the EUROCARE studies, a deficit in CRC survival was noted in Denmark and the United Kingdom compared with Sweden, Norway, and Finland (6). The increased mortality was attributed to inadequate patient management, poor diagnostic capabilities, and comorbidities.

Fecal Occult Blood Test

Fecal occult blood test (FOBT) is noninvasive; bowel preparation is not required, and the examination can be conducted by family practitioners in their offices. This test is cost-effective; however, FOBT requires annual testing and multiple sample testing. Patients with intermediate or small adenomas do not necessarily bleed either intermittently or at all; thus, FOBT might not be thorough enough to detect small cancers. It is also important to note that the dietary restrictions required for the test can lead to a false negative. There are two major technologies that are available to perform the FOBT: the first is guaiac based, and the second is immunologically based, using the antibody directed against the protein moiety. The latter option is more specific and more sensitive than the guaiac-based FOBT for occult blood. At this time, none of the guidelines has recommended one method over the other.

■ CURRENT SCREENING OPTIONS

There are multiple options for screening CRC. The recommended strategies (7) for persons of average risk include:

Flexible Sigmoidoscopy

The flexible sigmoidoscopy (FS) is an office-based procedure that requires a technician and not necessarily a gastroenterologist. This test is more

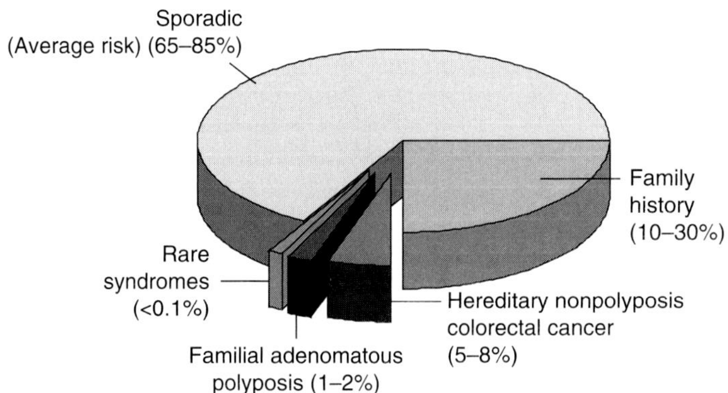

FIGURE 1 Colorectal cancer risk groups. (Adapted from Ref. 3.)

effective than FOBT and does not require sedation. Preparation for this test is easier than it is for a colonoscopy. The FS also carries a risk of perforation (1 in 10,000) and it is less effective (and less comfortable) than a colonoscopy because it does not examine all parts of the colon.

Single-Contrast Barium Enema (SCBE)

The single contrast barium enema (SCBE) test has poor sensitivity compared with endoscopy and very poor patient tolerance. The optimal interval that should be performed with regard to follow-up screenings with the DCBE has not been determined. In addition, radiologists are less experienced in interpreting results of the DCBE.

Colonoscopy

Finally, colonoscopy is currently the most accurate test available, not only for CRC but also for polyps, with a sensitivity ranging from 90% to 95%. This test has both diagnostic and therapeutic value. It provides the longest protective interval (every 10 years in patients with an average risk) and has been shown to reduce CRC mortality based on indirect evidence (8) and has resulted in higher patient satisfaction than sigmoidoscopy, despite the extensive bowel preparation and possible limitation of activities resulting from sedation. Colonoscopy, however, is also very expensive and a high-risk procedure (diagnostic perforation risk, 0.03% to 0.61%; therapeutic perforation risk, 0.07% to 0.72%) (9). In addition, the endoscopist might not detect flat lesions and lesions obscured by suboptimal bowel preparation.

Virtual Colonoscopy

Computed tomographic (CT) colonography (also known as virtual colonoscopy) is a less-invasive imaging technique. This procedure takes only 10 minutes and does not require sedation. CT colonography has been shown to have a high sensitivity and specificity for polyps ≥10 mm (10).

A key factor in the efficacy of CT colonography seems to be whether primary 2D or primary 3D evaluation is used. In late 2007, Pickhardt et al. reported the results of a study that evaluated several large CT colonography trials (10). At the ≥6-mm polyp size threshold, 2D sensitivity was 44.1%, compared with 3D sensitivity of 85.7% (P = 0.001); at the ≥10-mm polyp size threshold, 2D sensitivity was 75%, compared with 3D sensitivity of 92.2% (P = 0.027). However, there was little difference in by-patient specificity: the 2D evaluation at the ≥10-mm threshold level was 98.1%, compared with 97.4% for the 3D evaluation (P = 0.336). The researchers also noted that another critical difference for obtaining improved sensitivity and specificity was the use of oral contrast tagging (10).

The risk of perforation with CT colonography is very low, though reports vary as to how low the risk actually is. Sosna et al. conducted a review of all patients who underwent CT colonography in 11 medical centers between the beginning of 2001 and the end of 2004. Out of 11,870 CT colonographies, there were 7 colorectal perforations, yielding a rate of 0.059% (11). A survey conducted by the Working Group on Virtual Colonoscopy evaluated 21,923 CT colonography studies performed between 1997 and 2005; there were only 2 perforations (12).

Besides low perforation rate, another benefit of CT colonography is that same-day colonoscopy can be performed in these patients because of the required bowel preparation. Also, while the CT scan is being conducted, patients can also be examined for other tumors.

The limitations of CT colonography include bowel preparation, scheduling, high cost, nonuniform results, lack of coverage by managed care organizations, additional requirement for a colonoscopy in the presence of an abnormality, such as polyps, and lack of support in guidelines.

■ SCREENING

Compliance and Conduction

Unfortunately, far fewer colonoscopies are conducted compared with mammography (13) (Fig. 2). A 1998 National Health Interview survey revealed that far fewer patients undergo either FOBT or sigmoidoscopy (10%–20% of patients, respectively) compared with mammograms (70% of women). In addition, far fewer women than men undergo either FOBT or sigmoidoscopy.

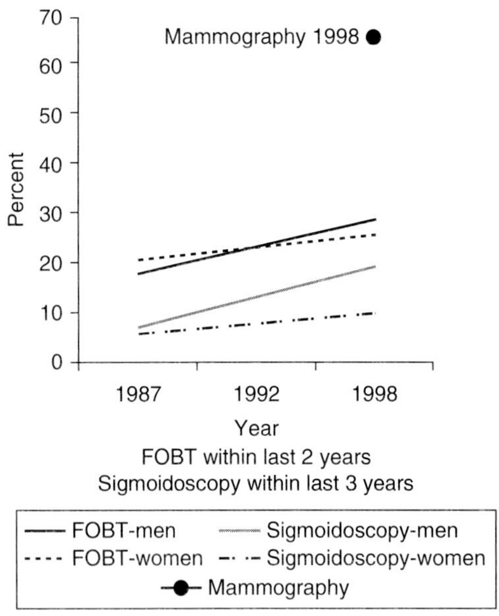

FIGURE 2 Colorectal cancer screening performance. (Adapted from Ref. 13.)

The American Cancer Society conducted a survey in 1998 to determine why patients did not undergo screening for CRC. Unfortunately, 88% of persons surveyed claimed that "it was not recommended by my doctor." It is a major responsibility of physicians to bring screening to the patient's attention, especially those over the age of 50. In addition, it is imperative to recommend the right method of screening for these patients and explain the procedure and what to expect. Patients should also be alerted that the removal of any polyps will necessitate additional screening for further evaluation.

Several screening campaigns have been conducted by the National Cancer Institute, the American Cancer Society, and the American Digestive Health Foundation, which seek to improve awareness and performance of screening for CRC in the United States.

In 2000, Medicare reimbursement was approved for FOBT and FS. This was followed in 2001 by Medicare's approval for screening colonoscopy. Screening for CRC is less than $20,000 per life saved, which is equivalent to the cost-effectiveness of conducting mammograms in breast cancer patients. Thus, the call to action is to screen patients for CRC.

Barriers to Screening

Lack of screening is a result of several factors. Cultural and economic disparities likely play a role in underscreening among African American patients compared with Hispanic, Asian, or white patients. Consequently, CRC is often diagnosed at a later stage in these patients. In one study, African American men were 25% less likely to undergo colonoscopy and 50% less likely to undergo testing with a flexible sigmoidoscope than were white patients (14). Disparities in outcomes among minority patients underscore the need for improving their access to care.

Lack of screening might also be related to lack of discussion about cancer between physicians and patients. Patients may be unaware of their risks or doubtful of the effectiveness of the methods examined here, or perhaps physicians are not clear about recommending testing for their patients. Other barriers to screening include poor acceptance by patients, underuse by providers, limited access resulting from capacity constraints, lack of insurance coverage, geographical limitations, high costs, and lack of understanding of the tests themselves.

To overcome these barriers, it is important to develop screening technologies that are more patient-friendly, less burdensome, and less invasive. Physician recommendations for screening must be increased as should public awareness of the need for screening, especially among those who are at high risk for CRC. In addition, a more effective support system should be established to help patients adhere to screening test orders and increase the consistency of repeat screening.

■ ETHNIC DISPARITIES

Recognizing that the incidence and mortality of CRC are greater in African Americans than whites, the American College of Gastroenterology (ACG) recommended in 2005 that African Americans be screened at the age of 45 years rather than 50 years (15). In its statement, the ACG reported that the mean age of CRC development in African Americans is younger than that of whites; moreover, there is a more proximal colonic distribution of cancers and adenomas among African Americans. The ACG urged gastroenterologists to take the lead in educating primary care physicians and developing culturally sensitive programs about CRC for African Americans (15).

■ FUTURE TECHNOLOGIES

Molecular diagnostics might help resolve some of the hesitancy among patients for screening. This technique takes advantage of the known genetic and epigenetic changes associated with CRC and polyp formation.

Stool DNA

A biologic rationale has been made with regard to DNA testing of the stool, based on the association between genetic alterations, CRC, and polyps; DNA is shed continuously and is stable in the stool, where it can be kept stable after collection. In a genetic model of CRC, a lag time has been demonstrated between late adenoma and early cancer of approximately 5 to 10 years (Fig. 3) (16), which can serve as an optimal phase for detection.

Stool-based DNA provides an assessment of the total colon. It is safe and noninvasive, does not require bowel preparation, and does not need stool manipulation. The test can be done every 3 years or alternated with other methods. Quality assurance can be maintained by centralizing analysis to provide high quality control. The test is not only convenient, but also cost-effective, ranging from $4000 to $14,000 quarterly (16,17). The stool-based DNA test is estimated to have a sensitivity of 65% to 70% (specificity 95%). In a recent study of version 1.1

panel on 40 patients with CRC and 122 normal patients, the test showed a sensitivity of 73% and a specificity of 89%. Version 2.0 panel showed a sensitivity of 88% and a specificity of 82% (18). This method, however, is less effective than colonoscopy and is not yet broadly covered by managed care organizations, nor is it covered in guidelines.

Several new technologies are emerging, including the supersensitive high-throughput molecular techniques: digital polymerase chain reaction and digital protein truncation assay.

Blood-Based Tests

In addition, blood-based tests are also being developed that target newly identified nuclear matrix proteins, cancer-associated metabolites, and circulating DNA. Imaging technology such as the colon version of the small intestinal *pill camera* is also being developed. Thus far, digital methods are more sensitive and provide more accurate quantification and genotyping. Conversely, they are more labor-intensive and expensive.

APC Stool Test

An adenomatous polyposis coli (APC) stool test has also been developed. This study requires no special bowel preparation or diet. In a study by Traverso

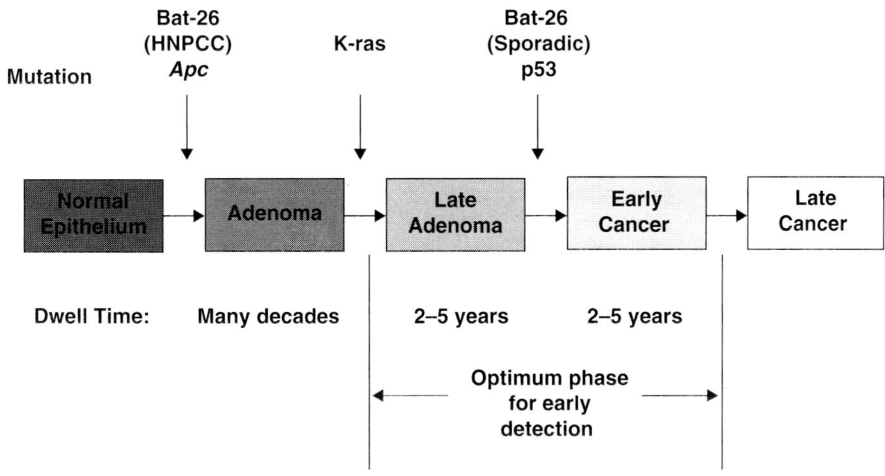

FIGURE 3 Genetic model of colorectal cancer. (Adapted from Ref. 16.)

and colleagues, stool samples were collected from 28 patients with early CRC disease, 18 patients with adenomas ≥1 cm in diameter, and 28 disease-free controls with confirmed negative colonoscopies (19). APC mutations were found in 26 of the 46 patients (57%) with neoplasia, including Duke's B CRC adenomas. None of the 28 controls had the APC mutation, whereas mutant APC genes made up 0.4% to 14.1% of all APC genes in the stool of patients with adenomas. The theoretical maximum sensitivity of this test was determined to be 75%. The remaining 25% undetectable sensitivity can be overcome by overlaying other fecal DNA assays such as BAT26 and PIK3CA.

Circulating Mutant APC Molecules

Blood tests, such as circulating mutant APC molecules, have also been developed. Approximately 63% of patients with Duke's A and B disease were found to have 0.04% and 1.28% APC DNA molecules, respectively, whereas 100% of patients with Duke's D disease had 8.05% mutant APC DNA molecules (20).

CRC Antigen

CRC antigen has been developed through the proteomic method. Two independent epitopes of novel colon cancer-specific antigen (CCSA)—CCSA-3 and CCSA-4—have been found. Both are highly specific and sensitive for detecting CRC and advanced adenomas. These antigens can be assayed through the serum enzyme-linked immunosorbent assay (ELISA). A recent study has shown that mapping CCSA-3 and CCSA-4 together can increase the sensitivity of the test to almost 91% (21).

■ SUMMARY

In short, the best screening is the one that can be done and can get done. Physicians should open discussions on screening with their patients and explore with them the most effective and cost-effective methods. Patients and their physicians should further be encouraged to follow up on results. In the near future, tests for CRC will be simpler and more accurate in identifying high-risk patients and detecting

CRC at earlier stages of disease. Doing so will not only reduce the burden on resources but also increase knowledge of the biology of CRC.

■ REFERENCES

1. American Cancer Society. Cancer Facts & Figures 2007. Atlanta, GA: American Cancer Society; 2007. http://www.cancer.org/downloads/STT/CAFF2007PWSecured.p Accessed February 4, 2008.
2. Metropolitan Area Planning Council. Population Projection 2010–2030. http://www.mapc.org/data_gis/data_center/2006_Projections/Projection_Pop_013106.pdf. Accessed February 12, 2008.
3. Winawer SJ, Schottenfeld D, Flehinger BJ. Colorectal cancer screening. *J Natl Cancer Inst* 1991;83(4):243–253.
4. Winawer SJ, Zauber AG, Fletcher RH, et al. Guidelines for colonoscopy surveillance after polypectomy: a consensus update by the US Multi-Society Task Force on Colorectal Cancer and the American Cancer Society. *CA Cancer J Clin* 2006;56(3):143–59; quiz 184.
5. Iversen LH, Pedersen L, Riis A, Friis S, Laurberg S, Sørensen HT. Population-based study of short- and long-term survival from colorectal cancer in Denmark, 1977–1999. *Br J Surg* 2005;92(7):873–880.
6. Engholm G, Kejs AM, Brewster DH, et al. Colorectal cancer survival in the Nordic countries and the United Kingdom: excess mortality risk analysis of 5 year relative period survival in the period 1999 to 2000. *Int J Cancer* 2007;121(5):1115–1122.
7. Byers T, Levin B, Rothenberger D, Dodd GD, Smith RA. American Cancer Society guidelines for screening and surveillance for early detection of colorectal polyps and cancer: update 1997. American Cancer Society Detection and Treatment Advisory Group on Colorectal Cancer. *CA Cancer J Clin* 1997;47(3):154–160.
8. Winawer S, Fletcher R, Rex D, et al. Gastrointestinal Consortium Panel. Colorectal cancer screening and surveillance: clinical guidelines and rationale-Update based on new evidence. *Gastroenterology* 2003;124(2):544–560.
9. U.S. Preventive Task Force. Screening for Colorectal Cancer: Recommendations and Rationale. Rockville, MD: Agency for Healthcare Research and Quality; 2002.
10. Pickhardt PJ, Lee AD, Taylor AJ, et al. Primary 2D versus primary 3D polyp detection at screening CT colonography. *AJR Am J Roentgenol* 2007;189(6):1451–1456.
11. Sosna J, Blachar A, Amitai M, et al. Colonic perforation at CT colonography: assessment of risk in a multicenter large cohort. *Radiology* 2006;239(2):457–463.
12. Pickhardt PJ. Incidence of colonic perforation at CT colonography: review of existing data and implications for screening of asymptomatic adults. *Radiology* 2006;239(2):313–316.
13. Subramanian S, Amonkar MM, Hunt TL. Use of colonoscopy for colorectal cancer screening: evidence

from the 2000 National Health Interview Survey. *Cancer Epidemiol Biomarkers Prev* 2005;14(2):409–416.

14. Richards RJ, Reker DM. Racial differences in use of colonoscopy, sigmoidoscopy, and barium enema in Medicare beneficiaries. *Dig Dis Sci* 2002;47(12):2715–2719.

15. Agrawal S, Bhupinderjit A, Bhutani MS, et al. Committee of Minority Affairs and Cultural Diversity, American College of Gastroenterology. Colorectal cancer in African Americans. *Am J Gastroenterol* 2005;100(3):515–23; discussion 514.

16. Parekh M, Fendrick AM, Ladabaum U. As tests evolve and costs of cancer care rise: reappraising stool-based screening for colorectal neoplasia. *Aliment Pharmacol Ther* 2008;27(8):697–712.

17. Ness RM, Holmes AM, Klein R, Dittus R. Cost-utility of one-time colonoscopic screening for colorectal cancer at various ages. *Am J Gastroenterol* 2000;95(7):1800–1811.

18. Itzkowitz SH, Jandorf L, Brand R, et al. Improved fecal DNA test for colorectal cancer screening. *Clin Gastroenterol Hepatol* 2007;5(1):111–117.

19. Traverso G, Shuber A, Levin B, et al. Detection of APC mutations in fecal DNA from patients with colorectal tumors. *N Engl J Med* 2002;346(5):311–320.

20. Diehl F, Li M, Dressman D, et al. Detection and quantification of mutations in the plasma of patients with colorectal tumors. *Proc Natl Acad Sci USA* 2005;102(45):16368–16373.

21. Leman ES, Schoen RE, Weissfeld JL, et al. Initial analyses of colon cancer-specific antigen (CCSA)-3 and CCSA-4 as colorectal cancer-associated serum markers. *Cancer Res* 2007;67(12):5600–5605.

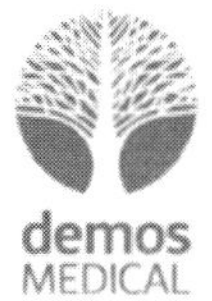

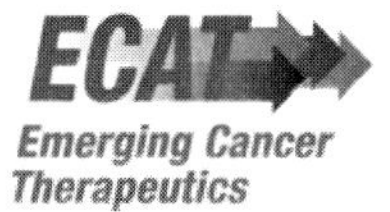

Assessment of KRAS and BRAF Mutations in Metastatic Colorectal Cancer: A Step Toward Personalized Medicine

Richard Kim[a]*, Brooke Phillips[a], and M. Wasif Saif[b]

[a]Taussig Cancer Center, Cleveland Clinic, Cleveland, OH
[b]Yale Cancer Center, Yale University School of Medicine, New Haven, CT

■ ABSTRACT

Discovery of biomarkers that would predict response to certain drugs now have become big part of treatment of metastatic colorectal cancer (mCRC). KRAS mutations are found up to 40 % and BRAF mutations are found up to 10% in patients with mCRC. Mutations in KRAS and BRAF appear to be mutually exclusive. From recent trials, predictive role of KRAS has been well validated. On the other hand, available data for BRAF mutations predicting response to anti epidermal growth factor receptor (anti-EGFR) therapy is limited by retrospective analysis and small numbers of patients with BRAF mutations.

Other than KRAS and BRAF, there are other potential targets/pathways in treatment of mCRC such as Insulin Growth Factor -1 Receptor (IGF-1R) or mammalian target of rapamycin(mTOR) pathway. In the future comprehensive dissection of the EGFR or other signaling pathways maybe needed to select appropriate therapies for mCRC patients.

■ INTRODUCTION

The advent of target-specific cancer therapeutics has remarkably improved the outcomes of patients with colorectal cancer (CRC). Commercially there are three monoclonal antibodies that are FDA approved in the treatment of advanced CRC. Cetuximab (Erbitux, Bristol-Myers Squibb) and panitumumab (Vectibix, Amgen) are monoclonal antibodies against epidermal growth factor receptor (EGFR) and bevacizumab (Avastin, Genentech) is a monoclonal antibody against vascular endothelial growth factor (VEGF) receptor. The molecular mechanisms underlying the clinical response to these drugs are not fully understood. Recent studies have shed some light on the effect of intracellular signaling pathways involving KRAS and BRAF on the safety and efficacy of the above drugs. In this chapter, we will review the association of KRAS and other important pathways and their clinical implication in the treatment of metastatic colorectal cancer (mCRC).

---

*Corresponding author, Taussig Cancer Center, Cleveland Clinic, Cleveland, OH

E-mail address: KIMR3@ccf.org

Emerging Cancer Therapeutics 1 (2010) 09–18.

DOI: 10.5003/2151–4194.1.1.9

■ EGFR

EGFR is a receptor tyrosine kinase and is composed of an extracellular ligand binding domain, a lipophilic transmembrane domain, and an intracellular tyrosine kinase domain. EGFR is the link between the extracellular space and the intracellular signal transduction, which regulates nuclear process involved in cell growth, differentiation, survival, cell cycle progression, and angiogenesis (1). Immunohistochemistry (IHC) of colorectal tumors indicates that EGFR protein expression occurs in 60% to 80% of colorectal tumors (2). The Bowel Oncology with Cetuximab Antibody (BOND) study, which compared irinotecan plus cetuximab with cetuximab alone in irinotecan-refractory patients, showed response rates were 22.9% and 10.8% in the combination and monotherapy group, respectively (3). Entry criteria for this study required EGFR expression by IHC in the primary tumor or metastatic lesion. From the BOND study, it was determined that the degree of EGFR expression determined by staining intensity or percentage of staining cells did not correlate with response. In addition, studies have shown a response rate of up to 25% in EGFR-negative colorectal patients indicating that analysis of IHC does not have predictive value (4,5).

Evidence from several studies has indicated that EGFR gene amplification as determined by EGFR gene copy number (GCN) is associated with clinical response (6–9). Other studies were not able to reproduce these results (5,10). The discrepant results can be explained by the lack of standardization in EGFR GCN measurement. Studies have used fluorescence in situ hybridization (FISH), chromogenic in situ hybridization (CISH), and polymerase chain reaction (PCR); the comparability of these methods is not defined. Thus, standardization and further studies need to be performed before the utility of EGFR gene amplification in CRC can be determined.

■ KRAS

KRAS protein is a GTPase and is an early player in many signal transduction pathways. KRAS is usually tethered to cell membranes because of the presence of an isoprenyl group on its C-terminus (11). It acts as a molecular on/off switch: once it is turned on it recruits and activates proteins necessary for the propagation of growth factor and other receptors' signal, such as c-Raf and PI 3-kinase. When EGFR pathway is activated, small G-protein RAS, which in concert with the protein kinase RAF activates the mitogen-activated protein kinase cascade (12).

KRAS mutations are found in up to 40 % of CRC tumors (13). Point mutations have been identified most commonly in codons 12 and 13 of the KRAS gene and less commonly in codon 61 (14). These mutations occur early in the course of oncogenesis and are preserved throughout the course of tumor progression. There is preclinical evidence that KRAS mutations are a predictor of resistance to EGFR therapy and are associated with a worse prognosis (7).

■ IMPORTANCE OF KRAS IN DETERMINING RESPONSE TO ANTICANCER DRUGS IN COLORECTAL CANCER

There are many randomized controlled trials of cetuximab or panitumumab with or without bevacizumab, which have evaluated outcomes for patients with metastatic colorectal carcinoma harboring KRAS mutation (15,16) (Table 1).

Cetuximab and KRAS

The phase III CRYSTAL trial evaluated the efficacy of irinotecan-based regimen with or without cetuximab in first-line advanced CRC (17). The results showed that the cetuximab plus FOLFIRI arm had superior median progression-free survival (PFS) compared to FOLIRI arm alone (8.9 vs 8 months; $P = .0479$). A retrospective analysis of this study looked at the impact of KRAS status. In patients with a wild-type KRAS, the addition of cetuximab to FOLFIRI significantly improved the median PFS to 9.9 months ($P = .017$) as well as the overall response rate (ORR) to 59% ($P = .0025$). However, patients with mutant KRAS did not derive any clinical benefit with the addition of cetuximab.

Similarly a first-line phase II study using oxaliplatin-based regimen with or without cetuximab came to similar conclusion (18). Primary endpoint was response rate (RR) and there was a trend toward high response rate (45.6% vs 35.7%; $P = .063$) in the cetuximab-containing arm. A retrospective analysis of the study investigated 233 patients who were evaluable for KRAS status. In patients with wild-type KRAS, the addition of cetuximab to FOLFOX resulted in a longer median PFS ($P = .016$) and a significant improvement in ORR ($P = .011$). Patients with mutant KRAS getting cetuximab had a decreased median PFS compared to the control (5.5 vs 8.6 months; $P = .0192$) and a trend toward decrease in ORR (32.7% vs 48.9%; $P = .106$).

Anther phase III trial by Karapetis et al. evaluated the link between cetuximab and KRAS status (19). In this trial, patients who were heavily pre-treated were randomized to cetuximab alone or best supportive care (BSC). In this trial, 394 of 572 patients (68.9%) with CRC had KRAS mutational status analyzed. In patients with wild-type KRAS tumors, treatment with cetuximab as compared with supportive care alone significantly improved overall survival (median, 9.5 vs 4.8 months; $P < 0.001$) and PFS (median, 3.7 months vs 1.9 months; $P < 0.001$). Among patients with mutated KRAS tumors, there was no significant difference between those two groups.

Panitumumab and KRAS

A phase III trial compared panitumumab, a fully human monoclonal antibody directed against the EGFR, plus BSC to that of BSC alone in patients with mCRC who progressed after standard chemotherapy (20). In this trial, there was PFS benefit (8 vs 7.3 weeks; $P < .0001$) in the panitumumab arm but there was difference in overall survival (OS) as crossover was allowed in this study. Then Amado and colleagues examined the KRAS status and the effectiveness of panitumumab (21). In the group of patients receiving panitumumab, benefits were only seen in patients with wild-type KRAS shown by the increase in PFS (12.3 vs 7.3 weeks $P < .0001$) and OS (8.1 vs 7 months).

Another similar study by Hecht et al. looked at interaction of KRAS status and efficacy of panitumumab in chemorefractory mCRC patients with low (1%–9%) or negative (<1%) EGFR tumor cell expression by IHC (22). In this study there was response observed to panitumumab in both EGFR negative and EGFR low cohorts. When KRAS analysis was examined, there was clear advantage to patients with wild-type KRAS as PFS (15 vs 7.1 months) and OS (54.0 vs 29.1 months), both doubled compared with KRAS mutant population.

Bevacizumab and KRAS

Bevacizumab is a monoclonal antibody to VEGF, which has shown PFS and overall survival benefit in combination with irinotecan- or oxaliplatin-based regimen (23,24). The correlation between KRAS status and bevacizumab was evaluated retrospectively by Hurwitz et al. (25). KRAS status was assessed in 230 patients in a phase III trial in which patients were randomized to irinotecan, fluorouracil, and leucovorin (IFL) in combination with either bevacizumab or placebo. The median PFS was significantly longer in bevacizumab-treated patients with wild-type (13.5 vs 7.4 months; $P < .0001$) and mutant KRAS (9.3 vs 5.5 months; $P = .0008$). Also there was a trend toward OS regardless of KRAS status. Thus, it can be concluded that KRAS testing is not warranted in patient selection for treatment of mCRC patients with bevacizumab.

■ DUAL BIOLOGIC THERAPY

There are at least two phase III trials that have looked at dual biologic therapy (anti-VEGF and anti-EGFR). A large phase III study known as the Panitumumab Advanced Colorectal Cancer Evaluation (PACCE) study investigated the role of panitumumab in first-line therapy of mCRC (26). Patients were randomized to FOLFOX or FOLIRI with bevacizumab with or without panitumumab. Results showed that addition of panitumumab to FOLFOX in combination with bevacizumab worsened PFS and increased toxicity. A retrospective analysis of tumor samples available for KRAS mutation analysis revealed that 57 of 103 patients (55%) treated in the panitumumab arm and 58 of 97 (60%) patients in the control arm had wild-type KRAS. As expected, the response was lower in the panitumumab arm among patients with a mutant KRAS relative to those in the control arm (30% vs 38%). In patients with wild-type KRAS, the response rate was higher in the panitumumab arm compared with the control arm (54% vs 47%). Thus, looking at the impact of KRAS status on outcome, these results were consistent with previous trials.

CAIRO 2 was a randomized phase III trial, which also investigated the efficacy of dual therapy in the treatment of mCRC (27). In this trial, patients were randomized to capecitabine, oxaliplatin, and bevacizumab, with or without cetuximab. The addition of cetuximab did not alter OS (20.3 vs 20.4 months; $P = .21$) or RR (44% vs 44%; $P = .88$).

TABLE 1 Clinical trial evidence of the response of anti-EGFR monoclonal antibodies as related to KRAS mutational status

			KRAS Wild Type		KRAS Mutated	
Reference	Treatment	Variable	Antibody Arm	Control Arm	Antibody Arm	Control Arm
Van Cutsem et al.	FOLFIRI ± cetuximab	No of patients	172	176	105	87
CRYSTAL (17)		Response rate,%	59.3	43.2	36.2	40.2
		P-value	0.0025		0.46	
	First line	Median PFS, months	9.9	8.7	7.6	8.1
		P-value	0.017		0.47	
Bokemeyer et al.	FOLFOX ± cetuximab	No of patients	61	73	52	47
OPUS (18)		Response rate,%	61	37	33	49
		P-value	0.011		0.106	
	First line	Median PFS, months	7.7	7.2	5.5	8.6
		HR; P-value	0.57; $P = .016$		1.83; $P = .0192$	
Karapetis et al. (19)	Cetuximab vs. supportive care	No of patients	117	113	81	83
		Response rate,%	13	0	0	0
		Median PFS months	3.7	1.9	1.8	1.8
	Chemorefractory	HR	0.4		0.99	
		95% CI; P-value	0.3–0.54; $P<.001$		0.73–1.35; $P = .96$	
		HR for death	0.55		0.98	
		95% CI; P-value	0.41–0.74; $P<.001$		0.70–1.37; $P = .89$	

Amado et al. (21)	Panitumumab vs. supportive care	No of patients	124	119	84	100
		Response rate, %	17	0	0	0
		Median PFS, weeks	12.3	7.3	7.4	7.3
	Chemorefractory	HR; *P*-value	0.45; <0.0001		0.99	
Hecht et al. (22)	Panitumumab	No. of patients	94	N/A	76	N/A
		Median PFS, months	15		7.1	
	Chemorefractory	OS, months	54		29	
Hurwitz et al. (25)	Irinotecan, fluorouracil, leucovorin, ± bevacizumab	No of patients	85	67	44	34
		Response rate, %	60	37	43	41
		Median PFS, months	13.5	7.4	9.3	5.5
		P-value	0.0001		0.0008	
	First line	OS, months	27.7	17.6	19.9	13.6
		P-value	0.04		0.26	
Hecht et al.	FOLFOX or FOLFIRI ± bevacizumab ± panitumumab First line	No. of patients	57	58	46	39
PACCE study (26)		Response rate, %	54	47	30	38

continued

TABLE 1 Clinical trial evidence of the response of anti-EGFR monoclonal antibodies as related to KRAS mutational status (continued)

Reference	Treatment	Variable	KRAS Wild Type		KRAS Mutated	
			Antibody Arm	Control Arm	Antibody Arm	Control Arm
Tol et al.	Capecitabine, oxaliplatin, bevacizumab, ± cetuximab	Response rate, %	44		44	
CAIRO2 study (27)		Median PFS, months	10.5	10.7	8.7	12.5
		P-value	0.1		0.043	
		Median OS, months	22.2	23	19.1	24.9
		P-value	0.49		0.35	

CRYSTAL, cetuximab combined with irinotecan in first-line therapy for metastatic colorecal cancer; FOLFIRI, fluorouracil, leucovorin, and irinotecan; PFS, progression-free survival; OPUS, oxaliplatin and cetuximab in first-line therapy for mCRC; FOLFOX, fluorouracil, leucovorin, and oxaliplatin; HR, hazard ratio; CI, confernece interval; OS, overall survival; PACCE, Panitumumab Advanced Colorectal Cancer Evaluation Study; CAIRO2, capecitabine, oxaliplatin, and bevacizumab with or without cetuximab in first-line advanced colorectal cancer.

Subset analysis was done to determine outcome depending on the KRAS status. Interestingly, in patients with wild-type KRAS there was no difference in PFS or OS. However, patients with KRAS mutant tumor who received cetuximab had shorter median PFS (8.6 months) than patients who received no cetuximab (12.5 months; P = .043).

■ BRAF

BRAF is a protein which is involved in sending signals within cells and has a role in cell growth. It is also a principal downstream effector of KRAS. Even though oncogenic activation of KRAS has been studied somewhat extensively, BRAF has been only marginally investigated. There are data showing that BRAF mutation in the primary tumor carries a poor prognosis, regardless of the specific treatment regimen (28). Also BRAF mutations account for a measurable fraction of patients whose wild-type KRAS tumors do not respond to cetuximab or panitumumab. The V600E is the most common oncogenic mutation of BRAF in cancer. The V600E amino acid change results in constitutive activation of the BRAF kinase and promotes cell transformation (29).

Di Nicolantonio et al. looked retrospectively at 113 patients with mCRC who had received either cetuximab or panitumumab (30). In this study, KRAS mutation was detected in 30% of the patients. The BRAF V600E mutation was detected in 11 of 79 patients who had wild-type KRAS. None of the BRAF-mutated patients responded to treatment, whereas none of the responders carried BRAF mutations (P =.029). In this study, BRAF mutation was a poor prognostic marker as patients had shorter PFS and OS (Table 2).

Similar to this study, Loupakis et al. looked retrospectively at BRAF status in patients receiving irinotecan and cetuxmab (31). Among the 87 patients in the study population, BRAF was mutated in 13 cases and none of those patients responded to chemotherapy compared to 24% response rate in patients with wild type. Once again, BRAF mutation was associated with a trend toward shorter PFS (HR, 0.59; P = 0.073).

Based on this data, the role of BRAF mutations in patients treated with EGFR-targeted drugs is similar to that played by mutated KRAS. We propose that the combined mutational analysis of both KRAS and BRAF could be used to prospectively select mCRC patients eligible for EGFR-targeted monoclonal antibody treatment, with evident medical and economic implications. However, these findings need to be formally confirmed in a randomized clinical trial comparing an experimental arm containing cetuximab or panitumumab with a control arm without this targeted therapy.

■ FUTURE TARGETS/DIRECTIONS

Insulin Growth Factor-1 Receptor

There are preclinical data suggesting that insulin growth factor-1 receptor (IGF-1R) plays an important role in multiple mechanisms that mediate the growth, angiogenesis, and metastasis of colorectal carcinoma and thus makes it a valid target for therapy (32). Furthermore, there is evidence that switching to the IGF-1R pathway is a common mechanism to promote resistance to anti-EGFR therapy and that inhibition of the IGF-1R transduction cascade augments the antiproliferative and proapoptotic effects of EGFR inhibition in CRC cells (33,34). Thus, clinical application of combination therapy targeting both EGFR and IGF-1R could be a promising therapeutic strategy especially in patients with KRAS or BRAF mutations.

Mammalian Target of Rapamycin Pathway

The mammalian target of rapamycin (mTOR) is an intracellular protein that acts as a central regulator of multiple signaling pathways (IGF, EGF, platelet deriving growth factor [PDGF], VEGF, amino acids) that mediate abnormal growth, proliferation, survival, and angiogenesis in cancer (35). mTOR is a critical component of the PI3K/AKT pathway, a key signaling pathway that is frequently dysregulated in many cancers. A group in Italy showed that everolimus (RAD001), mTOR inhibitor, alone or in combination with cetuximab, has activity on human cancer cell lines sensitive and resistant to EGFR inhibitors, both in vitro and in vivo (36). Furthermore, synergistic activity has been shown between mTOR inhibitors and epidermal growth inhibitors in colon cell lines with KRAS mutations (37). Therefore, targeting the mTOR pathway may overcome resistance to EGFR inhibitors and produces a cooperative effect with EGFR inhibitors, providing a valid therapeutic strategy to be tested in a clinical setting.

TABLE 2 Clinical trial evidence of the response of anti-EGFR monoclonal antibodies as related to BRAF mutational status in advanced colorectal carcinoma

Reference	Treatment	Variable	BRAF WT	BRAF Mutated
DiNicolantonio et al. (30)	Panitumumab or cetuximab	No. of patients	68/79	11/79
		Response rate	22/68 (3%)	0/11 (0%)
		P-value	0.029	
		PFS P-value	0.001	
		OS P-value	<0.0001	
Loupakis et al. (31)		No. of patients	74/87	13/87
		Response rate	24/74 (32%)	0/13 (0%)
	Irinotecan + cetuximab	P-value	0.016	
		HR; P-value	0.59; P=0.073	

PFS, progression-free survival; OS, overall survival; HR, hazard ratio.

■ CONCLUSION

While targeted therapies have contributed to improvements in outcome for patients with mCRC, these agents also have a downside including potential drug toxicity. Biomarkers can play a pivotal role in predicting response rate, sparing the toxicity, monetary costs, and treatment delay of futile therapy. It is clear from evidence from multiple trials that all patients with mCRC who are candidates for anti-EGFR monoclonal antibody therapy should have their tumor tested for KRAS mutation and even for BRAF mutation. The current guideline from the American Society of Oncology recommends KRAS testing prior to starting on anti-EGFR therapy. However, there is still more work to do as not all wild-type patients respond or have improved survival, and some mutant patients experience long-term disease control. Therefore, the identification of additional genetic determinants or other pathway of primary resistance to EGFR-targeted therapies in mCRC is important in future trials.

■ REFERENCES

1. Heinemann V, Stintzing S, Kirchner T, Boeck S, Jung A. Clinical relevance of EGFR- and KRAS-status in colorectal cancer patients treated with monoclonal antibodies directed against the EGFR. *Cancer Treat Rev* 2009;35(3):262–271.
2. Goldstein NS, Armin M. Epidermal growth factor receptor immunohistochemical reactivity in patients with American Joint Committee on Cancer Stage IV colon adenocarcinoma: implications for a standardized scoring system. *Cancer* 2001;92(5):1331–1346.
3. Cunningham D, Humblet Y, Siena S, et al. Cetuximab monotherapy and cetuximab plus irinotecan in irinotecan-refractory metastatic colorectal cancer. *N Engl J Med* 2004;351(4):337–345.
4. Chung KY, Shia J, Kemeny NE, et al. Cetuximab shows activity in colorectal cancer patients with tumors that do not express the epidermal growth factor receptor by immunohistochemistry. *J Clin Oncol* 2005;23(9):1803–1810.
5. Lenz HJ, Van Cutsem E, Khambata-Ford S, et al. Multicenter phase II and translational study of cetuximab in metastatic colorectal carcinoma refractory to irinotecan, oxaliplatin, and fluoropyrimidines. *J Clin Oncol* 2006;24(30):4914–4921.
6. Moroni M, Veronese S, Benvenuti S, et al. Gene copy number for epidermal growth factor receptor (EGFR) and clinical response to antiEGFR treatment in colorectal cancer: a cohort study. *Lancet Oncol* 2005;6(5):279–286.
7. Lièvre A, Bachet JB, Le Corre D, et al. KRAS mutation status is predictive of response to cetuximab therapy in colorectal cancer. *Cancer Res* 2006;66(8):3992–3995.
8. Cappuzzo F, Varella-Garcia M, Finocchiaro G, et al. Primary resistance to cetuximab therapy in EGFR FISH-positive colorectal cancer patients. *Br J Cancer* 2008;99(1):83–89.
9. Sartore-Bianchi A, Moroni M, Veronese S, et al. Epidermal growth factor receptor gene copy number and clinical outcome of metastatic colorectal cancer treated with panitumumab. *J Clin Oncol* 2007;25(22):3238–3245.
10. Khambata-Ford S, Garrett CR, Meropol NJ, et al. Expression of epiregulin and amphiregulin and K-ras

mutation status predict disease control in metastatic colorectal cancer patients treated with cetuximab. *J Clin Oncol* 2007;25(22):3230–3237.

11. Kranenburg O. The KRAS oncogene: past, present, and future. *Biochim Biophys Acta* 2005;1756(2):81–82.

12. Yarden Y, Sliwkowski MX. Untangling the ErbB signalling network. *Nat Rev Mol Cell Biol* 2001;2(2):127–137.

13. Raponi M, Winkler H, Dracopoli NC. KRAS mutations predict response to EGFR inhibitors. *Curr Opin Pharmacol* 2008;8(4):413–418.

14. Poehlmann A, Kuester D, Meyer F, Lippert H, Roessner A, Schneider-Stock R. K-ras mutation detection in colorectal cancer using the Pyrosequencing technique. *Pathol Res Pract* 2007;203(7):489–497.

15. Jimeno A, Messersmith WA, Hirsch FR, Franklin WA, Eckhardt SG. KRAS mutations and sensitivity to epidermal growth factor receptor inhibitors in colorectal cancer: practical application of patient selection. *J Clin Oncol* 2009;27(7):1130–1136.

16. Saif MW, Shah M. K-ras mutations in colorectal cancer: a practice changing discovery. *Clin Adv Hematol Oncol* 2009;7(1):45–53, 64.

17. Van Cutsem E, Köhne CH, Hitre E, et al. Cetuximab and chemotherapy as initial treatment for metastatic colorectal cancer. *N Engl J Med* 2009;360(14):1408–1417.

18. Bokemeyer C, Bondarenko I, Makhson A, et al. Fluorouracil, leucovorin, and oxaliplatin with and without cetuximab in the first-line treatment of metastatic colorectal cancer. *J Clin Oncol* 2009;27(5):663–671.

19. Karapetis CS, Khambata-Ford S, Jonker DJ, et al. K-ras mutations and benefit from cetuximab in advanced colorectal cancer. *N Engl J Med* 2008;359(17):1757–1765.

20. Van Cutsem E, Peeters M, Siena S, et al. Open-label phase III trial of panitumumab plus best supportive care compared with best supportive care alone in patients with chemotherapy-refractory metastatic colorectal cancer. *J Clin Oncol* 2007;25(13):1658–1664.

21. Amado RG, Wolf M, Peeters M, et al. Wild-type KRAS is required for panitumumab efficacy in patients with metastatic colorectal cancer. *J Clin Oncol* 2008;26(10):1626–1634.

22. Hecht JR ME, Baranda J, et al. Panitumumab efficacy in patients with metastatic colorectal cancer with low or undetectable levels of epidermal growth factor receptor: final efficacy and K-RAS analysis [abstract 343]. *Program and abstracts of the 2008 Gastrointestinal Cancers Symposium (GCS)*. 2008.

23. Hurwitz H, Fehrenbacher L, Novotny W, et al. Bevacizumab plus irinotecan, fluorouracil, and leucovorin for metastatic colorectal cancer. *N Engl J Med* 2004;350(23):2335–2342.

24. Saltz LB, Clarke S, Díaz-Rubio E, et al. Bevacizumab in combination with oxaliplatin-based chemotherapy as first-line therapy in metastatic colorectal cancer: a randomized phase III study. *J Clin Oncol* 2008;26(12):2013–2019.

25. Hurwitz HI, Yi J, Ince W, Novotny WF, Rosen O. The clinical benefit of bevacizumab in metastatic colorectal cancer is independent of K-ras mutation status: analysis of a phase III study of bevacizumab with chemotherapy in previously untreated metastatic colorectal cancer. *Oncologist* 2009;14(1):22–28.

26. Hecht JR ME, Chidiac T. Interim results from PACCE: irinotecan (Iri)/bevacizumab (bev) ± panitumumab (pmab) as first-line treatment (tx) for metastatic colorectal cancer (mCRC) [abstract 279]. *Gastrointestinal Cancers Symposium (GCS)*; 2008.

27. Tol J, Koopman M, Rodenburg CJ, et al. A randomised phase III study on capecitabine, oxaliplatin and bevacizumab with or without cetuximab in first-line advanced colorectal cancer, the CAIRO2 study of the Dutch Colorectal Cancer Group (DCCG). An interim analysis of toxicity. *Ann Oncol* 2008;19(4):734–738.

28. Souglakos J, Philips J, Wang R, et al. Prognostic and predictive value of common mutations for treatment response and survival in patients with metastatic colorectal cancer. *Br J Cancer* 2009;101(3):465–472.

29. Frattini M, Ferrario C, Bressan P, et al. Alternative mutations of BRAF, RET and NTRK1 are associated with similar but distinct gene expression patterns in papillary thyroid cancer. *Oncogene* 2004;23(44):7436–7440.

30. Di Nicolantonio F, Martini M, Molinari F, et al. Wild-type BRAF is required for response to panitumumab or cetuximab in metastatic colorectal cancer. *J Clin Oncol* 2008;26(35):5705–5712.

31. Loupakis F, Ruzzo A, Cremolini C, et al. KRAS codon 61, 146 and BRAF mutations predict resistance to cetuximab plus irinotecan in KRAS codon 12 and 13 wild-type metastatic colorectal cancer. *Br J Cancer* 2009;101(4):715–721.

32. Reinmuth N, Fan F, Liu W, et al. Impact of insulin-like growth factor receptor-I function on angiogenesis, growth, and metastasis of colon cancer. *Lab Invest* 2002;82(10):1377–1389.

33. Jones HE, Gee JM, Hutcheson IR, Knowlden JM, Barrow D, Nicholson RI. Growth factor receptor interplay and resistance in cancer. *Endocr Relat Cancer* 2006;13(suppl 1):S45–S51.

34. Kaulfuss S, Burfeind P, Gaedcke J, Scharf JG. Dual silencing of insulin-like growth factor-I receptor and epidermal growth factor receptor in colorectal cancer cells is associated with decreased proliferation and enhanced apoptosis. *Mol Cancer Ther* 2009;8(4):821–833.

35. Wullschleger S, Loewith R, Hall MN. TOR signaling in growth and metabolism. *Cell* 2006;124(3):471–484.

36. Bianco R, Garofalo S, Rosa R, et al. Inhibition of mTOR pathway by everolimus cooperates with EGFR inhibitors in human tumours sensitive and resistant to anti-EGFR drugs. *Br J Cancer* 2008;98(5):923–930.

37. Buck E, Eyzaguirre A, Brown E, et al. Rapamycin synergizes with the epidermal growth factor receptor inhibitor erlotinib in non-small-cell lung, pancreatic, colon, and breast tumors. *Mol Cancer Ther* 2006;5(11):2676–2684.

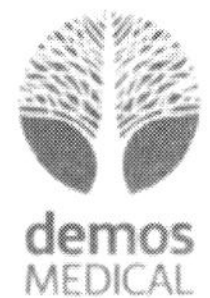

demos
MEDICAL

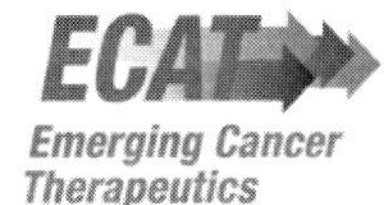

Emerging Cancer
Therapeutics

Esophageal Cancer

Advances in Surgical Therapy for Esophageal Cancer

Heather Yeo, Amir Shariff, and Charles Cha*

Yale Cancer Center, Yale University School of Medicine, New Haven, CT

■ ABSTRACT

Esophageal cancer remains a common malignancy worldwide and is the fastest growing cancer in the United States. The role of surgical therapy for esophageal cancer continues to evolve, but it still remains the gold standard for curative therapy. Outlined in this article are the major surgical techniques used for esophageal cancer, as well as some of the surgical debate regarding the extent of lymph node dissection necessary, role of minimally invasive or non-invasive techniques and technologies as well as the role of surgery in relation to other combination therapies. Though there have been significant advancements in the therapy of esophageal cancer over the past two decades, cure of this disease continues to be a challenge.

■ BACKGROUND

Esophageal cancer is the fastest growing cancer in the United States. It remains the sixth most common malignancy with an incidence of 20 per 100,000 and represents 4% of newly diagnosed cancers in North America. It is estimated that there will be over 14,500 deaths and 16,470 new cases in 2009 (1). Worldwide, esophageal cancer is even more prevalent, reaching an incidence of 160 per 100,000 in parts of South Africa and China and 540 per 100,000 in Kazakhstan (2).

Although worldwide squamous cell carcinoma accounts for most esophageal cancers, in the United States, esophageal adenocarcinoma is noted in up to 70% of patients presenting with esophageal cancer. The

distribution of esophageal cancer across gender, age, and race is affected by cell type. The male-to-female ratio for squamous cell cancer is 3:1; in contrast, the male-to-female ratio for adenocarcinoma is 15:1 (3,4).

Despite advances in surgical, anesthetic, and intensive care techniques, hospital morbidity and mortality are still substantial. Surgery is currently the only hope for definitive cure of esophageal cancer. The overall survival rate at 5 years is poor but increased from 4% in the 1970s to 14% in 2009 (5). After complete surgical removal of the tumor, the 5-year survival rate exceeds 95% for stage 0 disease, is 50% to 80% for stage I disease, 30% to 40% for stage IIA disease, 10% to 30% for stage IIB disease, and 10% to 15% for stage III disease. Median survival for patients with metastatic (stage IV) disease treated with palliative chemotherapy is less than 1 year (4,6,7).

Esophagectomy remains the gold standard for curative treatment of esophageal cancer. But a

---

*Corresponding author, Yale University School of Medicine, New Haven, CT

E-mail address: Charles.cha@yale.edu

Emerging Cancer Therapeutics 1 (2010) 19–34.

DOI: 10.5003/2151–4194.1.1.19

number of newer approaches have been introduced in an attempt to decrease morbidity and mortality (see Table 1). As well as careful patient selection, standardized postoperative pathways, and thoracic epidural analgesia, minimal invasive esophagectomy (MIE) has been advocated as a safe technique with comparable results to open esophagectomy such as the Ivor Lewis operation or the open cervico-thoracoabdominal approach (8–11).

Most recently, advances have been made in minimally invasive techniques (8,11). Commonly, this entails thoracoscopic mobilization of the esophagus in either the prone or left lateral decubitus position, with or without laparoscopic-assisted mobilization of the stomach, followed by an anastomosis in the neck. Alternatively, a transhiatal laparoscopic approach has been described, again with an anastomosis in the neck (12).

In addition there have been several newly described procedures, including endoscopic mucosal resection (EMR) and various forms of ablative therapy (13–15). While long-term results are still pending on these modalities, they offer potential for treatment in patients with significant comorbidities who may not be able to tolerate a more aggressive surgical treatment.

Clearly, curing esophageal cancer is a challenge. The clinical biology and presentation of esophageal cancer have changed dramatically in the past two decades. This has had an impact on the intent of treatment, resulting in a marked trend favoring curative therapy whenever possible. The rising use of upper endoscopy to evaluate upper gastrointestinal symptoms and the widespread adoption of Barrett's surveillance programs have markedly increased the proportion of patients in whom the cancer is found confined to the mucosa or submucosa. Trends also

TABLE 1 Surgical and endoscopic treatment options

Transhiatal (abdominal–cervical)
Transthoracic (Ivor Lewis)
En bloc three-field (right thoracic–abdominal–cervical/McKeown)
Vagal-sparing esophagectomy
Minimally invasive esophagectomy
Ablative therapy
Endoscopic mucosal resection

document an increasing prevalence of adenocarcinoma of the esophagus in younger patients.

The morbidity and mortality associated with esophageal resection have declined such that dedicated centers routinely achieve 1% to 2% 30-day mortality (6). Taken together, these changes support highly individualized treatment decisions in which each patient receives the treatment with the best chance of eliminating all disease.

■ SURGICAL RESECTION

Fewer than half the patients presenting with esophageal cancer are eligible for surgical resection (16). In patients for whom a cure is possible, treatment may include chemotherapy, radiation therapy (RT), surgical resection, or a combination of these modalities. In patients with a local tumor that does not involve other vital structures, who have no evidence of distant disease, and whose clinical and nutritional status are adequate, curative treatment is implemented. In patients with significant comorbidities, the evidence of advanced or distant disease or poor nutritional status is considered for palliation. Using the AJCC staging system (Table 2), surgery may be considered for any patient presenting in stage I through stage III. Patients with stage IV cancer are recommended to undergo definitive treatment with chemoradiotherapy.

While significant controversy surrounds both the medical and surgical treatment of esophageal cancer, there are some general guidelines upon which most physicians agree. The treatment for patients presenting with stage I cancer, T1 N0, is surgical resection only. If the surgical specimen reveals more advanced disease, adjuvant chemotherapy is considered. The treatment of patients presenting with stage II disease (T2 Nx, T3 N0) is the most controversial. Surgical resection is clearly indicated, but opinions vary as to the type of surgical resection that is best and if there is a need for chemotherapy. If chemotherapy is recommended, it is given in the neoadjuvant setting. Treatment of patients presenting with stage III disease (T3 N1, T4 N0) is also debated, but a little less so. Most physicians agree that multimodality therapy is needed, but the timing and type of surgical resection remains unresolved. Advocates of aggressive surgical resection (three-field en bloc esophagectomy with a radical thoracic and

TABLE 2 Esophageal cancer staging

T	Stage
Tis Carcinoma in situ	**I**
T1 Tumor invades lamina propria or submucosa	T1N0M0
T2 Tumor invades muscularis propria	**IIA**
T3 Tumor invades adventia	T2N0M0
T4 Tumor invades adjacent structures	T3N0M0
N	**IIB**
N0 No regional node metastases	T1N1M0
N1 Regional node metastases	T2N1M0
M	**III**
M0 No distant metastases	T3N1M0
M1 Distant metastases	T4 Any N M0
Tumors of the lower esophagus	**IV**
M1a Metastasis in celiac lymph nodes	Any T Any N M1
M1b Other distant metastasis	**IVA**
Tumors of the midthoracic esophagus	Any T Any N M1a
M1a Not applicable	**IVB**
M1b Nonregional lymph nodes and/or other distant metastasis	Any T Any N M1b
Tumors of the upper thoracic esophagus	
M1a Metastasis in cervical nodes	
M1b Other distant metastasis	

abdominal lymphadenectomy) stand in opposition to those who advocate multimodal therapy with neoadjuvant chemoradiotherapy followed by a more conservative surgical approach (transhiatal or transthoracic esophagectomy). Scientific evidence supporting the benefit of one over the other is lacking.

■ SURGICAL OPTIONS

While there are a multitude of esophageal resections that are used to treat esophageal cancer, no one technique has established dominance. With better understanding of tumor biology, improved chemotherapy, and advanced technology, more surgical techniques are emerging. Because of the morbidity of the disease and the variety among practitioners, there are no prospective trials randomizing surgical resection options. All the data used to guide surgical therapy come from retrospective reviews or clinical experience. Because fewer than 50% of patients are resectable at the time of diagnosis and many institutions have biases based on surgical experience and skill, developing evidence-based data is difficult. There are several factors that affect surgical decision making and subsequent operative and long-term outcomes. Patient health status and life expectancy, location of the tumor, surgical approach, location of the anastamosis, anastamotic type, type of conduit, and position of conduit placement must all be taken into account to determine what methodology will suit a patient best (17,18).

■ TRANSHIATAL ESOPHAGECTOMY

The first blunt transmediastinal esophagectomy without thoracotomy was reported by Denk in 1913 using a vein stripper to avulse the esophagus in cadavers (19). In 1933, Turner performed the first successful transhiatal esophagectomy for carcinoma (20). After the development of endotracheal anesthesia, however, transthoracic esophagectomy could be performed under direct vision, and transhiatal esophagectomy was only used occasionally.

In 1975, Orringer and Sloan (21) described the use of substernal gastric bypass and thoracic esophageal exclusion for palliation of dysphagia for incurable esophageal carcinoma. Their results and that of others (22–24) have demonstrated that few patients undergoing esophagectomy for benign or malignant disease require a thoracotomy.

Indications and Contraindications

All patients being evaluated for an esophagectomy for benign or malignant disease should be considered potential candidates for transhiatal esophagectomy (THE). Absolute contraindications include bronchoscopic evidence of tracheobronchial invasion in patients who have upper or middle esophageal carcinomas. THE is possible after RT and with periesophageal adhesions from caustic injuries, previous operations, or achalasia (24–26). Carcinomas of the cardia and proximal stomach can also be resected by THE, avoiding the intrathoracic anastomosis required after a traditional proximal hemigastrectomy. Patients who have biopsy-proven distant metastatic disease are considered unresectable. Although various imaging modalities (computed tomography [CT], endoscopic ultrasound [EUS], thoracoscopic and laparoscopic staging) are useful in evaluating for metastatic disease, the most important assessment is the surgeon's palpation through the hiatus and determination of esophageal fixation. If a safe transhiatal resection cannot be performed, one must be prepared to perform a thoracotomy.

Operative Technique

Abdominal Phase

The abdominal phase of the procedure is performed through a midline supraumbilical incision. After the triangular ligament is divided, the stomach is carefully examined for significant tumor involvement or scarring from previous surgery or disease. The right gastroepiploic artery is identified early and protected, especially with a history of previous abdominal surgery. The left gastroepiploic and short gastric vessels are ligated. The esophagogastric junction is mobilized, and the left gastric artery is ligated near its origin at the celiac axis. In carcinoma cases, the celiac lymph nodes are sent for pathological staging. Large celiac nodal metastases indicate incurable disease and are biopsied. The right gastric artery is protected as the dissection is continued along the lesser curvature. A Kocher maneuver is then performed to allow mobilization of the pylorus to the level of the xiphoid process. A pyloromyotomy is performed to decrease the incidence of postvagotomy delayed gastric emptying.

The distal 5 to 10 cm of esophagus is mobilized through the hiatus. The mobility of the esophageal tumor is then assessed to ensure that it is not fixed to the prevertebral fascia, aorta, or surrounding mediastinal structures. Deaver retractors inserted into the hiatus allow long right-angle clamps to be used to ligate the periesophageal tissues to the level of the carina under direct vision. A jejunostomy tube may be placed at this time.

Cervical Phase

An oblique incision is made along the anterior border of the sternocleidomastoid muscle. Care must be taken to avoid retraction on the recurrent laryngeal nerve in the tracheoesophageal groove. The middle thyroid vein and inferior thyroid artery may be ligated as needed. After dissecting to the prevertebral fascia, blunt finger dissection is continued into the superior mediastinum. Sharp dissection is used along the anterolateral surface of the esophagus, staying posterior to the recurrent laryngeal nerve. The upper thoracic esophagus is mobilized almost to the level of the carina, using blunt dissection and keeping the fingers directly against the esophagus.

Mediastinal Dissection

One hand is inserted through the diaphragmatic hiatus posterior to the esophagus while a half-sponge stick is placed through the cervical incision dissecting the esophagus off the prevertebral fascia. The blood pressure is carefully monitored to prevent prolonged hypotension. The anterior mobilization is performed from both the abdominal and cervical incisions, with the fingers directly against the anterior esophagus to avoid injury to the posterior membranous trachea. The esophagus is then held in the superior mediastinum, between the index and middle fingers of the hand inserted through the hiatus, and the remaining attachments are lysed with a downward motion. The upper esophagus is then divided obliquely, leaving some redundancy, and the thoracic esophagus is delivered through the diaphragmatic hiatus. The posterior mediastinum is inspected through the hiatus for hemostasis. If the pleural cavities have been entered, which occurs in two-thirds of cases, chest tubes are placed. The posterior mediastinum is packed to tamponade minor bleeding.

A partial proximal gastrectomy 4 to 6 cm distal to the tumor is performed using a gastrointestinal anastomosis (GIA) stapler. For benign disease or tumors of the middle esophagus, the amount of stomach resected is minimized to preserve collateral circulation to the fundus. The staple line is then oversewn. The mobilized stomach is passed through the hiatus and is delivered 4 to 5 cm above the clavicles, primarily by pushing the stomach up through the mediastinum. Traction sutures and suction devices to pull the stomach through the mediastinum are avoided to minimize trauma to the gastric tip. "Suspension sutures" to the prevertebral fascia are also avoided, due to the risk of vertebral osteomyelitis. The stomach is then palpated to ensure that there is no torsion.

The abdominal phase is then completed to avoid contamination with oral bacteria from the cervical esophagus. The diaphragm is reapproximated so that the hiatus permits three fingers to pass alongside the stomach. The anterior gastric wall is approximated to the edge of the hiatus, and the triangular ligament is sutured over the hiatus to prevent hiatal hernia.

Cervical Esophagogastric Anastomosis

A traction suture is placed in the anterior gastric wall to elevate the stomach into the wound. A vertical gastrotomy is made in the anterior gastric wall, far enough below the gastric fundus to allow the stapler to be fully inserted into the stomach. The cervical esophageal staple line is then obliquely amputated, with enough redundancy to ensure a tension-free anastomosis and sent to pathology as the proximal esophageal margin. After placing two stay sutures to align the stomach and esophagus, the stapler is inserted and closed. After firing the stapler, a

nasogastric tube is placed across the anastomosis, and the anterior wall of the anastomosis is then completed in two layers. Finally, the wound is closed over a drain.

Complications

Intraoperative complications include pneumothorax, hemorrhage, and tracheal tear. Early complications that occur within 10 days include hoarseness or difficulty swallowing due to recurrent laryngeal nerve injury, disruption of the anastomosis, arrhythmias, chylothorax, and sympathetic pleural effusion. Early complications that occur in less than 1% of patients are epidural abscess, vertebral osteomyelitis, tracheogastric anastomotic fistula, pulmonary microabscesses from an internal jugular vein abscess, and gastric tip necrosis. An inadequate gastric drainage procedure, narrowing of the hiatus, or tumor recurrence can also lead to delayed gastric emptying. Late complications are relatively uncommon and include diaphragmatic hernia and cervical anastomotic stricture.

Aortic esophageal arteries are small branches and generally thrombose if avulsed during esophagectomy (27). The average intraoperative blood loss is less than 1,000 mL if patients are properly selected. Patients who have tumors fixed to the aorta or periesophageal tissues should not undergo THE. If intraoperative hemorrhage occurs, efforts should be made to identify the bleeding source and control it. If the point of bleeding cannot be identified, the mediastinum is packed for 5 to 10 minutes with volume resuscitation. If bleeding continues, the procedure is converted to a thoracotomy.

One of the many advantages of a cervical esophagogastric anastomosis over an intrathoracic anastomosis is that a cervical esophagogastric anastomotic leak is relatively easy to treat. The published rate of leak is between 9% and 14% (24, 28) and this may prolong hospital stay and lead to other complications (29). Up to 40% (30) of anastomotic leaks can be diagnosed clinically. They can also be diagnosed by screening radiographic swallow studies with contrast. Barium is preferred in the screening test for anastomotic leak because it has a higher sensitivity for detecting a leak than thinner water-soluble contrast agents such as Gastrografin (31,32). In addition, Gastrografin poses a risk of pneumonitis if aspirated (33). Management involves opening the neck incision at the bedside, and the wound is irrigated both with saline and by having the patient drink tap water. The wound is packed as necessary with saline moistened gauze. To prevent an anastomotic stricture and to maintain an intraluminal path of least resistance, the anastomosis is dilated at the bedside by passing 30F, 36F, and 46F Maloney esophageal dilators within 1 week of opening the neck wound. With the above regimen, the majority of anastomotic cutaneous fistulas seal within 2 weeks (34). Long-term management of the anastomotic stricture is more of a challenge and may require that the patient learn the technique of self-esophageal dilation (35).

Cooke et al. published a study of 1,133 patients who underwent a transhiatal esophagectomy and demonstrated positive smoking history as a risk factor for an astomotic leak (30). They further showed that diabetes mellitus, heart disease, chronic renal insufficiency, hypertension, previous stroke, and chronic obstructive pulmonary disease were not independent risk factors; however, in aggregate, the increasing number of comorbid conditions was a risk factor for experiencing a leak. Advanced pathologic stage was also a risk factor. Relative ischemia of the tip of the newly mobilized gastric conduit has long been implicated in the cause of a leak. Those who experienced postoperative arrhythmias had a higher leak rate which they postulate to be a result of the postoperative arrhythmia causing a low-flow state, putting an already mildly ischemic anastomosis at additional risk. However, an arrhythmia may be a manifestation of a leak rather than a contributor, secondary to cardiac excitability as a result of the leak. Finally, a stapled anastomosis has been shown to be protective against anastomotic leaks (28,36,37).

Chest tube drainage greater than 200 to 400 mL per shift for greater than 48 hours should lead one to suspect a thoracic duct injury. Chest tube drainage will be serous until an oral diet of fats has been started. The diagnosis is confirmed by milky chest tube drainage after administering cream through the jejunostomy tube. Most patients are nutritionally compromised and do not tolerate the loss of protein-rich chyle. Unless the leak improves within 3 to 5 days of elemental tube feedings, a thoracotomy or video-assisted thoracoscopic surgery should be performed with ligation of the thoracic duct. Conservative treatment by lymphography and embolization has also been described (38,39).

Sympathetic pleural effusion may occur during the first postoperative week because of mediastinal dissection. Generally, asymptomatic stable effusions are observed and usually resolve spontaneously. Symptomatic patients are treated with thoracentesis or tube thoracostomy, and if the condition persists, injury to the thoracic duct should be considered. Our current practice is to place bilateral chest tubes at the time of surgery as prophylaxis.

■ TRANSTHORACIC ESOPHAGECTOMY

Transthoracic esophagectomy for esophageal disease was presented on January 10, 1946, when Ivor Lewis gave the Hunterian Lecture to the Royal College of Surgeons in London (40). At the time of this lecture, successful resections of the esophagus with primary anastomosis were a rarity. Lewis described an operation in which the esophagus was resected via a thoracic approach in two stages. The first stage was done through an abdominal incision, and freed the stomach, basing it on the right gastric and right gastroepiploic arteries. He also placed a jejunostomy tube during this first stage for nutritional support. The second stage was done 1 to 2 weeks later and involved resecting the esophagus and performing an anastomosis between the esophagus and stomach in the chest. Despite the simplicity of the pre- and postoperative care of the time, the operation was successful in five of seven patients.

The Ivor Lewis esophagectomy, or transthoracic esophagectomy, has been modified in subsequent years and is currently performed as a single-stage procedure. This approach allows complete visualization of all perigastric and periesophageal lymph tissue. It also allows direct visualization and dissection of the thoracic esophagus, thus virtually eliminating the uncommon but potentially disastrous damage to adjacent structures that can occur with transhiatal esophagectomy. The procedure remains an excellent technique for patients who have mid- and distal esophageal carcinomas.

Indications and Contraindications

Indications for performing a transthoracic esophagectomy, other than esophageal carcinoma, include high-grade dysphagia in Barrett's esophagus (BE), destruction of the lower two-thirds of the esophagus by caustic ingestion, complex strictures following multiple antireflux operations, end-stage motility disorders, and rarely, a perforated esophagus.

The transthoracic approach is not indicated for high thoracic or cervical esophageal carcinomas and can be difficult to perform in patients who have had a previous right thoracotomy.

Operative Technique

Abdominal Portion

A double-lumen endotracheal tube is placed. The patient is placed supine on the table and prepared from the chin to the pubis. An upper midline incision is begun just to the left of the xyphoid process and extended just cephalad to the umbilicus. Abdominal exploration is performed, carefully assessing for metastatic disease. The costal arch is lifted with retractors and the patient is placed in a reverse Trendelenburg position.

The gastroesophageal junction is mobilized to determine if the tumor is adherent to or invading the vertebral column, aorta, or pericardium. The left lobe of the liver is mobilized and retracted laterally, and the pharyngoesophageal ligament is divided. With blunt dissection, being careful not to transgress the tumor, the esophagus is circled with a Penrose drain. A portion of the crus and diaphragm can be resected with the tumor if necessary. Using manual palpation, adherence to mediastinal structures is assessed. If the tumor is mobile, the resection is begun.

The goal of the abdominal portion of the operation is to mobilize the stomach. With the stomach retracted cephalad and the colon caudad, the lesser sac is entered through the mesocolon, below the right gastroepiploic arcade. The omentum is then divided, carefully preserving the right gastroepiploic vessels. The short gastric vessels are divided. The stomach is then mobilized from the spleen, taking all short gastric vessels until the hiatus is reached. With the greater curve of the stomach lifted cephalad and the pancreas and celiac axis retracted caudad, the left gastric artery and vein are exposed, ligated, and divided. All nodal tissue found along the cephalad border of the pancreas is swept up with these vessels. The remaining tissue along the aorta cephalad to the hiatus is freed with the specimen. The stomach is then retracted laterally, allowing division of the hepatic branches of the vagal nerves and associated vessels. The hiatus is enlarged by dividing a portion of the right crus. The lesser curve area is prepared by dividing all of the blood vessels to the level between the third and fourth branches of the left gastric artery. The resulting bare area is where the stomach tube ends up in the chest. A pyloromyotomy or a pyloroplasty is performed to conclude the abdominal portion of the operation. Abdominal wall closure is then performed.

Right Thoracotomy

The patient is placed in the left lateral decubitus position and the right lung collapsed. A fourth interspace incision is made over the fifth rib. Exploration of the chest is performed, looking for any metastatic disease.

The mediastinal pleura overlying the esophagus is divided laterally along the hemiazygos vein, across the hiatus, then back cephalad along the pericardium and to the azygos vein. The entire envelope of tissue around the esophagus, including lymph nodes, fatty tissue, and the thoracic duct, is freed by developing a plane along the aorta. The thoracic duct is doubly clipped and divided. A Penrose drain is placed around the esophagus for traction. Separate lymph nodes are sampled from the low paraesophageal, inferior pulmonary ligament, subcarinal, and high paraesophageal/paratracheal areas. The azygos vein is ligated and divided at the level of the hemiazygos, disconnecting it from the superior vena cava. A pleural flap is incised up to the apex of the chest. The proximal esophagus is then freed to the apex of the chest, staying close to the wall of the esophagus to avoid injury to both the right and left recurrent laryngeal nerves. When the esophagus has been freed to the apex of the thoracic cavity, it is divided at this level. The surgical margins are sent for frozen-section inspection.

The stomach is transposed through the hiatus into the chest. Once the proximal esophageal margin is pathologically cleared, a gastric tube is made based on the greater curvature of the stomach. The fundus of the stomach is stretched out, and the distance to the anastomosis is measured along the greater curve. A stomach tube is then fashioned by stapler applications parallel to the greater curvature to a site at the bare area on the lesser curve. The fundus of the stomach is removed, along with a good portion of the lesser curve and the lymph nodes in this area. A handsewn end-to-side anastomosis is performed placing the stomach tube posterior to the esophagus. The anastomosis is covered with a mediastinal pleural flap.

A nasogastric is placed down to the level of the hiatus. The incision is closed in the usual fashion after placement of one chest tube.

Complications

Surgical treatment of esophageal cancer using an Ivor Lewis procedure carries a mortality rate of up to 9.2% and a complication rate between 27.3% and 57% (41,42). Most postoperative deaths arise from pulmonary complications (43,44). Other complications include bleeding, anastomotic leakage, necrosis of the gastric tube, chylothorax, pleural effusions, and esophagotracheal/bronchial fistulae.

There is a wide variation in reported anastomotic leakage rate, and much of this variation can be contributed to the different techniques and sites of the anastomosis. Management of leaks is more complicated than for transhiatal esophagectomy and can often by fatal, most commonly as a result of severe mediastinitis. The key to lowering morbidity and mortality after an intrathoracic anastomotic leakage is early and stringent complication management. Previously this may have included rethoracotomy and mediastinal lavage. However, the new treatment option of using endoscopically placed long covered stents within the gastric tube combined with CT-guided drainage of the mediastinum does allow conservative management of anastomotic leakages with favorable outcome in most cases (45).

■ COMPARISON OF TRANSHIATAL AND TRANSTHORACIC ESOPHAGECTOMIES

In studies comparing these two modalities, analysis of early outcomes demonstrate a 30-day mortality of approximately 10% for both approaches (46) despite the additional observations that postoperative pneumonia and myocardial infarction occurred more frequently among patients undergoing transthoracic esophagectomy.

Chang et al. (47) published one of the largest nationwide population-based studies assessing long-term outcome after esophagectomy for esophageal cancer using a cohort of 868 patients undergoing esophagectomy for cancer between 1992 and 2002. They found a 5-year survival advantage for transhiatal esophagectomy of 30.5% versus 22.7%

for transthoracic esophagectomy. However, they found no advantage to a transhiatal approach compared with transthoracic operations with regard to long-term survival after adjustment for tumor stage, patient, and provider factors. They did note that patients undergoing transhiatal esophagectomy were more likely to have earlier stage malignancy. This may be due to the fact that the extent of lymph node dissection may be greater for patients undergoing a transthoracic approach. Wolff et al. (48) in a series of 517 esophagectomies found that there not only was a statistically significant difference in the number of lymph nodes retrieved, but there were twice as many lymph nodes retrieved with the transthoracic as opposed to the transhiatal approach. This provides greater opportunity to determine esophageal cancer staging in the transthoracic approach. Such "stage migration" has also been proposed as a reason for differences previously observed in long-term survival between transthoracic and transhiatal esophagectomy (49).

■ EN BLOC ESOPHAGECTOMY

The concept of en bloc resection, as originally proposed by Logan (50) and later reintroduced by Skinner (51), aims to maximize local tumor control by resecting the tumor-bearing esophagus within a wide envelope of surrounding tissues. Thus, for tumors of the middle or lower thoracic esophagus, the en bloc specimen would include, in addition to the tumor-bearing organ, the pericardium anteriorly and both pleural surfaces laterally, as well as the thoracic duct and all other lymphoareolar tissue wedged posteriorly between the esophagus and the spine. Additionally, for tumors traversing the diaphragm, a 1-inch. cuff of diaphragm is excised circumferentially around the esophagus.

The associated two-field lymphadenectomy includes en bloc resection of all nodal groups between the tracheal bifurcation superiorly to the celiac axis inferiorly. The concept of three-field lymph node dissection for esophageal cancer was developed by Japanese surgeons in the 1980s. The additional third field of dissection includes excision of the nodes along both recurrent nerves as they course through the mediastinum and neck, as well as a modified cervical node dissection. The latter includes the nodes posterior and lateral to the internal jugular vein and an infraomohyoid node dissection bilaterally.

Indications

En bloc esophagectomy (EBE) is well indicated for middle and lower thoracic esophageal and cardia cancers because the upper esophagus is anatomically adherent to the surrounding vital organs (tracheobronchial trees) where EBE is quite impossible to perform.

Indications for EBE were limited initially and were restricted to patients with localized stage I or II disease (51) and to patients with no lymph-node metastasis (52). These indications have since been extended to all patients who have adequate cardiopulmonary reserve without visceral metastasis (M0) and locally advanced (T4) disease (53–57).

Operative Technique

Before the procedure begins, routine endoscopy is performed to examine the tumor and airway. Then nasogastric and double-lumen endotracheal tubes are placed.

Right Thoracotomy

The patient is turned to the left lateral decubitus position and the procedure initiated with a right posterolateral thoracotomy incision at the fifth interspace. The posterior mediastinal pleura is opened over the esophagus from the apex of the chest to the diaphragm at the level of the vertebral bodies. The azygos vein is divided and the tumor mobilized from above in a region of normal esophagus. As the dissection is continued superior to the azygos vein, only sparse periesophageal lymph node tissue is found and injury to the recurrent laryngeal nerve must be avoided. At the level of the thoracic inlet, finger dissection is used to define the plane between the trachea and the esophagus.

The operation proceeds distally using cautery dissection. All periesophageal nodal tissues remain with the esophagus. Adherent pericardium or contralateral pleura is incised and remains with the esophagus to ensure complete resection. A small cuff (2 cm) of diaphragm is left with the esophagus. The peritoneal cavity is entered posteriorly.

Any nodal tissue that has not been gathered up into the specimen, such as tissue in the subcarinal space or in the area of the inferior pulmonary ligament, is now dissected out separately. The chest is then closed following placement of a chest tube.

Abdominal Dissection

The patient is repositioned in the supine position. The double-lumen tube is converted back to a single-lumen tube to avoid the complications of performing this maneuver after the cervical anastomosis has been created.

An upper midline incision is created and the abdominal cavity is explored for evidence of metastatic disease. The short gastric vessels are then divided. The dissection begins at the level of the gastroesophageal junction, proceeds to the separation between the left and right gastroepiploic arcades, and is then continued 2 cm lateral to the right gastroepiploic pedicle. The greater omentum is divided. A liberal Kocher maneuver is performed and at this time a pyloromyotomy or pyloroplasty is completed. At this point, any nodal tissue is gathered up onto the specimen. The left gastric artery is then divided. The gastric conduit is now ready to be delivered to the neck.

Cervical Dissection

A left cervical incision is made obliquely along the anterior border of the sternocleidomastoid muscle starting at the sternal notch. The omohyoid muscle is mobilized or divided with electrocautery. Using gentle blunt finger dissection, the surgeon proceeds posteriorly to the level of the esophagus. Now the esophagus is divided using a stapler and the specimen is removed through the abdominal incision.

The gastric conduit is fashioned from the stomach using a stapler to divide the stomach, creating a tube-shaped gastric conduit. Maintaining a narrow conduit is important to ensure adequate emptying of the neoesophagus. The hiatus is dilated manually so that it will generously accommodate four fingers to fit within it transversely. The gastric conduit is then delivered to the cervical incision taking care to maintain its orientation. The abdomen is then closed.

A cervical side-to-side esophagogastric anastomosis is then created using a stapler. A nasogastric tube is placed and the neck incision closed over a drain.

Complications

The hospital mortality rate is quoted up to 10% (52,58,59). The overall morbidity rate is up to 40%. Pulmonary complications are the most common cause. Other complications include anastomotic leakage, empyema, chylothorax, and cardiac arrhythmias.

Outcomes

Though not unanimously accepted, some authors have reported excellent survival in patients with esophageal adenocarcinoma treated with primary en bloc resection. In similarly staged patients with limited lymph node involvement, they have shown that survival improved with the en bloc compared with the transhiatal esophagectomy (53,56,60,61). They postulate that the improved survival with an en bloc resection is likely due to the high frequency of involved lymph nodes both in the mediastinum and abdomen after neoadjuvant therapy and the fact that a systematic lymphadenectomy allows removal of both known and unknown (micrometastatic) disease. En bloc esophagectomies can therefore lead to "stage migration." In one series, this approach led to tumor upstaging in 23% of tumors, and another 20% were upstaged M1 because of positive distant abdominal nodes (62). They concluded that EBE upstaged 23% of tumors, mainly to M1, because of positive celiac nodes.

■ ENDOSCOPIC MUCOSAL RESECTION AND ABLATIVE THERAPY

There has been an increasing interest in endoscopic therapy of early esophageal cancer, where the risk of lymph node metastasis in early esophageal cancer, particularly in the setting of Barrett's adenocarcinoma, is lower than the surgical mortality rate (63). In contrast to surgical resection, which also allows for dissection of local lymph nodes, EMR is limited to the local removal of a lesion. The first endoscopic mucosal resection (EMR) procedures for early esophageal carcinoma were carried out in the early 1990s by Japanese endoscopists (64).

Indications and Contraindications

Pech et al. summarized the indications and contradictions as follows (65):

Absolute indications: BE, T1 m1–m3, no risk factors (lymphatic invasion [L1], venous infiltration [V1], poorly differentiated carcinoma [G3]), macroscopic elevated or flat

Intermediate indication: Tumor size >20 mm, multifocal cancer, T1 sm1 infiltration, no risk factors
Contraindication: T1 sm2 infiltration or deeper, T1 sm1 cancer with one risk factor, ulcerative lesion

Technique

There are varying approaches to EMR; however, there are two techniques that are particularly appropriate in the esophagus: in polypoid lesions, removal after injection under the lesion using the polypectomy technique, with loops adapted to the size of the lesion (the so-called strip biopsy or "lift-and-cut" technique); in flat lesions, the "suck-and-cut" technique with a ligation device or cap has proved its value.

A drawback of EMR is that only lesions with a diameter 20 mm or less can be resected en bloc. In addition, ulcerated lesions often have fibrosis, resulting in failure of the lesion to lift. In these cases, EMR is not advisable. Larger lesions can usually be resected completely using a piecemeal technique, but this method is associated with more recurrences because of small neoplastic residues resulting from insufficient overlapping of the resection areas. In addition, en bloc resection allows more accurate histologic evaluation of the neoplastic lesion, especially of the lateral and basal margins.

A new technique, endoscopic submucosal dissection (ESD), was therefore developed, which was initially described for early neoplastic lesions in the stomach (66). ESD is a method in which the submucosal layer underneath the carcinoma is dissected to obtain a larger mucosal specimen, with the neoplasm resected en bloc.

Outcomes

Data on EMR is currently limited. Das and colleagues (67) published a cohort of 742 patients of which 14% underwent endoscopic therapy (EMR alone or in combination with ablative therapy), whereas the remainder underwent surgical resection. They found no significant difference in the median cancer-free survival in these two groups of patients.

The results of EMR for early squamous cell neoplasia and early Barrett's neoplasia of the esophagus were summarized by Ono and colleagues (66). EMR of early squamous cell neoplasia has been proved safe and effective in several studies. Complete response in 10 reported series varied between 92% and 100%. Recurrent/metachronous lesions were seen in 0% to 26%. Risk factors for these lesions included piecemeal resection and multifocal lesions. Minor bleeding was seen in up to 23% of patients, stricture formation in up to 24%, and perforation in up to 7%. Perforations could be managed by endoscopic means.

Ablative Therapy

The most commonly used ablative techniques for BE have been photochemical destruction by photodynamic therapy (PDT) and thermal destruction by argon plasma coagulation. Other techniques include multipolar electrocoagulation and destruction of BE by liquid nitrogen or ultrasonic energy. These techniques are associated with local complications (such as strictures) due to deep thermal injury (mainly PDT) and the possibility of buried glandular mucosa (all methods).

PDT has been the best-studied ablative therapy. Pech and colleagues (65) reported the use of PDT with 5-aminolevulinic acid and demonstrated a long-term remission in 80% of patients with early mucosal cancer.

Recently, a balloon-based circumferential endoscopic radiofrequency device (HALO360) was introduced (BARRX Medical, Sunnyvale, California) (68). In a single trial, at 12 months follow-up, complete Barrett's eradication was achieved in 70% of patients with no strictures and no buried glandular mucosa (69).

The concept of a more individualized treatment using EMR with or without ablative therapy is interesting. For example, in the context of long segment Barrett's esophagus (LSBE), localized EMR is not an option because premalignant and malignant areas still may be present and new foci of dysplasia may develop over time (70). In addition, following circumferential EMR of LSBE, strictures may be long and difficult to treat. For such patients who have LSBE and early malignant changes, the combination of localized EMR and endoscopic ablation might be promising. So far, experience with this approach is limited.

Although new developments have made EMR technically easier, and despite promising new ablation techniques, it should be borne in mind that endoscopic treatment is only part of the overall management strategy of patients with early esophageal neoplasia. Apart from being skilled in endoscopic treatment, an endoscopist must be experienced in detecting and delineating early neoplasia and in selecting patients who are eligible for curative endoscopic treatment. In addition, adequate histopathological evaluation of EMR specimens may be difficult. Thus, to ensure optimal patient care, endoscopic treatment of early esophageal neoplasia should be centralized in centers with multidisciplinary experience in this field. Structured training aimed at improving endoscopic detection, endoscopic treatment, and histological evaluation of ER specimens is, therefore, necessary (71).

■ VAGAL-SPARING ESOPHAGECTOMY

Recently, vagal-sparing esophagectomy (VSE) has gained favor in a few centers in the United States. It was first described by Akiyama and colleagues as an effort to avoid the functional morbidity of standard esophagectomy by preserving the vagal trunks while removing all at-risk mucosa (72). It is similar to the transhiatal resection facilitating a limited nodal dissection and is advocated for treatment of intramucosal tumors. This approach is suitable only given confidence of the absence of regional nodal disease.

Procedure

The operation can be done with either open or laparoscopic techniques. The vagal nerves are identified and the proximal lesser curve is dissected similar to a highly selective vagotomy. Vessel loops are placed around the tissue bundles including both nerves. A gastric conduit is prepared and the stomach is divided below the esophagogastric junction. The left neck is dissected in a standard fashion exposing the cervical esophagus and it is divided at the level of thoracic inlet. A standard vein stripper is passed through the esophagus from abdomen to neck and is allowed to exit from the cut end of the cervical esophagus. A blunt "knob" is threaded onto its end and the esophagus is secured around the stripping device using an Endoloop. The stripper is slowly and gently pulled from the abdominal site progressively inverting the esophagus stripping it out of the posterior mediastinum. This maneuver strips the mucosa, circular, and most of the longitudinal muscle layer but preserves the vagal plexus intact, so that a pyloroplasty is not needed. Gastrointestinal continuity is restored by a gastric pull-up or colon interposition (21–23).

Outcomes and Comparison

Results from use of this technique show improved gastric function over esophageal resections that include a vagotomy and pyloroplasty. Incomplete resection of the esophagus is a concern, however, especially if multiple biopsies have been performed and scarring or tethering to surrounding structures has occurred. The morbidity and mortality are otherwise comparable to THE (73–75).

Banki and colleagues from the University of Southern California reported their initial results of VSE (76). Vagal function, assessed by increased acid output and pancreatic polypeptide levels after sham feeding and a preservation of normal gastric emptying, remained intact in 70% of the patients. Follow-up publications showed that the length of hospital stay and the incidence of major complications were significantly reduced when compared with transhiatal or en bloc transthoracic resection. Importantly, postvagotomy symptoms, such as dumping and diarrhea, were less common in the vagal-sparing group.

Peyre et al. describe their experience transitioning from en bloc esophagectomy to transhiatal esophagetomy to VSE in patients with Barrett's and high grade displasia (HGD) or intramucosal adenocarcinoma. In their series VSE is associated with significantly fewer major complications, a lower incidence of postvagotomy dumping syndrome, and less diarrhea than conventional esophagectomy. While the mortality was much lower in the VSE group (2%), the morbidity in these patients remained high (35%). The authors caution that for patients at high risk for lymph node metastasis, this is not an appropriate procedure (75). Jobe and colleagues reported minimally invasive vagal-sparing methods (77).

Candidates for vagal-sparing resection are relatively few and include those with high-grade dysplasia or nonvisible invasive cancer. The rationale includes the need for lifelong, meticulous, and intensive follow-up required after endoscopic techniques and the

small but real prevalence of failure, synchronous and metachronous cancer. VSE has the obvious advantage of removing all at risk mucosa, which obviates the need for rigorous follow-up.

■ MINIMALLY INVASIVE ESOPHAGECTOMY

With improved experience and skills for performing laparoscopic and thoracoscopic surgery, there have been a number of reports where these approaches have been used in association with the thoracic dissection of the esophagus or gastric mobilization, or both. These reports have confirmed that these approaches are possible, safe, and have reasonable outcomes when compared with the literature. As a result, over the past 10 years, minimally invasive esophagectomy (MIE) has gained significant popularity.

Indications and Contraindications

Relative contraindications include multiple previous laparotomies, massive ascites, previous major gastric resection, prior left pneumonectomy, or inability to tolerate single-lung anesthesia. Also, patients who have T4 lesions or bulky esophageal tumors are generally not candidates for resection.

Operative Technique

Thoracoscopy or transcervical mediastinoscopy are substituted for a thoracotomy, whereas laparoscopy is substituted for a laparotomy. The short-term outcomes have shown that the thoracoscopic-laparoscopic technique is safe and effective and offers comparable results to THE dissection with the benefits of less pain and a shorter hospital stay (78). Although these minimally invasive approaches are not aimed at achieving a radical resection, several recent studies have demonstrated the attempt of a hand-assisted minimally invasive approach to a radical thoracic lymphadenectomy. As these techniques are refined and taught in surgical training programs, the learning curves will fade and long-term outcomes will be established.

Outcomes and Comparisons

Recently, Luketich et al. reported their results of a series of 222 consecutive MIEs (10). MIE was successfully completed on 206 (92.8%) patients. The median lengths of stay were 1 day in the intensive care unit (ICU) and 7 days in the hospital. The operative mortality rate was 1.4%. Stage-specific survival was similar to open esophagectomy series.

Smithers et al. (11) describe patient outcomes from esophageal resection with respect to morbidity and cancer survival comparing open thoracotomy and laparotomy (open), with a thoracoscopic/laparotomy approach (thoracoscopic-assisted), and a total thoracoscopic/laparoscopic approach (total MIE): open, 114; thoracoscopic-assisted, 309; and total MIE, 23. The groups were comparable with respect to preoperative variables. There were no differences in lymph node retrieval for each of the approaches (11).

Recently, Zingg et al. retrospectively reviewed 56 patients who underwent MIE and 98 open esophagectomy (OE) from 1999 to 2007 (8). They concluded that MIE incorporating thoracoscopic esophageal dissection is comparable with OE in terms of morbidity, mortality, and oncologic survival. They suggest potential benefits for the minimally invasive approach in terms of less blood loss, shorter ICU stay, and possibly a shorter length of hospital stay.

Braghetto and colleagues describe their experience with MIE. They reported 166 patients who underwent surgery between 1990 and 2003. Open transthoracic surgery was performed on 60 patients. In this group of patients, postoperative mortality was observed in 11% of the cases. Major, minor, and late complications were observed in 61.6% of the patients, and the 3-year survival rate was 30% for this group. Open transhiatal surgery was performed on 59 patients. The morbidity, mortality, and 3-year rate were almost the same as for the transthoracic surgery group. For the 47 patients submitted to minimally invasive procedures (thoracoscopic and laparoscopic), the complications and mortality rates were significantly reduced (38.2% and 6.4%, respectively). For patients submitted to minimally invasive surgery, the 3-year survival rate was 45.4%. It is important to clarify that the patients submitted to minimally invasive surgery manifested early stages of the diseases, and morbidity and mortality and survival rates were better (9).

Berrisford et al. describe their experience with totally MIE being attempted on 77 patients, completed successfully on 70, abandoned in 6 patients (8%) with unsuspected metastatic disease, and converted to a thoracoscopic anastomosis in 1 patient. There was one in-hospital death (1%). Complications occurred in 33 patients (47%), including 9 gastric conduit-related complications

(13%). They report the median lymph node harvest was 21 (range 7–48) nodes. The mean overall and disease-free survival times were 35 and 33 months, respectively. Median disease-free survival for patients with stage III disease was 26 months. The authors expressed surprise that there was more morbidity here related to gastric tube ischemia than was expected (27).

A phase II study is currently in progress by the Eastern Cooperative Oncology Group (ECOG 2002) to evaluate the results of MIE in a multiinstitutional setting.

■ ROBOTIC-ASSISTED ESOPHAGECTOMY

Robotic surgery has generated much excitement and interest since the da Vinci Surgical System was approved in 2000. The da Vinci system offers the potential for more control and a more accurate nodal dissection than can be carried out by a traditional minimally invasive approach. Recent case series have described the first use of the da Vinci system to aid in esophagectomy (16,80).

The data on robotic-assisted esophagectomy suggest that the procedure is safe, feasible, and associated with perioperative outcomes similar to open esophagectomy and MIE. No data, however, demonstrate improved outcomes in terms of operative morbidity, pain, length of stay, operative time, or total costs.

■ EXTENT OF LYMPHADENECTOMY

The appropriate extent of lymphadenectomy during esophageal cancer surgery is debated. The minimum number of lymph nodes that should be removed during potentially curative esophagectomy has not been established.

Many high-volume surgical centers routinely perform en bloc esophagectomy with two-field (mediastinal, upper abdomen) lymph node dissection in the belief that this contributes to better locoregional control because of removal of metastatic lymph nodes. As noted above, however, surgical results from THE and transthoracic esophagectomy are comparable, despite the more extensive lymphadenectomy (mediastinal and all upper abdominal lymph nodes) that is typically performed as a component of transthoracic esophagectomy. An even more extensive lymphadenectomy, three-field lymphadenectomy of the mediastinal, abdominal and cervical nodes, is commonly practiced in Japan (81). In skilled hands, it can be performed with relatively low mortality and comparative morbidity to other techniques, but the long-term benefit of this approach compared to less extensive lymphadenectomy is controversial (82).

Proponents of extended lymphadenectomy emphasize the relationship between total lymph node count and prognosis and quote impressive long-term survival rates as evidence of its therapeutic benefit (83). For example, in one American series of 80 patients undergoing this technique in conjunction with en bloc esophagectomy, the overall 5-year survival rate was 51% (88% for node-negative and 33% for node-positive patients). Since the extent of lymph node dissection can affect the assignment of the final stage of disease, however, this resulting stage migration phenomenon hampers a stage-by-stage comparison between different forms of surgical resection. Furthermore, although unsuspected metastases in the recurrent laryngeal or cervical nodes were detected in 36% of patients in the above-noted series, others report a low incidence of cervical nodal recurrence following a two-field lymphadenectomy. The location of the tumor (upper vs middle to lower-third) may also have an influence on the frequency of finding cervical nodal metastases (82,84).

At least two randomized trials have compared different extents of lymphadenectomy during esophageal cancer surgery, although neither provides a conclusive result as to the benefit of extended lymphadenectomy (85).

A prospective trial from the Netherlands randomly assigned 220 (of 263 potentially eligible) patients with mid- to lower esophageal adenocarcinoma to THE (with celiac nodes dissected only if clinically suspicious and no cervical or mediastinal lymphadenectomy) or a transthoracic resection with an extended en bloc lymphadenectomy of mediastinal and upper abdominal nodes, and as a separate specimen, nodes in the aorticopulmonary window. Patients who received neoadjuvant chemotherapy or RT were excluded from the trial.

Perioperative morbidity was higher after transthoracic resection (mainly due to pulmonary complications). But in-hospital mortality was not significantly different (5% vs 2%). With a median follow-up of 4.7 years, there was a trend toward better disease-free (39% vs 27%) and overall survival (39% vs 29%) for the group undergoing transthoracic en

bloc esophagectomy, but neither reached the level of statistical significance.

A second prospective trial that directly compared extended (cervical and superior mediastinal) versus conventional lymphadenectomy in patients undergoing esophageal cancer resection was flawed because of the randomization of only 73 of a potential 264 eligible patients, raising the issue of selection bias. Following surgery, this small number of patients was randomly assigned to one of three groups for adjuvant therapy (none in 5, aggressive chemoradiotherapy in 32, and chemotherapy alone in 24). Although the authors concluded that 5-year survival (68% vs 44%) and local recurrence rates (20% vs 24%) favored extended lymphadenectomy, the heterogeneity in postoperative therapy makes it impossible to know whether the results were attributable to the extended lymphadenectomy.

In the United States, en bloc resection of the mediastinal and upper abdominal lymph nodes is considered a standard component of transthoracic esophagectomy, and a three-field lymphadenectomy has not been considered a standard treatment for patients with esophageal cancer. If a lymph node dissection is not done, however, then lymph node sampling should be carried out to accurately stage the patient and to gauge the response to induction treatment in patients enrolled in trials using neoadjuvant therapy.

■ PERIOPERATIVE CHEMOTHERAPY

The value of preoperative chemotherapy (usually consisting of cisplatin and fluorouracil) has been assessed in several large multiinstitutional trials, and the outcomes are conflicting. In contemporary practice, many patients with esophageal or gastroesophageal junction (GEJ) cancer are offered induction therapy with chemotherapy plus RT prior to attempted surgical resection. Although this is a preferred approach for patients who present with N1 or T3/4 disease, it is not universally accepted due to the lack of definitive data from randomized trials proving a survival benefit for neoadjuvant therapy followed by surgery over surgery alone (85–87).

In the United States, Intergroup 113 trial (also known as RTOG 8911), a randomized study involving 440 North American patients showed no benefit, with 35% of patients in the chemotherapy plus surgery group alive after 2 years as compared with 37% of patients in the surgery-alone group (86). Authors report that delivery of postoperative therapy was difficult.

Using a similar strategy, the Medical Research Council (MRC) enrolled 802 patients with esophageal cancer (EC) to surgery alone versus two cycles of chemotherapy followed by surgery. The latter group had better outcomes (overall survival [OS], 16.8 vs 13.3 months; 2-year survival, 43% vs 34%) (85).

Although the British study included almost twice as many patients, it did not require preoperative CT staging or stipulate the surgical technique. The North American study required CT staging, prescribed the operative technique, and used a longer and more intensive course of chemotherapy.

Node-positive (stage IIB and III) esophageal cancers are associated with high rates of recurrence and death. The optimal management of patients with esophageal and GEJ cancer who have persistently node-positive disease following neoadjuvant therapy is unclear. In patients who are found to have node-positive disease after undergoing surgery alone, the addition of postoperative chemotherapy with or without RT may be considered in an effort to improve outcomes.

■ CONCLUSION

Over the past two decades significant strides have been made in understanding the biology and mechanisms of treatment of esophageal cancer. Modern therapies strive to be less invasive and reduce the morbidity of traditional esophagectomy.

However, cure of this disease continues to pose a challenge and modern therapies will continue to evolve as does understanding of the disease.

■ REFERENCES

1. Institute, N.C. 2009 Available at http://www.cancer.gov/cancertopics/tvpes/esophageal/.
2. Parkin DM, Pisani P, Ferlay J. Estimates of the worldwide incidence of 25 major cancers in 1990. *Int J Cancer* 1999;80(6):
3. Posner MC, Forastiere AA, Minsky BD. Cancer of the esophagus. In Govindan, Ramaswamy, ed. *Cancer: Principles & Practice of Oncology*, 2005:Lippincott Williams and Wilkins.
4. Reed CE. Surgical management of esophageal carcinoma. *Oncologist* 1999;4(2):95–105.
5. American Cancer Society. *Cancer Facts and Figures 2009*.
6. Enzinger PC, Mayer RJ. Esophageal cancer. *N Engl J Med* 2003;349(23):2241–2252.
7. Hofstetter W, Swisher SG, Correa AM, et al. Treatment outcomes of resected esophageal cancer. *Ann Surg* 2002;236(3):376–84; discussion 384.
8. Zingg U, McQuinn A, DiValentino D, et al. Minimally invasive versus open esophagectomy for patients with esophageal cancer. *Ann Thorac Surg* 2009;87(3):911–919.
9. Braghetto L, Csendes A, Cardemil G, et al. Open transthoracic or transhiatal esophagectomy versus minimally invasive esophagectomy in terms of morbidity, mortality and survival. Surg Endosc 2006;20(11):1681–1686.
10. Luketich JD, Alvelo-Rivera M, Buenaventura PO, et al. Minimally invasive esophagectomy: outcomes in 222 patients. *Ann Surg* 2003;238(4):486–94; discussion 494.
11. Smithers BM, Gotley DC, Martin I, Thomas JM. Comparison of the outcomes between open and minimally invasive esophagectomy. *Ann Surg* 2007;245(2):232–240.
12. Kitagawa H, Akimori T, Okabayashi T, et al. Total laparoscopic gastric mobilization for esophagectomy. *Langenbecks Arch Surg* 2009;394(4):617–621.
13. Miura A, Momma K, Yoshida M. Endoscopic resection for Tla-MM and Tlb-SMl squamous cell carcinoma of the esophagus. *J Clin Gastroenterol* 2009;1–5.
14. Shimizu Y, Kato M, Yamamoto J, et al. EMR combined with chemoradiotherapy: a novel treatment for superficial esophageal squamous-cell carcinoma. *Gastrointest Endosc* 2004;59(2):199–204.
15. Ell C, May A, Gossner L, et al. Endoscopic mucosal resection of early cancer and high-grade dysplasia in Barrett's esophagus. *Gastroenterology* 2000;118(4):670–677.
16. Horgan S, Berger RA, Elli EF, Espat NJ. Robotic-assisted minimally invasive transhiatal esophagectomy. *Am Surg* 2003;69(7):624–626.
17. Koshy M, Esaiashvilli N, Landry JC, et al. Multiple management modalities in esophageal cancer: Epidemiology, presentation and progression, work-up, and surgical approaches. *Oncologist* 2004;9:137–146.
18. Khushalani NL. *Cancer of the Esophagus and Stomach*: Mayo Clinic Proceedings June 2008;83(6):712–722.
19. Denk W, Zur Radikahperation des osophaguskarfzentralbiChirurg 1913;40:1065.
20. Turner G, Excision of thoracic esophagus for carcinoma with construction of extrathoracic gullet. *Lancet* 1933;2:836–851.
21. Orringer MB, Sloan H. Substernal gastric bypass of the excluded thoracic esophagus for palliation of esophageal carcinoma. *J Thorac Cardiovasc Surg* 1975;70(5):836–851.
22. Barbier PA, Becker CD, Wagner HE. Esophageal carcinoma: patient selection for transhiatal esophagectomy. A prospective analysis of 50 consecutive cases. *World J Surg* 1988;12(2):263–269.
23. Daniel TM, Fleischer KJ, Flanagan TL, Tribble CG, Kron IL. Transhiatal esophagectomy: a safe alternative for selected patients. *Ann Thorac Surg* 1992;54(4):686–9; discussion 689.

24. Orringer MB, Marshall B, Iannettoni MD. Transhiatal esophagectomy: clinical experience and refinements. *Ann Surg* 1999;230(3):392–400; discussion 400.

25. Orringer MB. Transhiatal esophagectomy for benign disease. *J Thorac Cardiovasc Surg* 1985;90(5):649–655.

26. Orringer MB, Stirling MC. Esophageal resection for achalasia: indications and results. *Ann Thorac Surg* 1989;47(3):340–345.

27. Liebermann-Meffert DM, Luescher U, Neff U, Rüedi TP, Allgöwer M. Esophagectomy without thoracotomy: is there a risk of intramediastinal bleeding? A study on blood supply of the esophagus. *Ann Surg* 1987;206(2):184–192.

28. Orringer MB, Marshall B, Chang AC, Lee J, Pickens A, Lau CL. Two thousand transhiatal esophagectomies: changing trends, lessons learned. *Ann Surg* 2007;246(3):363–72; discussion 372.

29. Iannettoni MD, Whyte RI, Orringer MB. Catastrophic complications of the cervical esophagogastric anastomosis. *J Thorac Cardiovasc Surg* 1995;110(5): 1493–1500; discussion 1500–1501.

30. Cooke DT, Lin GC, Lau CL , *et al* . Analysis of cervical esophagogastric anastomotic leaks after transhiatal esophagectomy: risk factors, presentation, and detection. *Ann Thorac Surg* 2009;88(1):177–185; discussion 184.

31. Buecker A, Wein BB, Neuerburg JM, Guenther RW. Esophageal perforation: comparison of use of aqueous and barium-containing contrast media. *Radiology* 1997;202(3):683–686.

32. Levine MS. What is the best oral contrast material to use for the fluoroscopic diagnosis of esophageal rupture? *AJR Am J Roentgenol* 1994;162(5):1243.

33. Reich SB. Production of pulmonary edema by aspiration of water-soluble nonabsorbable contrast media. *Radiology* 1969;92(2):367–370.

34. Orringer MB, Lemmer JH. Early dilation in the treatment of esophageal disruption. *Ann Thorac Surg* 1986;42(5):536–539.

35. Chang AC, Orringer MB. Management of the cervical esophagogastric anastomotic stricture. *Semin Thorac Cardiovasc Surg* 2007;19(1):66–71.

36. Ercan S, Rice TW, Murthy SC, Rybicki LA, Blackstone EH. Does esophagogastric anastomotic technique influence the outcome of patients with esophageal cancer? *J Thorac Cardiovasc Surg* 2005;129(3):623–631.

37. Raz DJ, Tedesco P, Herbella FA, Nipomnick I, Way LW, Patti MG. Side-to-side stapled intra-thoracic esophagogastric anastomosis reduces the incidence of leaks and stenosis. *Dis Esophagus* 2008;21(1):69–72.

38. Binkert CA, Yucel EK, Davison BD, Sugarbaker DJ, Baum RA. Percutaneous treatment of high-output chylothorax with embolization or needle disruption technique. *J Vasc Interv Radiol* 2005;16(9):1257–1262.

39. Cope C, Kaiser LR. Management of unremitting chylothorax by percutaneous embolization and blockage of retroperitoneal lymphatic vessels in 42 patients. *J Vasc Interv Radiol* 2002;13(11):1139–1148.

40. Allen MS. Ivor Lewis esophagectomy. *Semin Thorac Cardiovasc Surg* 1992;4(4):320–323.

41. Junemann-Ramirez M, Awan MY, Khan ZM, Rahamim JS. Anastomotic leakage post-esophagogastrectomy for esophageal carcinoma: retrospective analysis of predictive factors, management and influence on longterm survival in a high volume centre. *Eur J Cardiothorac Surg* 2005;27(1):3–7.

42. Karl RC, Schreiber R, Boulware D, Baker S, Coppola D. Factors affecting morbidity, mortality, and survival in patients undergoing Ivor Lewis esophagogastrectomy. *Ann Surg* 2000;231(5):635–641.

43. Dumont P, Wihlm JM, Hentz JG, Roeslin N, Lion R, Morand G. Respiratory complications after surgical treatment of esophageal cancer. A study of 309 patients according to the type of resection. *Eur J Cardiothorac Surg* 1995;9(10):539–543.

44. Ott K, Bader FG, Lordick F, Feith M, Bartels H, Siewert JR. Surgical factors influence the outcome after Ivor-Lewis esophagectomy with intrathoracic anastomosis for adenocarcinoma of the esophagogastric junction: a consecutive series of 240 patients at an experienced center. *Ann Surg Oncol* 2009;16(4):1017–1025.

45. Kauer WKH., Stein HJ, Dittler H, et al. Stent implantation as a treatment option in patients with thoracic anastomotic leaks after esophagectomy. *Surg Endosc* 2008;22(1):50–53.

46. Rentz J, Bull D, Harpole D, et al. Transthoracic versus transhiatal esophagectomy: a prospective study of 945 patients. *J Thorac Cardiovasc Surg* 2003;125(5):1114–1120.

47. Chang AC, Ji H, Birkmeyer NJ, Orringer MB, Birkmeyer JD. Outcomes after transhiatal and transthoracic esophagectomy for cancer. *Ann Thorac Surg* 2008;85(2):424–429.

48. Wolff CS, Castillo SF, Larson DR, et al. Ivor Lewis approach is superior to transhiatal approach in retrieval of lymph nodes at esophagectomy. *Dis Esophagus* 2008;21(4):328–333.

49. Block MI. Transthoracic vs. transhiatal esophagectomy: Stage migration muddies the water. *J Surg Oncol* 2006;93(7):519–520.

50. LOGAN A. The surgical treatment of carcinoma of the esophagus and cardia. *J Thorac Cardiovasc Surg* 1963;46:150–161.

51. Skinner DB. En bloc resection for neoplasms of the esophagus and cardia. *J Thorac Cardiovasc Surg* 1983;85(1):59–71.

52. DeMeester TR, Zaninotto G, Johansson KE. Selective therapeutic approach to cancer of the lower esophagus and cardia. *J Thorac Cardiovasc Surg* 1988;95(1):42–54.

53. Altorki N, Skinner D. Should en bloc esophagectomy be the standard of care for esophageal carcinoma? *Ann Surg* 2001;234(5):581–587.

54. Collard JM. Exclusive radical surgery for esophageal adenocarcinoma. *Cancer* 2001;91(6):1098–1104.

55. Collard JM, Otte JB, Fiasse R, et al. Skeletonizing en bloc esophagectomy for cancer. *Ann Surg* 2001;234(1):25–32.

56. Hagen JA, DeMeester SR, Peters JH, Chandrasoma P, DeMeester TR. Curative resection for esophageal adenocarcinoma: analysis of 100 en bloc esophagectomies. *Ann Surg* 2001;234(4):520–30; discussion 530.

57. Siewert JR, Stein HJ, Feith M, Bruecher BL, Bartels H, Fink U. Histologic tumor type is an independent prognostic parameter in esophageal cancer: lessons from more than 1,000 consecutive resections at a single center in the Western world. *Ann Surg* 2001;234(3):360–7; discussion 368.

58. Lerut T, De Leyn P, Coosemans W, Van Raemdonck D, Scheys I, LeSaffre E. Surgical strategies in esophageal carcinoma with emphasis on radical lymphadenectomy. *Ann Surg* 1992;216(5):583–590.

59. Lund O, Kimose HH, Aagaard MT, Hasenkam JM, Erlandsen M. Risk stratification and long-term results after surgical treatment of carcinomas of the thoracic esophagus and cardia. A 25-year retrospective study. *J Thorac Cardiovasc Surg* 1990;99(2):200–209.

60. Johansson J, DeMeester TR, Hagen JA, et al. En bloc vs transhiatal esophagectomy for stage T3 N1 adenocarcinoma of the distal esophagus. *Arch Surg* 2004;139(6):627–31; discussion 631.

61. Portale G, Hagen JA, Peters JH, et al. Modern 5-year survival of resectable esophageal adenocarcinoma: single institution experience with 263 patients. *J Am Coll Surg* 2006;202(4):588–96; discussion 596.

62. Hulscher JB, Van Sandick JW, Offerhaus GJ, Tilanus HW, Obertop H, Van Lanschot JJ. Prospective analysis of the diagnostic yield of extended en bloc resection for adenocarcinoma of the oesophagus or gastric cardia. *Br J Surg* 2001;88(5):715–719.

63. Stein HJ, Feith M, Bruecher BL, Naehrig J, Sarbia M, Siewert JR. Early esophageal cancer: pattern of lymphatic spread and prognostic factors for long-term survival after surgical resection. *Ann Surg* 2005;242(4):566–73; discussion 573.

64. Inoue H, Endo M, Takeshita K, et al. Endoscopic resection of carcinoma in situ of the esophagus accompanied by esophageal varices. *Surg Endosc* 1991;5(4):182–184.

65. Pech O, May A, Rabenstein T, Ell C. Endoscopic resection of early oesophageal cancer. *Gut* 2007;56(11):1625–1634.

66. Ono H, Kondo H, Gotoda T, et al. Endoscopic mucosal resection for treatment of early gastric cancer. *Gut* 2001;48(2):225–229.

67. Das A, Singh V, Fleischer DE, Sharma VK. A comparison of endoscopic treatment and surgery in early esophageal cancer: an analysis of surveillance epidemiology and end results data. *Am J Gastroenterol* 2008;103(6):1340–1345.

68. Ganz RA, Overholt BF, Sharma VK, et al.. U.S. Multicenter Registry. Circumferential ablation of Barrett's esophagus that contains high-grade dysplasia: a U.S. Multicenter Registry. *Gastrointest Endosc* 2008;68(1):35–40.

69. Sharma VK, Wang KK, Overholt BF, et al. Balloon-based, circumferential, endoscopic radiofrequency ablation of Barrett's esophagus: 1-year follow-up of 100 patients. *Gastrointest Endosc* 2007;65(2):185–195.

70. Shaheen NJ, Sharma P, Overholt BF, et al. Radiofrequency ablation in Barrett's esophagus with dysplasia. *N Engl J Med* 2009;360(22):2277–2288.

71. Siersema PD. Esophageal cancer. *Gastroenterol Clin North Am* 2008;37(4):943–964.

72. Akiyama H, Hiyama M, Miyazono H. Total esophageal reconstruction after extraction of the esophagus. *Ann Surg* 1975;182(5):547–552.

73. Horváth OP, Kalmár K. Early-stage adenocarcinoma in Barrett's esophagus: aspects of surgical therapies. *Dig Dis* 2009;27(1):45–53.

74. Pech O, Ell C. Is vagal-sparing esophagectomy ideal for Barrett's esophagus with intramucosal adenocarcinoma or high-grade dysplasia? *Nat Clin Pract Gastroenterol Hepatol* 2008;5(6):302.

75. Peyre CG, DeMeester SR, Rizzetto C, et al. Vagal-sparing esophagectomy: the ideal operation for intramucosal adenocarcinoma and barrett with high-grade dysplasia. *Ann Surg* 2007;246(4):665.

76. Banki F, Mason RJ, DeMeester SR, et al. Vagal-sparing esophagectomy: a more physiologic alternative. *Ann Surg* 2002;236(3):324–35; discussion 335.

77. Jobe BA, Kim CY, Minjarez RC, O'Rourke R, Chang EY, Hunter JG. Simplifying minimally invasive transhiatal esophagectomy with the inversion approach: Lessons learned from the first 20 cases. *Arch Surg* 2006;141(9):857–65; discussion 865.

78. Gemmill EH, McCulloch P. Systematic review of minimally invasive resection for gastro-oesophageal cancer. *Br J Surg* 2007;94(12):1461–1467.

79. Berrisford RG, Wajed SA, Sanders D, Rucklidge MW. Short-term outcomes following total minimally invasive oesophagectomy. *Br J Surg* 2008;95(5):602–610.

80. van Hillegersberg R, Boone J, Draaisma WA, Broeders IA, Giezeman MJ, Borel Rinkes IH. First experience with robot-assisted thoracoscopic esophagolymphadenectomy for esophageal cancer. *Surg Endosc* 2006;20(9):1435–1439.

81. Kajitani T. The general rules for the gastric cancer study in surgery and pathology. Part I. Clinical classification. *Jpn J Surg* 1981;11(2):127–139.

82. Wilson M, Rosato EL, Chojnacki KA, et al. Prognostic significance of lymph node metastases and ratio in esophageal cancer. *J Surg Res* 2008;146(1):11–15.

83. Greenstein AJ, Litle VR, Swanson SJ, Divino CM, Packer S, Wisnivesky JP. Prognostic significance of the number of lymph node metastases in esophageal cancer. *J Am Coll Surg* 2008;206(2):239–246.

84. Peyre CG, Hagen JA, DeMeester SR, et al. The number of lymph nodes removed predicts survival in esophageal cancer: an international study on the impact of extent of surgical resection. *Ann Surg* 2008;248(4):549–556. 10.1097/SLA.0b013e318188c474.

85. Group MRCOCW. Surgical resection with or without preoperative chemotherapy in oesophageal cancer: a randomised controlled trial. *Lancet* 2002;359: 1727–1733.

86. Kelsen DP, Ginsberg R, Pajak TF, et al. Chemotherapy followed by surgery compared with surgery alone for localized esophageal cancer. *N Engl J Med* 1998;339(27):1979–1984.

87. Urschel JD, Vasan H. A meta-analysis of randomized controlled trials that compared neoadjuvant chemoradiation and surgery to surgery alone for resectable esophageal cancer. *Am J Surg* 2003;185(6):538–543.

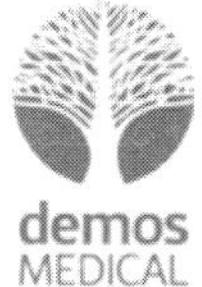

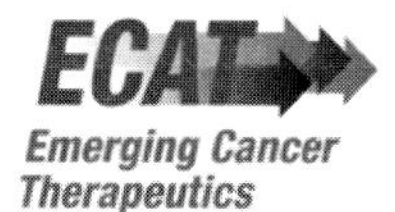

Esophageal Cancer

New Developments in Combined-Modality Therapy

Bryan Chang*

Yale Cancer Center, Yale University School of Medicine, New Haven, CT

■ **ABSTRACT**

Although the exact benefit over surgery alone is controversial, preoperative chemoradiation with cisplatin, 5-fluorouracil (5-FU), and radiation to 50–50.4 Gy followed by surgical resection has emerged as the standard treatment for locally advanced esophageal cancer in the United States. Patients with localized disease who are inoperable are typically treated with the same regimen minus surgery, and approximately 25% will be long-term survivors. The significant toxicity of this regimen and local failure rates of up to 40% have prompted investigators to study combined-modality regimens for esophageal cancer incorporating novel systemic agents including taxanes, irinotecan, oxaliplatin, EGFR inhibitors, trastuzumab, and bevacizumab. Finally, results of two recent European randomized trials suggest that chemoradiation alone offers long-term survival equivalent to chemoradiation followed by surgery in localized squamous cell cancers of the esophagus.

■ **INTRODUCTION**

Modern surgical series performed in cooperative group settings have demonstrated that over 80% of patients who undergo surgery alone for apparently localized esophageal cancer will ultimately suffer disease recurrence and death from cancer (1,2). The high rates of local recurrence and distant metastases seen in these trials indicate that there is a significant risk of persistent local tumor as well as micrometastatic disease, even in patients who undergo margin-negative resection.

Preoperative concurrent chemoradiation has been studied as a way to improve outcomes by increasing locoregional control, improving resectability, and

decreasing distant metastases. Several randomized phase 3 trials have tested preoperative chemoradiation followed by surgery against surgery alone for localized esophageal cancer (Table 3).

Walsh and colleagues conducted a randomized trial of preoperative chemoradiation with cisplatin and 5-fluorouracil (5-FU) and concurrent radiotherapy versus surgery alone. Patients with localized adenocarcinoma of the esophagus and gastric cardia were eligible, and staging included chest radiography, abdominal ultrasound, and upper endoscopy. The median survival of the combined modality group was 16 months, compared to 11 months for the surgery arm, and the 3-year survival was also improved (32% vs 6%). The rate of pathological complete response (pCR) was 25%, and the rate of nodal involvement at surgery was significantly lower in the combined modality arm (42% vs 82%, $P < 0.001$). However,

---

*Corresponding author, Department of Therapeutic Radiology, Yale University School of Medicine, New Haven, CT
  E-mail address: bryan.chang@yale.edu

Emerging Cancer Therapeutics 1 (2010) 35–58.

DOI: 10.5003/2151–4194.1.1.37

TABLE 3 Randomized clinical trials of trimodality therapy versus surgery for esophageal cancer

Reference	Patients	Chemo	RT	pCR	Survival	Notes
Irish (3)	CRTS— 58 S—55	F 15 mg/kg days 1–5, 36–40 C 75 mg/m^2 days 1, 36	40 Gy in 15 fx beginning day 1	CRTS—22%	3 YS: CRTS—32% S—6% $P = 0.01$	ACA only No routine EUS or CT
EORTC (4)	CRTS— 143 S—138	C 80 mg/m^2 given 0–2 days before first day of each RT cycle	37 Gy in 10 fx, split course	CRTS—20%	3 YS: CRTS—33% S—36% $P = NS$	SCC only No EUS Single-agent chemo w/ hypofractionated RT
University of Michigan (5)	CRTS—50 S—50	F 300 mg/m^2 days 1–21 C 20 mg/m^2 days 1–5, 17–21 VB 1 mg/m^2 days 1–4, 17–20	45 Gy in 30 fractions, given bid, beginning day 1	CRTS—28%	3 YS: CRTS—30% S—16% $P = NS$	SCC and ACA
Australian (6)	CRTS—128 S—128	F 800 mg/m^2 days 1–4 C 80 mg/m^2 day 1	35 Gy in 15 fractions, beginning day 1	CRTS—16%	5 YS: CRTS—35% S—31% $P = NS$	SCC and ACA Low doses of chemo and RT R0 surgery achieved in 80% of CRTS vs 59% of S patients ($P = 0.0002$)
CALGB (7)	CRTS—30 S—26	F 1 g/m^2 days 1–4, 29–32 C 100 mg/m^2 days 1, 29	50.4 Gy in 28 fractions	CRTS—40%	5 YS: CRTS—39% S—16% $P = 0.008$	SCC and ACA MS 4.48 years in CRTS arm vs 1.79 years in S arm

ACA, adenocarcinoma; C, cisplatin; chemo, chemotherapy; CRTS, neoadjuvant chemoradiation followed by surgery; CT, staging computed tomography scan; EUS, staging endoscopic ultrasound; F, 5-fluorouracil; fx, fractions; Gy, gray; MS, median survival; NS, difference not significant at $P < 0.05$; pCR, pathological complete response; RT, radiation; S, surgery alone arm; SCC, squamous cell carcinoma; VB, vinblastine; YS, years survival.

the outcomes in the surgical arm are generally regarded as unexpectedly poor, leading to questions about the adequacy of the staging procedures (3).

In 1997, Bosset et al. published results of an EORTC trial comparing preoperative treatment with cisplatin and split-course hypofractionated radiation with surgery alone. Stage I and II patients with squamous cell carcinoma were included, although endoscopic ultrasound was not used in staging. In contrast to the Walsh results, the EORTC trial resulted in a median survival of 18.6 months for both arms. The rate of postoperative mortality was 12.3% in the combined-modality arm, compared to 4% in the surgery-alone arm. Preoperative chemoradiation did lead to significantly improved disease-free survival and local control and a higher rate of curative resection. The use of split-course hypofractionated radiation and single-agent cisplatin as opposed to standard radiation and two-drug chemotherapy may have hindered the performance of the combined modality arm (4).

Two smaller studies have also addressed the question of whether adding preoperative chemoradiation improves outcomes in localized esophageal cancer. Urba et al. randomized patients to surgery versus preoperative cisplatin, 5-FU, and vinblastine with radiation delivered in 1.5 Gy fractions, twice a day, to 45 Gy. Chemoradiation was followed by a transhiatal esophagectomy. A total of 100 patients were randomized, and the pCR rate was 28%. Although locoregional control was better in the combined modality arm, there was no decrease in distant metastases. The median survival was not significantly different (16.9 months) compared to the surgery-alone arm (17.6 months), although the trial was only powered to detect an increase in median survival from 1 to 2.2 years (5). More recently, Tepper et al. published the results of CALGB 9781, a randomized phase 3 trial designed to compare trimodality therapy with cisplatin, 5-FU, and 50.4 Gy followed by surgery to surgery alone. Due to poor accrual, the trial was closed after only 56 patients were enrolled. The median survival was 4.48 years in the combined modality arm and 1.79 years in the surgery-alone arm (7).

A metaanalysis comparing preoperative chemoradiation to surgery alone for esophageal cancer found a nonsignificant trend toward improved survival for trimodality therapy. However, when analysis was confined to concurrent chemoradiation studies, there was a significant improvement in 3-year survival (odds radio [OR] for mortality 0.45, 95% confidence interval [CI] 0.26–0.79) (8). A second metaanalysis included 1,209 patients from 10 studies and found that trimodality therapy significantly decreased all-cause mortality at 2 years (hazard ratio [HR] 0.81, 95% CI 0.7–0.93) (9).

Despite the ongoing controversy, preoperative chemoradiation with cisplatin, 5-FU, and 50.4 Gy radiotherapy has been adopted as a standard practice in the United States for patients with T3–4 or node-positive localized esophageal cancers. Similarly, patients with localized disease who are medically inoperable or refuse surgery are typically treated with the same regimen. RTOG 85–01 convincingly demonstrated that adding two cycles of concurrent cisplatin (75 mg/m^2, day 1 or weeks 1 and 5) and 5-FU (1,000 mg/m^2/day, days 1–4 of weeks 1 and

5) to 50 Gy improves survival compared to radiation alone at a higher dose (64.8 Gy). Three-year survival was 26% in the combined modality arm, compared to 0% in the radiation-alone arm (10). A subsequent Intergroup trial comparing 50.4 Gy with concurrent cisplatin and 5-FU to 64.8 Gy with the same chemotherapy failed to show a benefit to increasing the dose of radiation (11). Current areas of investigation in combined modality treatment of localized esophageal cancer include intensified chemoradiation with newer chemotherapeutic agents, adding biologically targeted therapy to chemoradiation, and the possibility of omitting surgery following definitive chemoradiation.

■ CHEMORADIATION WITH TAXANES

Paclitaxel is a radiosensitizing agent (12) known to have single-agent activity in the setting of metastatic esophageal cancer (13). Numerous phase1 and 2 studies have evaluated paclitaxel-based chemoradiation regimens in the neoadjuvant setting in an effort to improve pathological response rates and survival; results are summarized in Table 4. A single-arm study from Brown University enrolled 41 patients with locally advanced esophageal cancer, including 6 patients with celiac or portal adenopathy. A regimen of weekly paclitaxel, cisplatin, and 50.4 Gy was delivered. Only 5% of patients had grade 4 esophagitis, and the 2-year overall survival rate was 54% (14). Memorial Sloan-Kettering Cancer Center researchers treated 34 patients with escalating doses of paclitaxel up to 80 mg/m^2, 30 mg/m^2 weekly cisplatin, and 50.4 Gy radiation. The regimen was tolerable and 22 patients underwent resection, yielding a pCR rate of 24% (15). RTOG 0113 tested two taxane-based chemoradiation regimens in the cooperative-group setting. The protocol enrolled 84 patients with localized esophageal cancer who were unwilling or unable to undergo surgery. Patients were randomized to either induction chemotherapy with 5-FU, cisplatin, and paclitaxel followed by 5-FU, paclitaxel, and 50.4 Gy (Arm A) or induction with cisplatin and paclitaxel and chemoradiation with the same agents and 50.4 Gy (Arm B). Disappointingly, there was substantial toxicity. In Arm A, 27% of patients had grade 4 toxicity, and 3% died. In Arm B, 40% of patients had grade 4 toxicity, and 6% died. Median survival time was 28.7 months for Arm A and 14.9

TABLE 4 Two-drug taxane-based chemoradiation regimens for esophageal cancer

Reference	Study Type	Patients	Chemo	RT	Toxicity	Outcomes	Notes
Brown University (14)	Phase 2	$N = 41$ 29 ACA and 12 SCC; 6 M1a	P 60 mg/m^2/week C 25 mg/m^2/week days 1, 8, 15, 22	1.8 Gy/day, beginning day 1, to 50.4 Gy	G4 esophagitis 5% G3–4 neutropenia 24%	2 YS 54% CR 29%	
MSKCC (15)	Phase 1	34 LA 3 recurrent	P 10–80 mg/m^2/week C 30 mg/m^2/week days 1, 8, 15, 22, 28, 36	1.8 Gy/day, beginning day 1, to 50.4 Gy	DLT at P 80 mg/m^2/week	16/22 had R0 resection pCR 24%	P 60 mg/m^2/week safe and tolerable
RTOG 0113 (16)	Phase 2 RCT	$N = 84$ T1N1 or T2–4 localized; unresectable or unfit for surgery	Arm A Induction: F 700 mg/m^2 C 15 mg/m^2 days 1–5 P 200 mg/m^2 day 1 every 4 weeks × 2 Arm A CRT: P 50 mg/m^2 weekly F 300 mg/m^2/day w/RT Arm B Induction: C 75 mg/m^2 P 175 mg/m^2 every 3 weeks × 2 Arm B CRT: C 30 mg/m^2 weekly P 60 mg/m^2/day w/RT	1.8 Gy/day, beginning day 1 of CRT, to 50.4 Gy	Arm A: G3—54% G4—27% Death—3% Arm B: G3—43% G4—40% Death—6%	Arm A: 1 YS—75.7% 2 YS—56% MS—28.7 months Arm B: 1 YS, 2 YS—37% MS—14.9 months	No surgery permitted Both arms toxic
UC Davis (17)	Phase 2	$N = 50$ 16 stage II 8 stage III 26 stage IV 67% ACA 33% SCC	CB AUC 1.5/week P 30 mg/m^2 twice/week during RT and 2 cycles after RT if unresectable	1.8 Gy/day, beginning day 1, to 45 Gy; 50.4 Gy if unresectable	G3–4 nausea—19% G3–4 esophagitis—9% G3–4 neutropenia—4%	CR 26% PR 17% SD 41% stage II–III: CRTS—MS 44 months CRT—MS > 44 months stage IV: MS 12 months	

Vanderbilt (18)	Phase 2	N = 50 resectable unresectable	C 75 mg/m^2 P 175 mg/m^2 days 1, 29 Postop: P 175 mg/m^2 day 1 F 350 mg/m^2 days 1–3 every 28 days × 2	2 Gy/day beginning day 1, to 30 Gy; 60 Gy if unresectable	G3–4 leukopenia 34.8% G3–4 nausea 17.3% G3–4 dysphagia 15.2%	40 had surgery 25 completed all treatment pCR 17% MS 20.4 months 3 YS 23.2%	Preoperative treatment tolerable but not superior to standard of care
Taiwan (19)	Phase 2	N = 97 T3N0–1 or T1–3N1M0 95% SCC 90% T3N1	C 15 mg/m^2 day 2, 5 P 35 mg/m^2 days 1, 4 weekly	2 Gy/day beginning day 1, to 40 Gy; 60 Gy if unresectable	G3–4 leukopenia—30% G3–4 thrombocytopenia—10% G3–4 diarrhea—15%	61 had surgery pCR 25% MS 28.8 months	
Taiwan (20)	Phase 2	N = 56 30 T3N1 7 M1a 19 M1b All SCC	Induction: P 70 mg/m^2 or D 40 mg/m^2 C 15 mg/m^2 F 2 g day 1, 8 P 35 mg/m^2 day 1, 4 C 15 mg/m^2 day 2, 5 weekly	2 Gy/day beginning day 1, to 40 Gy; 60 Gy if unresectable	G3–4 leukopenia 30% G3–4 thrombocytopenia 10% G3–4 diarrhea 15%	pCR 20% 1 YS 76% 2 YS 57%	
University of Michigan (21)	Phase 2	N = 69	C 75 mg/m^2 day 1 P 60 mg/m^2 days 1, 8, 15, 22	1.5 Gy bid beginning day 1, to 45 Gy	G3–4 neutropenia—13% Feeding tube 17%	90% had R0 resection pCR 19% MS—24 months 1 YS—75% 2 YS—50% 3 YS—34%	
Italy (22)	Phase 2	N = 74 stage II–III 50% ACA	D 35 mg/m^2 P 25 mg/m^2 weekly × 8 F 180 mg/m^2 days 1–21 and 150 mg/m^2 days 29–64	2 Gy/day beginning day 29, to 50 Gy	G3–4 hematologic 13.5% G3–4 nonhematologic 30% Deaths 4%, including 2 postoperative	pCR 47% MS 50 months 3 YS 81% in pCR patients	High pCR rate and MS but toxic

ACA, adenocarcinoma; AUC, area under the curve; C, cisplatin; CB, carboplatin; CR, clinical complete response; D, docetaxel; DLT, dose-limiting toxicity; F, 5-fluorouracil; G, toxicity grade; Gy, gray; I, irinotecan; MS, median survival; MTD, maximum tolerated dose; P, paclitaxel; pCR, pathological complete response; PR, clinical partial response; SCC, squamous cell carcinoma; SD, stable disease; X, capecitabine; YS, years survival.

months for Arm B. The 75.7% 1-year survival rate for Arm A fell short of the 77.5% goal established for the trial (16).

Several groups have investigated three-drug paclitaxel-based neoadjuvant chemoradiation, as shown in Table 5. Meluch et al. reported results of a phase 2 study of 123 patients with resectable stage I to III esophageal cancer. Treatment consisted of paclitaxel 200 mg/m^2 and carboplatin area-under-the-curve (AUC) 6 on days 1 and 22 and 5-FU 225 mg/m^2/day on days 1 to 42 with radiation to 45 Gy beginning day 1. Seventy-four percent of patients were able to undergo resection, and the pCR rate was 38%. Six percent of patients died postoperatively. Three-year survival was 41% (23). Gannett and colleagues treated 24 patients with locally advanced esophageal cancer with weekly carboplatin and paclitaxel plus infusional 5-FU and 45 Gy, resulting in an impressive 12 patients with pCR and 48% 3-year survival (24). A study of preoperative carboplatin, paclitaxel, infusional 5-FU, and radiotherapy with amifostine produced a pCR rate of 35% but was highly toxic, with three treatment-related deaths, one of which was attributed to amifostine (25). Similarly, a small phase 1 trial of carboplatin, paclitaxel, and capecitabine with radiation showed significant toxicity (26).

Docetaxel was investigated as a single-agent radiosensitizer in esophageal and non–small cell lung cancer by Mauer et al. in 1998 (30). Patients were treated with 60 Gy and concurrent escalating doses of docetaxel. Esophagitis and neutropenia were the dose-limiting toxicities, and a weekly dose of 20 mg/m^2 was recommended for phase 2 studies. Two patients had fatal pulmonary infiltrates, and 5 of 29 patients experienced late esophageal strictures. Higuchi et al. performed a phase 1 study of escalating doses of docetaxel and cisplatin 40 mg/m^2 every 2 weeks with continuous infusion 5-FU and 61.2 Gy. Nineteen patients with T4 or M1a esophageal cancer were enrolled. Toxicities included myelosuppression and esophagitis, and a complete response rate of 42.1% was reported (29). There was one case of late grade 3 pneumonitis. The median survival was 20 months.

■ CHEMORADIATION WITH IRINOTECAN

Irinotecan is known to have activity against a variety of gastrointestinal (GI) cancers, including gastric, colorectal, and esophageal cancer. Ilson et al. enrolled 19 patients with stage II and III esophageal cancer onto a Memorial Sloan-Kettering Cancer Center phase 1 trial of weekly induction irinotecan 65 mg/m^2 with cisplatin 30 mg/m^2 during weeks 1 to 5 (31). Starting in week 8, patients received 50.4 Gy with concurrent weekly cisplatin 30 mg/m^2 and escalating doses or irinotecan. There was no grade 3 or 4 esophagitis, diarrhea, or stomatitis during chemoradiation. Fifteen patients underwent surgery, with a pCR rate of 27%.

Subsequently, the Eastern Cooperative Oncology Group protocol E1201 compared weekly cisplatin 30 mg/m^2 with irinotecan 50 mg/m^2 and 45 Gy followed by surgery and three cycles of postoperative cisplatin and irinotecan (Arm A) to weekly cisplatin 30 mg/m^2 with paclitaxel 50 mg/m^2 and 45 Gy followed by surgery and three cycles of postoperative cisplatin and paclitaxel. Staging was done with endoscopic ultrasound. The pCR rates were 14% for Arm A and 16% for Arm B, and median survival was 34.9 and 20.9 months, respectively (difference not significant). Overall, these results were not felt to be a significant improvement on standard neoadjuvant chemoradiation with cisplatin and 5-FU (32). Results of other irinotecan-based chemoradiation regimens are shown in Table 6. Results of a phase 2 Memorial Sloan-Kettering Cancer Center study evaluating induction irinotecan, docetaxel, and cisplatin followed by chemoradiation with irinotecan and docetaxel plus or minus cisplatin are pending.

■ CHEMORADIATION WITH OXALIPLATIN

Oxaliplatin has also shown promise in esophageal cancer in combination with continuous-infusion 5-FU and radiotherapy. Although neurotoxic, oxaliplatin compares favorably with cisplatin in terms of vomiting, nephrotoxicity, and myelosuppression, potentially making it more tolerable. In 2002, Khushlani et al. published results of a phase 2 study conducted at the Roswell Park Cancer Institute (39). Patients with stage II to IV adenocarcinoma or squamous cell carcinoma of the esophagus were enrolled and treated with weekly oxaliplatin at 85 mg/m^2. On day 8, patients received 5-FU 180 mg/m^2/day for 35 days and radiotherapy at 1.8 Gy/day to a total of 50.4 Gy. Patients then were restaged and some underwent surgery, while all patients received adjuvant oxaliplatin and 5-FU. Only 18% experienced grade 3

TABLE 5 Three-drug taxane-based chemoradiation regimens for esophageal cancer

Reference	Study Type	Patients	Chemo	RT	Toxicity	Outcomes	Notes
Minnie Pearl Cancer Research Network (23)	Phase 2	N = 129 stage I–III	CB AUC 6 days 1, 22 P 200 mg/m^2 days 1, 22 F 225 mg/m^2/day days 1–42	1.8 Gy/day beginning day 1, to 45 Gy	G3–4 leukopenia 73% G3–4 esophagitis 43% Hospitalization 57% 6% died after surgery	pCR—38% 1 YS—71% 2 YS—47% 3 YS 41%	No deaths due to CRT
Pacific Oncology Cancer Center (24)	Phase 2	N = 24 T2–4N0–1 M0–1a	P 45 mg/m^2 CB AUC 2 days 1, 8, 15, 22, 29 F 225 mg/m^2/day days 1–33	1.8 Gy/day beginning day 1, to 45 Gy	G3–4 esophagitis 33% G3–4 hypotension 29% G3–4 stomatitis 25% G3–4 neutropenia 13% G3–4 anemia 8%	pCR 57% 3 YS—48%	
Mayo Clinic (25)	Phase 2	N = 54	CB AUC 4 days 1, 22 P 200 mg/m^2 days 1, 22 F 225 mg/m^2/day days 1–42 Amifostine 500 mg SC before RT to first 19 patients	1.8 Gy/day beginning day 1, to 45 Gy	G3 or higher—94% Deaths—3 treatment related	pCR 35%	High rate of toxicity 1 death from amifostine
Duke University (26)	Phase 1	N = 13	Dose level 1 X 825 mg/m^2 bid w/RT CB AUC 2 weekly P 60 mg/m^2 weekly Dose level -1 X 600 mg/m^2 bid w/RT CB AUC 1.5 weekly P 45 mg/m^2 weekly	1.8 Gy/day beginning day 1, to 50.4 Gy	DLT, Dose level 1: G4 esophagitis 2/3 patients DLT, Dose level -1: 2/10 G3 esophagitis 1/10 G3 hypotension	Dose level 1: 2/3 had surgery pCR 2/2 Dose level -1: 6/10 had surgery pCR 2/6	Primary toxicity esophageal Use dose level -1 for phase 2

continued

TABLE 5 Three-drug taxane-based chemoradiation regimens for esophageal cancer (continued)

Reference	Study Type	Patients	Chemo	RT	Toxicity	Outcomes	Notes
Netherlands (27)	Phase 2	$N = 50$ stage II–III Resectable 84% ACA 16% SCC	P CB F	1.8 Gy/day beginning day 1, to 45 Gy	84% completed all treatment 8.5% died after surgery	96% had R0 resection pCR 38% 3 YS—56% (estimated)	Toxicity acceptable High pCR rate
Thomas Jefferson University (28)	Phase 2	$N = 54$	CB AUC 5 day 1, 29 P 50 mg/m^2 days 1, 8, 15, 22, 29 F 225 mg/m^2/day w/RT	1.8 Gy/day beginning day 1, to 45 Gy	G3 36% G4 5%	88% had surgery pCR 30% MS 23 months 5 YS 29%	67% developed metastases
Kitasato University (29)	Phase 1	$N = 19$ T4 and/or M1a	F 400 mg/m^2/day days 1–5, 15–19, 29–33, and 43–47 D 20–40 mg/m^2 C 40 mg/m^2 days 1, 15, 29, 43	1.8 Gy/day beginning day 1, to 61.2 Gy	DLT febrile neutropenia and G4 leukopenia in 3 of 4 patients at D 40 mg/m^2	CR 42.1%	D 35 mg/m^2 safe for Phase 2

ACA, adenocarcinoma; AUC, area under the curve; CB, carboplatin; C, cisplatin; CR, clinical complete response; D, docetaxel; DLT, dose-limiting toxicity; F, 5-fluorouracil; G, toxicity grade; Gy, gray; I, irinotecan; MS, median survival; pCR, pathological complete response; P, paclitaxel; SCC, squamous cell carcinoma; X, capecitabine; YS, years survival.

TABLE 6 Irinotecan-based chemoradiation regimens for esophageal cancer

Reference	Study Type	Patients	Chemo	RT	Toxicity	Outcomes	Notes
MSKCC (31)	Phase 1	$N = 19$ stage II–III	Induction: I 65 mg/m^2 C 30 mg/m^2 weekly × 5 Concurrent: I 40–80 mg/m^2 C 30 mg/m^2 weekly w/RT	1.8 Gy/day beginning day 1 of concurrent to 50.4 Gy	No G3–4 diarrhea, esophagitis, or stomatitis DLT myelosuppression in 2/6 at I 80 mg/m^2	15/19 had resection pCR 27%	Only 1 patient required feeding tube Use I 65 mg/m^2 for phase 2
E1201 (32,33)	Phase 2	$N = 86$ stage II–IVa	Arm A Concurrent: I 50 mg/m^2 C 30 mg/m^2 weekly w/RT Arm A Adjuvant: I 65 mg/m^2 C 30 mg/m^2 every 3 weeks × 3 Arm B Concurrent: C 30 mg/m^2 P 50 mg/m^2 weekly w/RT Arm B Adjuvant: C 75 mg/m^2 P 175 mg/m^2 every 3 weeks × 3	1.8 Gy/day beginning day 1, to 45 Gy	Arm A: G3–4 hematologic 43% G3–4 dysphagia 13% G3–4 diarrhea 9% Arm B: G3–4 hematologic 39% G3–4 dysphagia 20% G3–4 diarrhea 23%	pCR: Arm A—14% Arm B—16% MS: Arm A—34.9 months Arm B—20.9 months	EUS staging used <50% in each arm able to complete adjuvant treatment Neither arm is superior to standard therapy
French FFCD (34)	Phase 2	$N = 43$ stage I–III	I 60 mg/m^2 C 30 mg/m^2 weekly × 8	2 Gy/day beginning day 43, to 50 Gy	G3–4 23.3% Most toxicities hematologic (64.5%) One patient died of diarrhea	CR 58.1% 1 YS—62.8% 2 YS—27.9%	

continued

TABLE 6 Irinotecan-based chemoradiation regimens for esophageal cancer (continued)

Reference	Study Type	Patients	Chemo	RT	Toxicity	Outcomes	Notes
German (35)	Phase 2	$N = 14$	I 65 mg/m^2 C 30 mg/m^2 weekly × 2, then 1-week break, then weekly × 4 w/RT	2 Gy/day beginning day 29, to 40 Gy	G3 neutropenia 3/14 G 4 leukopenia 1/14 G3 anorexia 1/14 G3 fatigue 3/14	14/14 had R0 resection pCR 1/14	
University of Alabama (36)	Phase 2	$N = 14$ 10 ACA 4 SCC	Induction: I 50 mg/m^2 D 35 mg/m^2 weekly × 3 then 1 week break Concurrent: I 45 mg/m^2 D 30 mg/m^2 weekly × 3 w/RT	Beginning week 5	2/14 required feeding tubes 4/14 required dose-modification due to neutropenia	5 had resection pCR 2/5	
Brazilian (37)	Phase 2	$N = 26$ All SCC	I 65 mg/m^2 C 30 mg/m^2 weekly on weeks 1, 2, 4, 5, 8, 9, 11, 12	1.8 Gy/day beginning week 8, to 50.4 Gy	G3–4 vomiting 45% G3–4 diarrhea 33% G3–4 neutropenia 18% G3–4 thrombocytopenia 13% 5/26 died, mostly of infection	CR 40% 1 YS 34.6% MS 9.2%	Protocol closed due to toxicity
Roswell Park (38)	Phase 2	$N = 44$ 86% ACA stage II–IV	I 65 mg/m^2 C 30 mg/m^2 days 1, 8 every 3 weeks	1.8 Gy/day beginning day 1 to 45–50.4 Gy	Diarrhea 19/44 Fatigue 24/44 Vomiting 15/44 Hematologic 11/44 Constipation 11/44 Neurologic 7/44	All had R0 resection pCR 25% 3 YS 46% MS 34 months	Better efficacy than E1201

ACA, adenocarcinoma; C, cisplatin; chemo, chemotherapy; CR, clinical complete response; D, docetaxel; F, 5-fluorouracil; G, toxicity grade; Gy, gray; I, irinotecan; MS, median survival; pCR, pathological complete response; P, paclitaxel; RT, radiation; SCC, squamous cell carcinoma; YS, years survival.

toxicities. Five of thirteen patients had a pCR (38%) (39). Preliminary results of a follow-up study from Roswell Park utilizing neoadjuvant capecitabine, oxaliplatin, and radiation and two cycles of adjuvant chemotherapy indicate this regimen is tolerable, with three grade 4 toxicity events and one postoperative death in 18 patients (40). The pCR rate so far is 20%. A recent Italian phase 2 trial tested weekly oxaliplatin 60 mg/m^2 with continuous-infusion 5-FU (200 mg/m^2/day on days 1–22 and 29–64) and 45 Gy in 59 patients with unresectable locally advanced esophageal cancers. Toxicity was moderate, and the pCR rate was 18%, with a median survival of 18.5 months (41). Results of the Southwest Oncology Group (SWOG) protocol S0356 were recently presented in abstract form. Ninety patients with stage II to III esophageal cancer were treated with biweekly oxaliplatin 85 mg/m^2, continuous-infusion 5-FU, and 45 Gy followed by surgery and a cycle of adjuvant chemotherapy. There were four deaths (4.5%) attributed to treatment. The rates of grade 3 and 4 toxicities were 43% and 18%, respectively. Although survival data is not yet mature, the pCR rate was 33% (42).

Three-drug oxaliplatin-based chemoradiation regimens are also being investigated in locally advanced esophageal cancer. Meluch et al. utilized weekly oxaliplatin and docetaxel with capecitabine and 45 Gy. There were no treatment-related deaths or grade 3 to 4 hematologic toxicities, and the rate of grade 3 to 4 esophagitis was 16%. Two-thirds of patients analyzed were able to undergo surgery, with pCR documented in 17 (65%) (43). Noting that oxaliplatin and cisplatin show synergistic activity in platinum-refractory ovarian cancer, Maurel and colleagues tested escalating doses of oxaliplatin, cisplatin, and 5-FU with radiotherapy in 17 patients with esophageal cancer. Two of twelve patients who underwent surgery had pCRs (44). Phase 2 results from the same group were recently presented, with a 5% rate of toxic death and pCR rate of 17% (45). Results of protocols testing oxaliplatin-based chemoradiation regimens are summarized in Table 3.7.

■ NOVEL RADIOSENSITIZING AGENTS

Several new radiosensitizing drugs are currently in development for esophageal cancer. Paclitaxel poliglumex (PPX) is an investigational macromolecular conjugate consisting of paclitaxel linked to a biodegradable polyglutamate polymer that increases the water solubility of the conjugate and theoretically increases therapeutic index by exploiting the porous nature of tumor vasculature. Ng et al. reported the results of a small phase 2 study in which 23 patients with localized esophageal cancer were treated with 50 mg/m^2 PPX and 25 mg/m^2 cisplatin with 50.4 Gy. In the first 15 patients, there were 5 cases each of grade 3 to 4 dehydration and anorexia, and 2 hypersensitivity reactions. Five of the first eleven patients undergoing surgery had pCR (47). A phase 2 neoadjuvant trial of PPX with cisplatin and radiotherapy is now open. Oncogel is an injectable form of paclitaxel formulated in a biodegradable gel that provides controlled local release of paclitaxel with theoretically decreased systemic exposure. A phase 2 dose-escalation study enrolled 11 patients with inoperable esophageal cancer. A single dose of Oncogel was injected using endoscopic techniques, and patients then received 50.4 Gy. There were no dose-limiting toxicities, and subsequent biopsies were negative for tumor in four patients (48). A phase 2b trial of Oncogel with cisplatin, 5-FU, and radiation is open and ongoing.

S-1 is an oral fluoropyrimidine consisting of three drugs: the 5-FU prodrug ftorafur, chlorohydroxy dihydropyridine to inhibit catabolism of 5-FU, and oxonic acid, a compound which is thought to decrease intestinal phosphorylation of 5-FU, thereby reducing treatment-related diarrhea. S-1 is approved for use in gastric cancer in Japan but is not yet available in the United States, although trials are ongoing. A Korean trial of S-1, cisplatin, and radiation showed a pCR rate of 18.5% in operable patients (49), and a Korean phase 2 study is ongoing. Notably, S-1 appears to be metabolized differently in Asian and non-Asian patients, and it remains to be seen whether this will impact outcomes in Western trials.

■ BIOLOGICAL THERAPY TARGETING THE EPIDERMAL GROWTH FACTOR RECEPTOR

The epidermal growth factor receptor (EGFR) is a cell surface tyrosine kinase receptor encoded by the protooncogene c-erbB-1 (50). EGFR promotes a variety of oncogenic activities in human cells when overexpressed or activated inappropriately, including uncontrolled proliferation, angiogenesis, and inhibition of apoptosis (51). EGFR is overexpressed in approximately 50% to 70% of esophageal

TABLE 7 Oxaliplatin-based chemoradiation regimens for esophageal cancer

Reference	Study Type	Patients	Chemo	RT	Toxicity	Outcomes	Notes
Roswell Park (39)	Phase 2	$N = 38$ 84% ACA stage: II 8 III 8 IV 22	Concurrent: O 85 mg/m^2 days 1, 15, 29 F 180 mg/m^2 days 1–35 1 cycle w/RT and 1–2 cycles after CRT or S	1.8 Gy/day beginning day 8, to 50.4 Gy	No G4 hematologic G3–4 21%	13 had resection pCR 38%	Included stage IVB patients
Roswell Park (40)	Phase 2	$N = 20$ 85% ACA stage: II 3 III 13 IVa 4	Concurrent: O 85 mg/m^2 days 1, 15, 29 X 625 mg/m^2 bid w/RT 1 cycle w/RT and 2 cycles after S	1.8 Gy/day beginning day 1, to 50.4 Gy	G4 anemia 1 G4 lymphopenia 2 18 incidents of G3 toxicity seen, w/inclusion of S complications	15 had resection pCR 20%	
Italian (41)	Phase 2	$N = 59$	O 60 mg/m^2 weekly × 8 F 200 mg/m^2 days 1–22 and 29–64	1.8 Gy/day beginning day 29, to 45 Gy	68% completed regimen without modification Esophagitis G3 20% G4 5% Diarrhea G3 8.5% G4 8.5%	33 had resection 26 had R0 resection pCR 18% MS 18.5 months 1 YS 63%	Low hematologic toxicity
SWOG S0356 (42)	Phase 2	$N = 98$ stage II–III	O 85 mg/m^2 days 1, 15, 29 F 180 mg/m^2 days 8–43, 1 cycle w/RT and 1 cycle after S	1.8 Gy/day beginning day 8, to 45 Gy	G3 43% G4 18% Toxicities were 39% GI, 22% fatigue, 17% pulmonary, 16% hematologic	77 had resection pCR 33%	<50% had adjuvant chemo
(43)	Phase 1/2	$N = 43$ 74% ACA stage: I 8% II 45% III 47%	O 40 mg/m^2 D 20 mg/m^2 weekly × 5 X 1000 mg/m^2 po bid days 1–7, 15–21, 29–35	1.8 Gy/day beginning day 1, to 45 Gy	No G3–4 hematologic toxicities G3–4 Anorexia 21% Dehydration 16% Esophagitis 16%	CR 4 PR 18 26 had resection pCR 65% 1 YS 64%	

Spanish (44)	Phase 1	$N = 19$ 2 locally recurrent	O C days 1, 29 F days 1–4, 29–32	1.8 Gy/day beginning day 1, to 50.4 Gy	DLT diarrhea and asthenia at O 85 mg/m^2, C 55 mg/m^2, F 3000 mg/m^2/4 days	12 had resection pCR 16%	
Spanish (45)	Phase 2	$N = 41$ uT3–4N1 71% eso 39% gast	O 85 mg/m^2 P 55 mg/m^2 d 1, 29 F 750 mg/m^2 days 1–4, 29–32	1.8 Gy/day beginning day 1, to 45 Gy	2 toxic deaths G3–4 Asthenia 27% Infection 7% Diarrhea 7%	31 had resection pCR 17% MS 28.9 months	Most active in eso
Northwestern University (46)	Phase 2	$N = 41$ stage I–Iva	Induction O 70 mg/m^2 X 1 g bid days 1, 8 Concurrent O 50 mg/m^2 weekly × 6 X 825 mg bid w/RT	1.8 Gy/day beginning day 1 of concurrent to 45 Gy	2 toxic deaths G3–5 Lymphopenia 14 Dehydration 7 Diarrhea 6 Dysphagia 4	19 had resection pCR 38%	Most toxicity due to X

ACA, adenocarcinoma; C, cisplatin; chemo, chemotherapy; CR, clinical complete response; D, docetaxel; eso, esophageal cancer; F, 5-fluorouracil; gast, gastric cancer; G, toxicity grade; Gy, gray; MS, median survival; O, oxaliplatin; pCR, pathological complete response; RT, radiation; S, surgery; X, capecitabine; YS, years survival.

cancers, and overexpression has been correlated with decreased survival (52). A randomized phase 3 study in locally advanced head and neck squamous cell carcinoma showed a survival benefit to the addition of the monoclonal antibody EGFR inhibitor cetuximab to definitive radiation therapy (53). In light of these findings, both small molecule and monoclonal antibody inhibitors of EGFR are being intensively studied in hopes that they will improve outcomes in the neoadjuvant combined-modality setting.

Among small molecule inhibitors of EGFR, gefitinib has shown an acceptable safety profile but very modest single-agent activity in metastatic esophageal cancer, with partial response rates of 3% to 15% (54–56). A small phase 1 study of 1 year of oral gefitinib with biweekly oxaliplatin and 50.4 Gy was halted in 2005 when the Food and Drug Administration restricted the use of gefitinib. In six evaluable patients there was one complete response, one partial response, and three cases of progression. Biopsies taken after treatment did not show downregulation of EGFR, and there was no correlation between outcome and EGFR expression (57). A phase 2 study of concurrent gefitinib, cisplatin, 5-FU, and 60 Gy followed by maintenance gefitinib enrolled a mixed population of locally advanced and metastatic squamous cell and adenocarcinomas. Of 27 locally advanced patients, 21 had complete or partial response (78%). The doses of cisplatin and 5-FU were reduced after 10 patients due to concerns over neutropenia and mucositis. Diarrhea and rash (commonly seen with EGFR inhibitors) were mostly mild (58). Rodriguez et al. added concurrent gefitinib to continuous-infusion cisplatin, 5-FU, and 30 Gy delivered in 1.5 Gy bid fractions. Neoadjuvant therapy was followed by surgery, adjuvant chemoradiation, and 2 years maintenance gefitinib. Toxicity was not substantially increased when compared to a cohort of similar patients treated without gefitinib, and 75% of patients completed both chemoradiation cycles, although compliance with maintenance gefitinib was estimated at 50%. There was a trend toward improved survival in the gefitinib cohort (59). A phase 2 study of neoadjuvant gefitinib, cisplatin, and paclitaxel with radiation followed by surgery and maintenance gefitinib is ongoing at Johns Hopkins (NCT00493025).

Similar to gefitinib, the small molecule EGFR inhibitor erlotinib has shown modest single-agent activity in advanced esophageal cancer (60). A phase 1 study from the University of Alabama showed that erlotinib 150 mg/day was tolerable when given with standard neoadjuvant cisplatin, 5-FU, and radiation. Major toxicities included 55% with grade 1 rash, 18% with grade 2 diarrhea, and 27% with grade 3 dehydration (61). Studies are ongoing to evaluate erlotinib as a single agent with radiation in elderly patients (NCT00524121), and with a combination of carboplatin, paclitaxel, bevacizumab, 5-FU, and radiotherapy (NCT00393068). So far, results have been modest.

Results of chemoradiation protocols involving cetuximab are summarized in Table 3.8. Safran et al. published results of a phase 2 protocol combining cetuximab with weekly carboplatin, paclitaxel, and 50.4 Gy. A total of 60 patients with locally advanced esophageal or proximal gastric cancer were enrolled, although 3 were removed due to cetuximab hypersensitivity reactions. Other toxicities included 15% with grade 3 to 4 esophagitis, 23% with grade 3 acneiform rash. Seventy percent had a clinical complete response, and the pCR rate was 27% (62). Preliminary reports of several other early studies have been presented in abstract form. Agarwala and colleagues treated patients with 50.4 Gy and concurrent cetuximab followed by resection. Of the 26 patients who underwent surgery, 13 had pCR, including 5 with squamous cell carcinomas and 8 with adenocarcinomas. Grade 3 dysphagia occurred in only 6% of patients, but 56% had grade 3 rash (63). A phase 2 study from the Dana Farber Cancer Institute treated 17 patients with weekly cetuximab and cisplatin 30 mg/m^2, irinotecan 65 mg/m^2/week on weeks 1, 2, 4, and 5, and radiation to 50.4 Gy. After surgery, patients received an additional 6 months of cetuximab. Toxicity was considerable, and one patient died of a fungal infection. Of 15 patients to have surgery, only 2 had a pCR (13%) (64). At this time, results from SWOG protocol S0414, which tests induction cisplatin, irinotecan, and cetuximab followed by definitive chemoradiation with the same agents, are pending.

Particularly notable from these results is the high pCR rate and low toxicity seen in the Agarwala study, which used only cetuximab and radiotherapy, especially when compared to the Dana Farber three-drug regimen. Some groups have advocated simply adding biological agents onto existing chemoradiation regimens. A French phase 1–2 trial is evaluating addition of cetuximab to chemoradiation with 5-FU and cisplatin (NCT00544362). RTOG-0436 is expected to enroll 420 patients and will compare preoperative cisplatin, paclitaxel, and radiation to

TABLE 8 Cetuximab-based chemoradiation regimens for esophageal cancer

Reference	Study Type	Patients	Chemo	RT	Toxicity	Outcomes	Notes
Brown University (62)	Phase 2	$N = 60$ T2–4N0–1 included 3 gastric 75% ACA 25% SCC	C225 400 mg/m^2 day 1 then 250 mg/m^2 weekly P 50 mg/m^2 CB AUC 2 weekly × 6	1.8 Gy/day beginning day 1, to 50.4 Gy	G3 rash 23% G3 esophagitis 12% G4 esophagitis 3% 3 had C225 hypersensitivity	CR 70% 49 had surgery 8 medically inoperable pCR 27%	
Hoosier Oncology Group (63)	Pilot	$N = 40$ stage II–Iva 78% ACA 22% SCC	C225 400 mg/m^2 day -7 then 250 mg/m^2 weekly	1.8 Gy/day beginning day 1, to 50.4 Gy	G3 rash 56% G3 dysphagia 6% G3 infection 6% G3 GI bleed 3%	7 progressed 26 had surgery pCR 13/26	
Dana Farber (64)	Phase 2	N = 17	C225 400 mg/m^2 day -7 then 250 mg/m^2 weekly w/RT then for 6 months after surgery C 30 mg/m^2 I 65 mg/m^2 days 1, 8, 22, 29	1.8 Gy/day beginning day 1, to 50.4 Gy	G3–4 seen in all patients 1 death from infection	15 had surgery pCR 13%	Significant toxicity Low pCR rate
Swiss (65)	Phase 1b-2	$N = 20$ 11 ACA 9 SCC	Induction: D 75 mg/m^2 C 75 mg/m^2 every 3 weeks × 2 C225 250 mg/m^2 weekly Concurrent: D 20 mg/m^2 C 25 mg/m^2 C225 250 mg/m^2 weekly × 5	1.8 Gy/day beginning day 1 of CRT, to 45 Gy	G3 esophagitis 15% G3 rash 5% G3 pruritus 5% 1 pulmonary embolism	17 had surgery pCR or "near pCR" 65%	First 7 patients not treated w/D
Italian (66)	Phase 2	$N = 40$ T3N1 or T4 Resectable 12 ACA 28 SCC	Induction: FOLFOX-4 every 2 weeks × 4 C225 400 mg/m^2 day -7 then 250 mg/m^2 weekly Concurrent: C225 250 mg/m^2 weekly w/RT	1.8 Gy/day beginning day 1 of CRT, to 50.4 Gy	G3–4 dermatologic 32% G3–4 neutropenia 29% G3–4 esophagitis 9%	9 progressed 22 had surgery pCR 27%	

continued

TABLE 8 Cetuximab-based chemoradiation regimens for esophageal cancer (continued)

Reference	Study Type	Patients	Chemo	RT	Toxicity	Outcomes	Notes
German (67)	Phase 1	$N = 15$ T2–4M0–1a All SCC	C225 400 mg/m^2 day -15 then 250 mg/m^2 day -8 and weekly O 45–50 mg/m^2 days 1, 8, 22, 29 F 180–225 mg/m^2 days 1–5, 8–12, 15–19, 22–26, 29–33	1.8 Gy/day beginning day 1, to 45 Gy	G3 esophagitis 1/6 at highest dose 14/15 had "mild or moderate" rash No allergic reactions to C225	12 had surgery pCR 4/12	O and F dose escalation trial with C225
Danish (68)	Phase 1	$N = 11$	Induction: O 130 mg/m^2 day 1 Uftoral 300 mg/m^2 days 1–14 Concurrent: O 30 mg/m^2 every 2 weeks begin day 22 Uftoral 150–300 mg/m^2/day w/RT C225 400 mg/m^2 day 15 then 250 mg/m^2 weekly days 22–64 Adjuvant: O 130 mg/m^2 days 78, 99 Uftoral 300 mg/m^2 days 78–91, 99–112	1.8 Gy/day on days 22–64, to 59.4 Gy	2 G3–4 allergies to C225 G3 esophagitis 2/9; one developed fistula DLT of fistula and neuropathy seen in 2/3 at uftoral 300 mg/m^2 and O 30 mg/m^2 during RT	CR 3/9	Doses of uftoral and O escalated w/RT MTD: uftoral 150 mg/m^2 and O 30 mg/m^2 w/RT

ACA, adenocarcinoma; AUC, area under the curve; C225, cetuximab; CB, carboplatin; C, cisplatin; chemo, chemotherapy; CR, clinical complete response; D, docetaxel; DLT, dose-limiting toxicity; F, 5-fluorouracil; G, toxicity grade; Gy, gray; I, irinotecan; MS, median survival; MTD, maximum tolerated dose; pCR, pathological complete response; P, paclitaxel; PR, clinical partial response; RT, radiation; SCC, squamous cell carcinoma; SD, stable disease; X, capecitabine; YS, years survival.

the same regimen plus cetuximab (NCT00655876). However, the mechanisms of action for biological agents are still not well understood. It is possible that another approach, such as induction chemotherapy to suppress systemic disease, followed by radiation with cetuximab and then surgery for local control, might prove superior. A phase 2 study from the Netherlands is testing the addition of preoperative radiotherapy with cetuximab to the pre- and postoperative ECF regimen used in the MAGIC trial (69).

Finally, an objective response was seen in a phase 1 trial of panitumumab, a monoclonal antibody inhibitor of EFGR that is approved for metastatic colon cancer (70). Phase 1 studies of panitumumab in metastatic esophageal cancer, as well as with chemoradiation for localized disease, will begin enrolling shortly.

■ BIOLOGICAL THERAPY TARGETING HER2

Nineteen to forty-three percent of esophageal adenocarcinomas overexpress the transmembrane receptor tyrosine kinase human epidermal growth factor 2, or HER2 (71–73). Her2/neu gene amplification as detected by fluorescence in situ hybridization has been correlated with poor survival (74). Treatment with trastuzumab, a monoclonal antibody targeting HER2, significantly reduces disease recurrence in breast adenocarcinomas that overexpress HER2 (75,76).

The Brown group performed a phase 1–2 study of weekly trastuzumab, cisplatin, and paclitaxel with 50.4 Gy. Nineteen patients with esophageal adenocarcinomas with 2+ or 3+ expression of HER2 by immunohistochemistry were enrolled, including fourteen with celiac, portal, or retroperitoneal adenopathy. One year of maintenance trastuzumab was added for the last 13 patients. The radiation dose to the whole heart was limited to 40 Gy, but up to 45 Gy could be given to less than 50% of the heart. Trastuzumab has been noted to cause congestive heart failure, but in this study, there were no cardiac toxicities seen. Only two patients developed grade 3 to 4 esophagitis. Nine patients had clinical complete response, and six were surgically explored, revealing three pCR, two cases of microscopic residual disease, and two cases with metastases. The median survival was 24 months, with a 2-year survival of 50% (77). The survival data in this very small cohort of high-risk

patients is encouraging, and the regimen appears tolerable. Further phase 1 and 2 studies will be needed to substantiate the efficacy of trastuzumab-based combined modality therapy and to establish the pCR rate in a more uniform, less advanced population.

■ BIOLOGICAL THERAPY TARGETING THE VASCULAR ENDOTHELIAL GROWTH FACTOR

Vascular endothelial growth factor (VEGF) is a pleiotropic cytokine with potent proangiogenic effects. VEGF also promotes proliferation and migration of endothelial cells, survival of nascent vasculature, remodeling of extracellular matrix, and increased permeability of blood vessels (78). Bevacizumab, a monoclonal antibody inhibitor of VEGF, has been shown to increase survival in conjunction with chemotherapy in metastatic colon and non–small cell lung cancer, and progression-free survival in breast cancer. VEGF is overexpressed in approximately 30% to 60% of esophageal cancers, although the significance of overexpression is not clear (79,80).

Shah et al. evaluated bevacizumab with cisplatin and irinotecan in 47 patients with unresectable or metastatic adenocarcinoma of the stomach or gastroesophageal junction. The response rate in 34 patients with measurable disease was 65%, and median survival was 12.3 months. Possible bevacizumab-related toxicity included a 28% rate of grade 3 hypertension, two patients with gastric perforation, and one with a near-perforation, one myocardial infarction, and 25% of patients with grade 3 to 4 thromboembolic events (81). Enzinger et al. treated 20 patients with metastatic gastric or esophageal cancer with bevacizumab and docetaxel. In this mostly pretreated population, there were 4 partial responses among 15 evaluable patients (27%). Three patients died within 30 days of coming off the study. Grade 3 to 4 toxicities included GI bleed (15%) and arterial thrombosis (10%) (82). El-Rayes and colleagues treated eight previously untreated patients with bevacizumab, oxaliplatin, and docetaxel, resulting in four partial responses and four patients with stable disease. However, there were two GI perforations after the second cycle. Neither patient had had prior surgery. Grade 3 to 4 hypertension was seen in 13% of patients (83). Preliminary analysis of a phase 2 trial of induction and concurrent cisplatin, irinotecan, and bevacizumab with radiation showed no grade 3 to 4 hypertension or unexpected surgical complications (84). A number of studies combining bevacizumab with chemotherapy and radiation for locally advanced esophageal cancer are ongoing. Clinical experience has shown that even so-called targeted biological therapies can sometimes have unexpected toxicities. In the case of bevacizumab, the risk of GI perforation should not be minimized. Further phase 1 studies are required to evaluate the safety of this agent in esophageal cancer.

■ CYCLOOXYGENASE 2 INHIBITORS

Cyclooxygenase 2 (COX-2) is an inducible enzyme in the arachidonic acid cascade that catalyzes prostaglandin synthesis and has been implicated in angiogenesis, tumor cell invasion, and metastasis. Downstream products of COX-2 such as prostaglandin E2 (PGE2) are able to simulate VEGF production and upregulate matrix metalloproteinases, among other effects. Overexpression of COX-2 and PGE-2 has been reported in both squamous cell carcinomas and adenocarcinomas esophagus, although the significance of these findings is unclear (85,86). COX-2 inhibitors are widely used for a variety of clinical indications, but recent signs that they may be cardiotoxic (87) have dampened research interest in cancer.

Celecoxib, a nonsteroidal antiinflammatory drug that is selective for COX-2, has been approved for inhibition of intestinal polyp formation in familial adenomatous polyposis. However, chemoprevention trials of celecoxib in esophageal squamous dysplasia and Barrett's esophagus were not successful (88,89). Several early trials of chemoradiation combined with celecoxib have been reported. An Australian group combined escalating doses of celecoxib with standard doses of 5-FU, cisplatin, and 50 Gy. Thirteen patients were enrolled. No maximum tolerated dose was reached, and seven patients had radiographic complete responses (90). In a phase 2 study from the Dana Farber Cancer Institute, 36 patients with localized esophageal cancer received treatment with cisplatin, irinotecan, 50.4 Gy, and celecoxib, followed by surgery and maintenance celecoxib for 6 months. Twenty-five patients were able to undergo surgery, and eleven had pCR (44%). Two patients died within 30 days of surgery, but toxicity was otherwise moderate (60% grade 3–4), with only one case of severe esophagitis (91). Results from a Washington University protocol consisting of celecoxib with standard 5-FU, cisplatin, and radiotherapy showed a 70% rate of grade 3 to 4 toxicity and a 22% pCR rate (92). Given the lack of a clear benefit over standard therapy and the concerns over the safety of COX-2 inhibitors, interest has waned in COX-2 inhibition as a therapeutic modality.

■ CHEMORADIATION WITHOUT SURGERY

With the realization that chemoradiation alone resulted in a 5-year survival of 27% in RTOG 85–01, similar to that seen with surgery alone (93), combined with the fact that standard regimens can produce complete pathological sterilization of tumor in approximately 20% of cases, some investigators have proposed omitting surgery from treatment of locally advanced esophageal cancer. Results of two large European randomized phase 3 trials have recently been reported and are summarized in Table 9. Bedenne et al. enrolled 444 patients with T3N0–1M0 thoracic esophageal cancer (94). Treatment consisted of two cycles of cisplatin and 5-FU with either conventional radiation to 46 Gy in 1.8 Gy/day fractions or split course radiation to 30 Gy in 10 fractions given on days 1 to 5 and 22 to 26. The 259 patients who responded and had no contraindications to surgery were randomly assigned to either surgery (Arm A) or continued chemoradiation (Arm B) to a final dose of 66 Gy (conventional) or 60 Gy (split course). Eighty-nine percent of patients had squamous cell carcinoma. Two-year survival and median survival times were not significantly different at 34% and 17.7 months in Arm A versus 40% and 19.3 months in Arm B. Two-year local control was superior in Arm A (66.4% vs 57%), and esophageal stents were required in only 5% of patients, versus 32% in Arm B. The 3-month mortality rate was significantly higher in Arm A (9.3% vs 0.8%). The pCR rate in Arm A was 23%. Overall, the author concluded that there was no benefit to the addition of surgery after chemoradiation for squamous cell carcinoma of the esophagus (94).

Stahl et al. (95) randomized 172 patients with T3–4N0–1M0 esophageal squamous cell carcinoma to either three cycles of induction cisplatin, etoposide, and 5-FU and chemoradiation to 40 Gy in 20 fractions with cisplatin and etoposide followed by surgery (Arm A), or the same induction chemotherapy followed by chemoradiation to over 65 Gy with cisplatin

TABLE 9 Randomized clinical trials of trimodality therapy versus definitive chemoradiation for esophageal cancer

Reference	Patients	Chemo	RT	pCR	Local Control	Survival	Notes
German (95)	CRTS—86 CRT—86	Induction: F 500 mg/m^2 E 100 mg/m^2 P 30 mg/m^2 days 1–3 every 3 weeks Concurrent: E 80 mg/m^2 days 3–5 w/RT P 50 mg/m^2 days 2–8 w/RT	40 Gy in 20 fractions beginning d for CRTS 50 Gy in 25 fractions beginning d for CRT, then boost of 15 Gy in 10 fractions given bid or 8 Gy in 2 fractions w/HDR	CRTS—35%	2Y LPFS: CRTS—64.3% CRT—40.7% $P = 0.003$	2 YS: CRTS—39.9 % CRT—35.4 % P = NS MS: CRTS—16.4 months CRT—14.9 months P = NS	All SCC
French (4)	CRTS—129 CRT—130	P 15 mg/m^2 F 800 mg/m^2 days 1–5 every 3 weeks 2 cycles (days 1, 22) then 3 cycles if randomized to CRTS arm (days 43, 64, 92)	46 Gy in 26 fractions or 30 Gy in 10 fractions, split course for CRTS 66 Gy in 33 fractions or 45 Gy in 15 fractions, split course	CRTS—23%	2 YS LC: CRTS—66.4% CRT—57% $P = 0.03$	2 YS: CRTS—34% CRT—40% P = NS MS: CRTS—17.7 months CRT—19.3 months	89% SCC

ACA, adenocarcinoma; chemo, chemotherapy; C, cisplatin; CRT, definitive chemoradiation arm; CRTS, neoadjuvant chemoradiation followed by surgery; E, etoposide; F, 5-fluorouracil; fx, fractions; Gy, gray; LC, local control; LPFS, local progression-free survival; MS, median survival; NS, difference not significant at $P < 0.05$; pCR, pathological complete response; RT, radiation; SCC, squamous cell carcinoma; YS, years survival.

and etoposide (Arm B). Patients on Arm B with T4 or obstructing T3 tumors were treated to 50 Gy with 2 Gy/day fractions, followed by a 15 Gy boost in 1.5 Gy fractions delivered twice per day. Traversable T3 tumors were treated to 60 Gy with 2Gy/day fractions, followed by two 4 Gy boosts delivered by high dose-rate brachytherapy. Two-year survival and median survival were statistically equivalent at 39.9% and 16.4 months for Arm A and 35.4% and 14.9 months for Arm B. Local progression-free survival at 2 years was better in Arm A (65.4% vs 40.7%), but treatment-related mortality was also higher (12.8% vs 3.5%). The pCR rate in Arm A was 35%.

Taken together, these two large studies suggest that in squamous cell carcinoma of the esophagus, definitive chemoradiation offers equivalent long-term survival but lower local control, compared to trimodality therapy. The addition of surgery to chemoradiation also reduces the need for future palliative procedures, but at the cost of added perioperative morbidity and mortality. Of note, both studies used nonstandard radiation fractionation and higher doses than are typically employed in the United States, although it is not clear whether this was helpful or detrimental to the outcomes in the chemoradiation arms.

The German trial found that clinical response to induction chemotherapy was an important prognostic factor for overall survival, while the French trial randomized only patients who had an objective tumor response or improvement in dysphagia after induction chemoradiation. A subgroup analysis in the German trial revealed that nonresponders to induction therapy had improved long-term survival if a margin-negative resection could be achieved. Surgical salvage might therefore play an important role in the treatment of nonresponders to induction therapy. This approach was tested in RTOG 0246, in which induction therapy with paclitaxel, 5-FU, and cisplatin was followed by conventional chemoradiation with 5-FU, cisplatin, and 50.4 Gy. Surgery was performed only for patients with recurrent or residual disease. Of the 40 patients with localized esophageal cancer who were analyzed, 1 died during induction, 2 died prior to chemoradiation, and 1 died during chemoradiation. Two-thirds of patients experienced grade 3 to 4 toxicity. The 1-year survival rate was 71% (96).

Currently, there is no strong data to support omission of surgery in the treatment of esophageal adenocarcinomas. While squamous cell carcinomas tend to be located in the thorax, in close proximity to critical structures such as the aorta and the trachea, adenocarcinomas usual present more distally and can generally be resected with clear margins. At the Yale Cancer Center, the majority of our patients present with gastroesophageal junction adenocarcinomas, and we routinely recommend chemoradiation followed by surgery (97).

■ CONCLUSIONS

Current treatments for locally advanced esophageal cancer still leave much to be desired. Although one quarter of patients treated with combined-modality therapy will be long-term survivors, the median survival in most series is about 20 months. Even with surgery, nearly 40% of patients will have a component of local failure, with a similar number eventually developing metastases. Recent advances in multi-agent chemotherapy and biological targeted therapies have the potential to both improve outcomes and overwhelm clinicians with a bewildering variety of choices. Caution is in order when constructing multiagent regimens, since these can be quite toxic. Ultimately, progress will most likely come from an individualized approach to therapy, but this will require both methodical preclinical work to search for optimal combinations and sequences of drugs and radiation, and carefully constructed, randomized phase 2 studies comparing new regimens to standard doses of cisplatin, 5-FU, and radiotherapy. Given that esophageal cancer is not rare and that the prognosis is less than optimal, there should be no shortage of trial candidates.

■ REFERENCES

1. Kelsen DP, Ginsberg R, Pajak TF, et al. Chemotherapy followed by surgery compared with surgery alone for localized esophageal cancer. *N Engl J Med* 1998;339(27):1979–1984.
2. Medical Research Council Oesophageal Cancer Working Group. Surgical resection with or without preoperative chemotherapy in esophageal cancer: a randomized controlled trial. *Lancet*, 2002; 359, 1727–1733.
3. Walsh TN, Noonan N, Hollywood D, Kelly A, Keeling N, Hennessy TP. A comparison of multimodal therapy and surgery for esophageal adenocarcinoma. *N Engl J Med* 1996;335(7):462–467.
4. Bosset JF, Gignoux M, Triboulet JP, et al. Chemoradiotherapy followed by surgery compared with surgery alone in squamous-cell cancer of the esophagus. *N Engl J Med* 1997;337(3):161–167.

5. Urba SG, Orringer MB, Turrisi A, Iannettoni M, Forastiere A, Strawderman M. Randomized trial of preoperative chemoradiation versus surgery alone in patients with locoregional esophageal carcinoma. *J Clin Oncol* 2001;19(2):305–313.

6. Burmeister BH, Smithers BM, Gebski V, et al. Trans-Tasman Radiation Oncology Group; Australasian Gastro-Intestinal Trials Group. Surgery alone versus chemoradiotherapy followed by surgery for resectable cancer of the oesophagus: a randomised controlled phase III trial. *Lancet Oncol* 2005;6(9):635–637.

7. Tepper J, Krasna MJ, Niedzwiecki D, et al. Phase III trial of trimodality therapy with cisplatin, fluorouracil, radiotherapy, and surgery compared with surgery alone for esophageal cancer: CALGB 9781. *J Clin Oncol* 2008;26(7):1086–1092.

8. Urschel JD, Vasan H. A meta-analysis of randomized controlled trials that compared neoadjuvant chemoradiation and surgery to surgery alone for resectable esophageal cancer. *Am J Surg* 2003;185(6):538–543.

9. Gebski V, Burmeister B, Smithers BM, Foo K, Zalcberg J, Simes J. Australasian Gastro-Intestinal Trials Group. Survival benefits from neoadjuvant chemoradiotherapy or chemotherapy in oesophageal carcinoma: a meta-analysis. *Lancet Oncol* 2007;8(3):226–234.

10. Herskovic A, Martz K, al-Sarraf M, et al. Combined chemotherapy and radiotherapy compared with radiotherapy alone in patients with cancer of the esophagus. *N Engl J Med* 1992;326(24):1593–1598.

11. Minsky BD, Pajak TF, Ginsberg RJ, et al. INT 0123 (Radiation Therapy Oncology Group 94–05) phase III trial of combined-modality therapy for esophageal cancer: high-dose versus standard-dose radiation therapy. *J Clin Oncol* 2002;20(5):1167–1174.

12. Choy H, Rodriguez FF, Koester S, Hilsenbeck S, Von Hoff DD. Investigation of taxol as a potential radiation sensitizer. *Cancer* 1993;71(11):3774–3778.

13. Ajani JA, Ilson DH, Daugherty K, Pazdur R, Lynch PM, Kelsen DP. Activity of taxol in patients with squamous cell carcinoma and adenocarcinoma of the esophagus. *J Natl Cancer Inst* 1994;86(14):1086–1091.

14. Safran H, Gaissert H, Akerman P, et al. Paclitaxel, cisplatin, and concurrent radiation for esophageal cancer. *Cancer Invest* 2001;19(1):1–7.

15. Brenner B, Ilson DH, Minsky BD, et al. Phase I trial of combined-modality therapy for localized esophageal cancer: escalating doses of continuous-infusion paclitaxel with cisplatin and concurrent radiation therapy. *J Clin Oncol* 2004;22(1):45–52.

16. Ajani JA, Winter K, Komaki R, et al. Phase II randomized trial of two nonoperative regimens of induction chemotherapy followed by chemoradiation in patients with localized carcinoma of the esophagus: RTOG 0113. *J Clin Oncol* 2008;26(28):4551–4556.

17. Wang H, Ryu J, Gandara D, et al. A phase II study of paclitaxel, carboplatin, and radiation with or without surgery for esophageal cancer. *J Thorac Oncol* 2007;2(2):153–157.

18. Kim DW, Blanke CD, Wu H, et al. Phase II study of preoperative paclitaxel/cisplatin with radiotherapy in locally advanced esophageal cancer. *Int J Radiat Oncol Biol Phys* 2007;67(2):397–404.

19. Lin C, Hsu C, Cheng C, et al. Induction chemotherapy followed by concurrent chemoradiotherapy with/without esophagectomy for locally advanced esophageal squamous cell carcinoma. *Ann Oncol* 2007;18(1):93–98.

20. Lin C, Hsu C, Cheng C, et al. Induction chemotherapy followed by concurrent chemoradiotherapy with/without esophagectomy for locally advanced esophageal squamous cell carcinoma. *J Clin Oncol* 2009;27 (suppl; abst e15526).

21. Urba SG, Orringer MB, Ianettonni M, Hayman JA, Satoru H. Concurrent cisplatin, paclitaxel, and radiotherapy as preoperative treatment for patients with locoregional esophageal carcinoma. *Cancer* 2003;98(10):2177–2183.

22. Pasini F, de Manzoni G, Stierano L, et al. Effect of neoadjuvant combined modality therapy with weekly docetaxel, cisplatin, 5-Fu continuous infusion and radiotherapy on pathological response rate in esophageal cancer: a phase II study. *J Clin Oncol* 2009;27(abstr 4548).

23. Meluch AA, Greco FA, Gray JR, et al. Preoperative therapy with concurrent paclitaxel/carboplatin/infusional 5-FU and radiation therapy in locoregional esophageal cancer: final results of a Minnie Pearl Cancer Research Network phase II trial. *Cancer J* 2003;9(4):251–260.

24. Gannett DE, Wolf RF, Takahashi GW, et al. Neoadjuvant chemoradiotherapy for esophageal cancer using weekly Paclitaxel and Carboplatin plus infusional 5-Fluorouracil. *Gastrointest Cancer Res* 2007;1(4):132–138.

25. Jatoi A, Martenson JA, Foster NR, et al. North Central Cancer Treatment Group (N0044). Paclitaxel, carboplatin, 5-fluorouracil, and radiation for locally advanced esophageal cancer: phase II results of preliminary pharmacologic and molecular efforts to mitigate toxicity and predict outcomes: North Central Cancer Treatment Group (N0044). *Am J Clin Oncol* 2007;30(5):507–513.

26. Czito BG, Kelsey CR, Hurwitz HI, et al. A Phase I study of capecitabine, carboplatin, and paclitaxel with external beam radiation therapy for esophageal carcinoma. *Int J Radiat Oncol Biol Phys* 2007;67(4):1002–1007.

27. Van de Schoot L, Romme E, van der Sangen M, et al. A highly active and tolerable neoadjuvant regimen combining paclitaxel, carboplatin, 5-FU, and radiation therapy in patients with stage Ii and III esophageal cancer. *Ann Surg Oncol*, 2008; 15(1), 88–95.

28. Whiton M, Berger A, Mitchell E, et al. Long-term follow-up of a phase I/II clinical trial of neoadjuvant chemoradiation with paclitaxel, carboplatin, 5-fluorouracil, and radiation followed by surgery for locally advanced esophageal or gastric cancer. American Society for Clinical Oncology 2009 Gastrointestinal Cancers Symposium; abstract 54.

29. Higuchi K, Koizumi W, Tanabe S, et al. A phase I trial of definitive chemoradiotherapy with docetaxel, cisplatin, and 5-fluorouracil (DCF-R) for advanced esophageal carcinoma: Kitasato digestive disease & oncology group trial (KDOG 0501). *Radiother Oncol* 2008;87(3):398–404.

30. Mauer AM, Masters GA, Haraf DJ, et al. Phase I study of docetaxel with concomitant thoracic radiation therapy. *J Clin Oncol* 1998;16(1):159–164.

31. Ilson DH, Bains M, Kelsen DP, et al. Phase I trial of escalating-dose irinotecan given weekly with cisplatin and concurrent radiotherapy in locally advanced esophageal cancer. *J Clin Oncol* 2003;21(15):2926–2932.

32. Kleinberg L, Powell, M, Forastiere A, et al. Survival outcome of E1201: an Eastern Cooperative Oncology Group randomized phase II trial of neoadjuvant preoperative paclitaxel/cisplatin/irinotecan/radiotherapy (RT) of irinotecan/cisplatin/RT in endoscopy with ultrasound staged esophageal adenocarcinoma [Abstract 4532]. *J Clin Oncol*, 2008 (May 20 Suppl).

33. Kleinberg L, Powell M, Forastiere A, et al. E1201: An Eastern Cooperative Oncology Group randomized phase II trial of neoadjuvant preoperative paclitaxel/cisplatin/RT or irinotecan/cisplatin/RT in endoscopy with ultrasound-staged adenocarcinoma of the esophagus [Abstract 4533]. *J Clin Oncol*, 2007; 25(June 20 Suppl).

34. Michel P, Adenis A, Di Fiore F, et al. Induction cisplatin-irinotecan followed by concurrent cisplatin-irinotecan and radiotherapy without surgery in oesophageal cancer: multicenter phase II FFCD trial. *Br J Cancer* 2006;95(6):705–709.

35. Darling G, Knox J, Wong R, et al. A phase II study to assess the efficacy of combined preoperative chemotherapy with irinotecan and cisplatin and radiotherapy plus surgery for potentially resectable thoracic esophageal cancer. American Society for Clinical Oncology 2004 Gastrointestinal Cancers Symposium [Abstract 32].

36. Posey J, Thornton J, Russo S, et al. A phase II study of irinotecan and docetaxel with concurrent radiotherapy as preoperative treatment in resectable esophageal cancer. *J Clin Oncol*, 2004; 22(14S), 4245.

37. Geib G, Machado M, Pozzi B, et al. Mortality rate with irinotecan/cisplatin plus concomitant radiation therapy in patients in locally advanced esophageal squamous cell carcinoma [Abstract e15560]. *J Clin Oncol*, 2009; 27.

38. Sharma R, Yang G, Nava H, et al. A single institution experience with neoadjuvant chemoradiation with irinotecan and cisplatin in locally advanced esophageal carcinoma [Abstract e15619]. *J Clin Oncol*, 2009; 27.

39. Khushalani NI, Leichman CG, Proulx G, et al. Oxaliplatin in combination with protracted-infusion fluorouracil and radiation: report of a clinical trial for patients with esophageal cancer. *J Clin Oncol* 2002;20(12):2844–2850.

40. Khushlani N, Miecznikowski J, Wang D, et al. Capecitabine, oxaliplatin, and radiation in resectable esophageal cancer: a phase II trial with gene expression profiling [Abstract e15543]. *J Clin Oncol*, 2009; 27.

41. Chiarion-Sileni V, Innocente R, Cavina R, et al. Multicenter phase II trial of chemo-radiotherapy with 5-fluorouracil, leucovorin and oxaliplatin in locally advanced esophageal cancer. *Cancer Chemother Pharmacol* 2009;63(6):1111–1119.

42. Leichman L, Goldman B, Benedetti J, et al. Oxaliplatin plus protracted infusion 5-fluorouracil and external beam radiation prior to surgery for potentially curable esophageal adenocarcinoma: a Southwest Oncology Group phase II trial with molecular correlates [Abstract 4513]. *J Clin Oncol*, 2009; 27(15s).

43. Meluch A, Spigel D, Greco F, et al. Phase I/II trial of preoperative oxaliplatin, docetaxel, capecitabine and radiation for localized esophageal cancer. *J Clin Oncol*, 2007; 25(18S), 4595.

44. Maurel J, Cervantes A, Conill C, et al. Phase I trial of oxaliplatin in combination with cisplatin, protracted-infusion fluorouracil, and radiotherapy in advanced esophageal or gastric carcinoma. *Int J Radiat Oncol Biol Phys* 2005;62(1):91–96.

45. Pera M, Gallego R, Martin-Richard M, et al. Phase II study with preoperative oxaliplatin, cisplatin, 5-fluorouracil , and radiation in patients with esophageal, gastroesophageal, and gastric cancer [Abstract e15612]. *J Clin Oncol*, 2009; 27.

46. Ruch J, Mulcahy M, Small Jr. W, et al. Capecitabine and oxaliplatin as induction therapy and with radiation for resectable esophageal adenocarcinoma. American Society for Clinical Oncology 2009 Gastrointestinal Cancers Symposium [Abstract 84].

47. Ng T, DiPetrillo T, Sunthralingam M, et al. Neoadjuvant paclitaxel poliglumex, cisplatin, and radiation for esophageal cancer: a phase II trial. *J Clin Oncol*, 2009; 27(15S), e15542.

48. DuVall GA, Tarabar D, Seidel RH, et al. Phase 2: a dose-escalation study of OncoGel (ReGel/paclitaxel), a controlled-release formulation of paclitaxel, as adjunctive local therapy to external-beam radiation in patients with inoperable esophageal cancer. *Anticancer Drugs* 2009;20(2):89–95.

49. Cho SH, Shim HJ, Lee SR, et al. Concurrent chemoradiotherapy with S-1 and cisplatin in advanced esophageal cancer. *Dis Esophagus* 2008;21(8):697–703.

50. Mendelsohn J, Baird A, Fan Z, et al. *Growth factors and their receptors in epithelial malignancies.* In: The Molecular Basis of Cancer. Philadelphia: WB Saunders Co, 2001, 137–144.

51. Baselga J. Why the epidermal growth factor receptor? The rationale for cancer therapy. *Oncologist* 2002;7 (Suppl 4), 2–8.

52. Hackel PO, Zwick E, Prenzel N, Ullrich A. Epidermal growth factor receptors: critical mediators of multiple receptor pathways. *Curr Opin Cell Biol* 1999;11(2):184–189.

53. Bonner JA, Harari PM, Giralt J, et al. Radiotherapy plus cetuximab for squamous-cell carcinoma of the head and neck. *N Engl J Med*, 2006; 354, 367–378.

54. Janmaat ML, Gallegos-Ruiz MI, Rodriguez JA, et al. Predictive factors for outcome in a phase II study of gefitinib in second-line treatment of advanced esophageal cancer patients. *J Clin Oncol* 2006;24(10):1612–1619.

55. Adelstein D, Rybicki L, Carroll M, et al. Phase II trial of gefitinib for recurrent or metastatic esophageal or gastroesophageal junction cancer [Abstract 4054]. *J Clin Oncol*, 2005; 23(16S).

56. Ferry DR, Anderson M, Beddard K, et al. A phase II study of gefitinib monotherapy in advanced esophageal adenocarcinoma: evidence of gene expression, cellular, and clinical response. *Clin Cancer Res* 2007;13(19):5869–5875.

57. Javle M, Pande A, Iyer R, et al. Pilot study of gefitinib, oxaliplatin, and radiotherapy for esophageal adenocarcinoma: tissue effect predicts clinical response. *Am J Clin Oncol* 2008;31(4):329–334.

58. Sunpaweravong P, Sunpaweravong S, Sangthawan D, et al. Combination of gefitinib, cisplatin, and 5-FU chemotherapy, and radiation therapy in newly-diagnosed patients with esophageal carcinoma. *J Clin Oncol*, 2007;25(18S):4605.

59. Rodriguez C, Adelstein D, Rybicki L, et al. A phase II trial of perioperative concurrent chemoradiotherapy and gefitinib in locally advanced esophagus and gastroesophageal junction cancer [Abstract 4547]. *J Clin Oncol*, 2009; 26(May 20 Suppl).

60. Dragovich T, McCoy S, Fenoglio-Preiser CM, et al. Phase II trial of erlotinib in gastroesophageal junction and gastric adenocarcinomas: SWOG 0127. *J Clin Oncol* 2006;24(30):4922–4927.

61. Dobelbower M, Russo S, Raisch K, et al. Erlotinib as a radiosensitizer for patients with esophageal cancer. *Int J Radiat Oncol Biol Phys*, 2005; 63(2, suppl; abstract 2090).

62. Safran H, Suntharalingam M, Dipetrillo T, et al. Cetuximab with concurrent chemoradiation for esophagogastric cancer: assessment of toxicity. *Int J Radiat Oncol Biol Phys* 2008;70(2):391–395.

63. Agarwala A, Hanna N, McCollum A, et al. Preoperative cetuximab and radiation for patients with surgically resectable esophageal and gastroesophageal junction carcinomas: a pilot study from the Hoosier Oncology Group and the University of Texas Southwestern [Abstract 4557]. *J Clin Oncol*, 2009;27(May 20 Suppl).

64. Enzinger P, Yock T, Suh W, et al. Phase II cisplatin, irinotecan, cetuximab and concurrent radiation therapy followed by surgery for locally advanced esophageal cancer [Abstract 4064]. *J Clin Oncol*, 2006;24 (June 20 Suppl).

65. Ruhstahller T, Pless M, Schuller J, et al. Cetuximab in combination with chemoradiotherapy prior to surgery in patients with resectable, locally advanced esophageal carcinoma: a prospective, multicenter phase Ib-II trial of the Swiss Group for Clinical Cancer Research [Abstract 4570]. *J Clin Oncol*, 2009;27 (15s).

66. DeVita F, Orditura M, Innocente R, et al. A multicenter phase II study of induction CT with FOLFOX-4 and cetuximab followed by RT and cetuximab in locally advanced esophageal cancer [Abstract 4546]. *J Clin Oncol*, 2009; 27(15s).

67. Lordick F, Meyer zum Buschenfelde C, Thuss-Patience P, et al. Weekly cetuximab plus oxaliplatin, infusional 5-fluorouracil and radiation therapy as neoadjuvant treatment for esophageal squamous cell carcinoma: a phase I study of the Arbeitsgemeinschaft Internistische Onkologie [Abstract e15507]. *J Clin Oncol*, 2009; 27.

68. Baeksgaard L, Sorensen M, Albertsson P, et al. A phase I study of concomitant radiotherapy and oxaliplatin, uftoral, and cetuximab as first-line theraphy for locally advanced esophageal cancer. American Society of Clinical Oncology 2009. Gastrointestinal Cancers Symposium.

69. Cunningham D, Allum WH, Stenning SP, et al. Perioperative chemotherapy versus surgery alone for resectable gastroesophageal cancer. *N Engl J Med* 2006;355(1):11–20.

70. Stephenson JJ, Gregory C, Burris H, et al. An open-label clinical trial evaluating safety and pharmacokinetics of two dosing schedules of panitumumab in patients with solid tumors. *Clin Colorectal Cancer* 2009;8(1):29–37.

71. Al-Kasspooles M, Moore J, Orringer M, et al. Amplification and overexpression of EGFR and C-erb B-2 genes in human esophageal adenocarcinomas. *Int J Cancer*, 1993; 53, 213–219.

72. Fléjou JF, Paraf F, Muzeau F, et al. Expression of c-erbB-2 oncogene product in Barrett's adenocarcinoma: pathological and prognostic correlations. *J Clin Pathol* 1994;47(1):23–26.

73. Duhaylongsod FG, Gottfried MR, Iglehart JD, et al. The significance of c-erb B-2 and p53 immunoreactivity in patients with adenocarcinoma of the esophagus. *Ann Surg* 1995;221(6):677–683.

74. Brien TP, Odze RD, Sheehan CE, et al. HER-2/neu gene amplification by FISH predicts poor survival in Barrett's esophagus-associated adenocarcinoma. *Hum Pathol* 2000;31(1):35–39.

75. Piccart-Gebhart MJ, Procter M, Leyland-Jones B, et al. Trastuzumab after adjuvant chemotherapy in HER2-positive breast cancer. *N Engl J Med* 2005;353(16):1659–1672.

76. Romond EH, Perez EA, Bryant J, et al. Trastuzumab plus adjuvant chemotherapy for operable HER2-positive breast cancer. *N Engl J Med* 2005;353(16):1673–1684.

77. Safran H, Dipetrillo T, Akerman P, et al. Phase I/II study of trastuzumab, paclitaxel, cisplatin and radiation for locally advanced, HER2 overexpressing, esophageal adenocarcinoma. *Int J Radiat Oncol Biol Phys* 2007;67(2):405–409.

78. Ferrara N, Davis-Smyth T. The biology of vascular endothelial growth factor. *Endocr Rev* 1997;18(1):4–25.

79. Shih CH, Ozawa S, Ando N, et al. Vascular endothelial growth factor expression predicts outcome and lymph node metastasis in squamous cell carcinoma of the esophagus. *Clin Cancer Res* 2000;6(3):1161–1168.

80. Kulke MH, Odze RD, Mueller JD, et al. Prognostic significance of vascular endothelial growth factor and cyclooxygenase 2 expression in patients receiving preoperative chemoradiation for esophageal cancer. *J Thorac Cardiovasc Surg* 2004;127(6):1579–1586.

81. Shah MA, Ramanathan RK, Ilson DH, et al. Multicenter phase II study of irinotecan, cisplatin, and bevacizumab in patients with metastatic gastric or gastroesophageal junction adenocarcinoma. *J Clin Oncol* 2006;24(33):5201–5206.

82. Enzinger PC, Fidias P, Meyerhardt J, et al. Phase II study of bevacizumab and docetaxel in metastatic esophageal and gastric cancer. American Society for Clinical Oncology 2006 Gastrointestinal Cancers Symposium [Abstract 68].

83. El Rayes B, Hammad N, Philip P, et al. A phase II study of bevacizumab, docetaxel and oxaliplatin in gastric and gastroesophageal junction cancer [Abstract 15608]. *J Clin Oncol*, 2008; 26(May 20 Suppl).

84. Ilson D, Bains M, Rizk N, et al. Phase II trial of preoperative bevacizumab, irinotecan, cisplatin, and radiation in esophageal adenocarcinoma: preliminary safety analysis [Abstract 4573]. *J Clin Oncol*, 2009; 27(15S).

85. Kuo KT, Wang HW, Chou TY, et al. Prognostic role of PGE2 receptor EP2 in esophageal squamous cell carcinoma. *Ann Surg Oncol* 2009;16(2):352–360.

86. von Rahden BH, Stein HJ, Hartl SA, et al. Expression of prostaglandin E synthase in Barrett's cancer. *Dis Esophagus* 2008;21(4):304–308.

87. Solomon SD, McMurray JJ, Pfeffer MA, et al. Cardiovascular risk associated with celecoxib in a clinical trial for colorectal adenoma prevention. *N Engl J Med* 2005;352(11):1071–1080.

88. Heath EI, Canto MI, Piantadosi S, et al. Chemoprevention for Barrett's Esophagus Trial Research Group. Secondary chemoprevention of Barrett's esophagus with celecoxib: results of a randomized trial. *J Natl Cancer Inst* 2007;99(7):545–557.

89. Limburg PJ, Wei W, Ahnen DJ, et al. Randomized, placebo-controlled, esophageal squamous cell cancer chemoprevention trial of selenomethionine and celecoxib. *Gastroenterology* 2005;129(3):863–873.

90. Dawson SJ, Michael M, Biagi J, et al. A phase I/II trial of celecoxib with chemotherapy and radiotherapy in the treatment of patients with locally advanced oesophageal cancer. *Invest New Drugs* 2007;25(2):123–129.

91. Enzinger P, Mamon H, Choi N, et al. Phase II cisplatin, irinotecan, celecoxib and concurrent radiation therapy followed by surgery for locally advanced esophageal cancer. American Society for Clinical Oncology 2004 Gastrointestinal Cancers Symposium 2004 [Abstract 35].

92. Govindan R, McLeod H, Mantravadi P, et al. Cisplatin, fluorouracil, celecoxib, and RT in resectable esophageal cancer: preliminary results. *Oncology (Williston Park, NY)* 2004;18(14 Suppl 14):18–21.

93. Wu P, Posner M. The role of surgery in the management of esophageal cancer. *Lancet Oncol*, 2003;4:481–488.

94. Bedenne L, Michel P, Bouché O, et al. Chemoradiation followed by surgery compare with chemoradiation alone in squamous cancer of the esophagus: FFCD 9102. *J Clin Oncol* 2007;25(10):1160–1168.

95. Stahl M, Stuschke M, Lehmann N, et al. Chemoradiation with and without surgery in patients with locally advanced squamous cell carcinoma of the esophagus. *J Clin Oncol* 2005;23(10):2310–2317.

96. Swisher S, Winters K, Komaki R, et al. A phase II study of a paclitaxel based chemoradiation regimen with selective surgical salvage for resectable locoregionally advanced esophageal cancer: initial reporting of RTOG 0246. *Int J Radiat Oncol Biol Phys*, 2007; 69(3), S106.

97. Kleinberg L, Knisely J, Heitmiller R, et al. Mature survival results with preoperative cisplatin, protracted infusion 5-fluorouracil, and 44-Gy radiotherapy for esophageal cancer. *Int J Radiat Oncol Biol Phys* 2001;51(3):Suppl1:32.

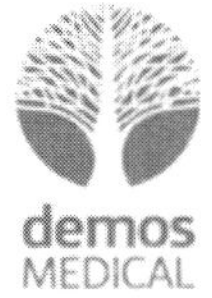

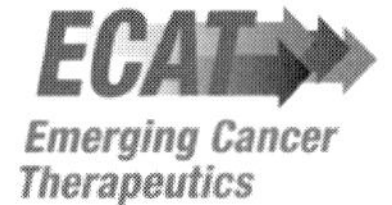

Esophageal Cancer

New Developments in Radiation Therapy Planning

Bryan Chang*

Yale Cancer Center, Yale University School of Medicine, New Haven, CT

■ ABSTRACT

Traditional radiation therapy fields for esophageal cancer are large and encompass a significant volume of normal tissue. Recent studies have significantly improved understanding of cardiac and pulmonary tolerance to therapeutic radiation, enabling clinicians to better define risk and minimize toxicity to these organs. Positron-emission (PET) scans have significant utility in staging of esophageal cancer, but it is not yet clear how this data should be incorporated into treatment planning. Likewise, it is not clear if there is a significant dosimetric benefit to intensity-modulated radiation therapy (IMRT) for esophageal cancer, and clinical experience is still limited. Tumors of the gastroesophageal junction can exhibit significant motion with respiration, and 4-dimensional (4D) treatment planning is a promising technique for tailoring fields to avoid a geographic miss.

■ INTRODUCTION

Surgical series have demonstrated that esophageal cancer is prone to extensive lymphatic involvement and submucosal spread up to 5 cm from the main tumor (1,2). Thus, both regional nodal basins and significant lengths of esophagus above and below the grossly visible tumor are theoretically at risk for potential microscopic involvement by tumor. Simulation for esophageal radiation is performed using a planning computed tomography (CT) with oral barium, incorporating data from endoscopy reports, endoscopic ultrasound (EUS), and diagnostic CT. The Herskovic trial (RTOG 85–01) specified that radiation be delivered to the entire length of the esophagus to a total of 30 Gy, followed by a "cone-down" to treat the gross tumor with a 5-cm margin in the superior/inferior direction and a 2-cm radial margin to a total of 50 Gy (3). Subsequently, the INT-0123 radiation dose-escalation trial called for 5-cm superior/inferior margins and 2-cm radial margins from the outset, omitting the whole-esophagus phase (4). If the tumor extends into the stomach clinically, 5 cm of stomach are included within the target volume. Typically, the supraclavicular fossae are treated electively for tumors above the carina, and the celiac axis is covered when the tumor is located distally, although some trials have shown reasonable outcomes without using elective nodal radiation (5–8).

Following the criteria outlined above typically results in very large treatment volumes that can pose a significant risk to the adjacent normal tissues, both in terms of acute and late toxicity. Distal esophageal

*Corresponding author, Department of Therapeutic Radiology, Yale University School of Medicine, New Haven, CT
E-mail address: bryan.chang@yale.edu

Emerging Cancer Therapeutics 1 (2010) 59–68.

DOI: 10.5003/2151–4194.1.1.61

tumors located posterior to the heart pose a particular challenge, as the radiation oncologist must weigh the need to cover the area at risk against the tolerances of the heart and lungs when devising a treatment plan (Figs 1A and B). Recently, data has emerged that will allow radiation oncologists to quantify better and define the risks of irradiating normal structures. Incorporating findings from positron-emission tomography CT (PET-CT) scans into treatment planning will allow physicians to more accurately define the extent of esophageal tumors. Finally, advances in intensity-modulated radiation therapy (IMRT) and 4D treatment planning enable radiotherapy to be delivered with increased precision, thereby sparing normal tissues.

■ NEW INSIGHTS INTO CARDIAC RADIATION TOLERANCE

Cardiac irradiation is associated with acute pericarditis, pericardial effusion, and decreased ejection fraction. Late toxicities include valvular damage and a risk of accelerated coronary atherosclerosis. Chemotherapy is thought to enhance the toxicity of cardiac irradiation, although precise data is lacking. RTOG-0436, activated in 6/08, stipulates that the whole heart should receive less than 40 Gy, two-thirds should receive less than 45 Gy, and one-third should receive less than 50 Gy. These values are derived from tables published by Emami nearly two decades ago (9).

Much of the data on late cardiac effects comes from studies of long-term survivors of Hodgkin's lymphoma and older breast cancer series. In esophageal cancer data so far has been limited with regard to the impact of radiotherapy on long-term cardiac health, in part due to the limited life expectancy of patients with locally advanced disease. A SEER-Medicare study of localized esophageal cancer patients diagnosed between 1992 and 2002 revealed 2,240 patients, of whom 69% received radiation as part of their treatment and 31% were treated with surgery alone. A multivariate analysis showed an increased risk of cardiac-related events in patients ($P < 0.001$, HR 1.50, 95% CI 1.16–1.95). In contrast, there was no increase in cerebrovascular events in patients treated with radiation. The median time to occurrence of a cardiac event was 0.53 years. Subset analysis showed that the increased risk was confined to patients treated with trimodality

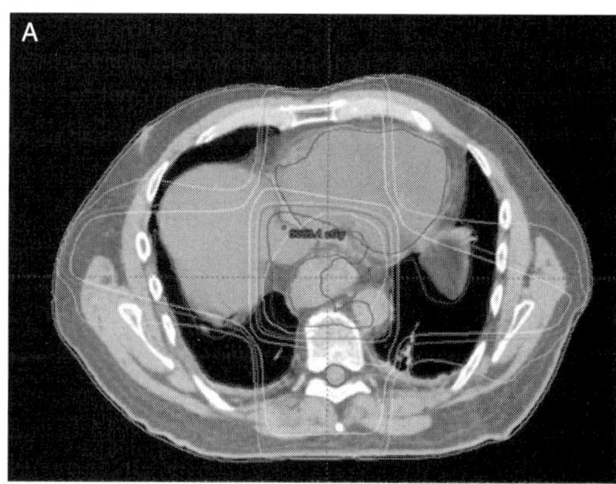

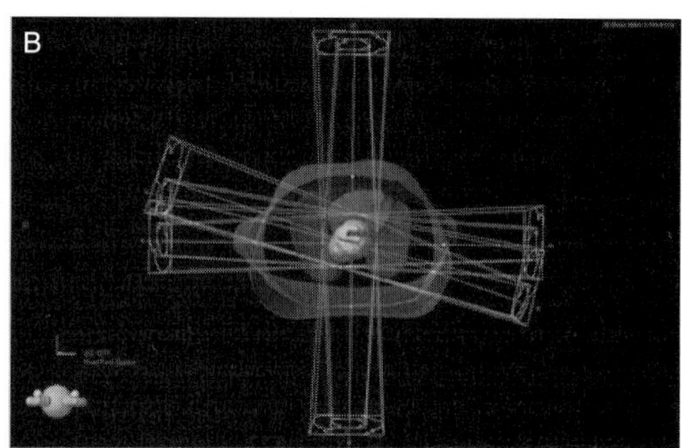

FIGURE 1 Gastroesophageal junction tumor radiation plan and field arrangement. A 73-year-old man with a history of gastroesophageal reflux disease presented with a T3N1 adenocarcinoma of the gastroesophageal junction. He was treated with definitive chemoradiation with cisplatin, 5-FU, and 50 Gy in 25 fractions. (A) Isodose curves from the six-field plan. (B) The beam arrangement. Anteroposterior, posteroanterior, left and right lateral, and left posterior oblique and right anterior oblique fields were used to provide good coverage of the PTV while sparing the normal heart (anterior) and lungs (lateral). The volume of lung receiving more than 20 Gy (V20) is 23%.

therapy. There was no increase in postoperative cardiac mortality in this group, but nonfatal late cardiac events were significantly increased, perhaps in part due to the fact that the trimodality group had the highest 1-year overall survival (10).

Hashimoto et al. analyzed dose–volume histogram parameters for 37 patients with thoracic esophageal squamous cell carcinoma treated with 5-FU, cisplatin, and 60 Gy without surgery, and cardiac toxicity was scored according to the Common Terminology Criteria for Adverse Events (CTC-AE) system. Grade 3 or higher toxicity was seen in eight patients (22%). The incidence of grade 3 or higher toxicity was 47% in patients with a mean heart dose (MHD) of 40 Gy or higher, and 10% in patients with an MHD of less than 40 Gy (11). Wei and colleagues analyzed 101 patients treated with definitive chemoradiation at the M.D. Anderson Cancer Center to identify clinical and dosimetric factors influencing the risk of pericardial effusion. The crude rate of effusion formation was 27.7%, with a median time to onset of 5.3 months. In multivariate analysis, volume of heart receiving over 30 Gy (V30) was the only significant predictor of pericardial effusion. V30 > 46% was associated with a 73% rate of effusion formation, while the rate with V30 < 46% was only 13% (12). In contrast, Tripp et al. published a retrospective series of 20 patients who were treated with definitive chemoradiation consisting of platinum-based chemotherapy and 50.4 Gy. By multiple gated acquisition scan, there was a clinically insignificant decline (59–54%, $P = 0.01$) in ejection fraction following chemoradiation. No significant association between radiation dose to different parts of the heart and decreased ejection fraction was found, possibly due to the small size of the series (13).

The available data suggests that chemoradiation increases the risk of late cardiac events, and that both dose and volume parameters play a role. Further research to validate these findings, and to explore the relationship between dose–volume parameters and cardiac toxicity in the setting of trimodality therapy, is indicated. Other issues for future consideration include possibly incorporating cardiac screening into follow-up and possible prophylactic pharmacologic intervention.

■ NEW INSIGHTS INTO PULMONARY RADIATION TOLERANCE

Acute pneumonitis occurs 4 to 6 weeks following radiation to the thorax and consists of a clinical syndrome of dyspnea, cough, low-grade fevers, and chest pain in the absence of infection, tumor recurrence, or other medical conditions (Figs 2A and B). After months to years, late fibrosis sets in, with scarring and contraction of the affected lung and a decrease in carbon monoxide diffusing capacity (Dlco). Dose–volume histogram data has been extensively

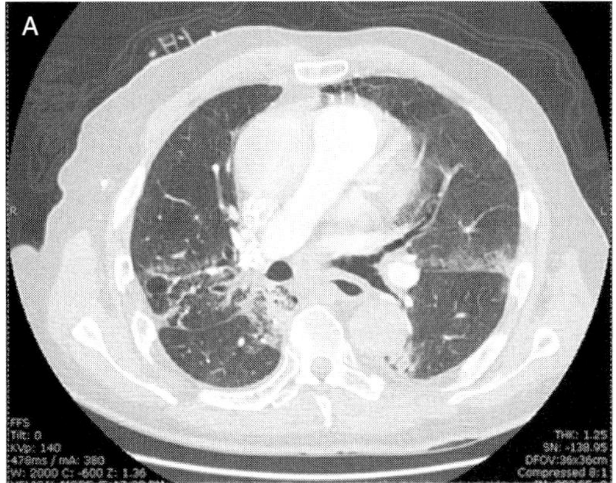
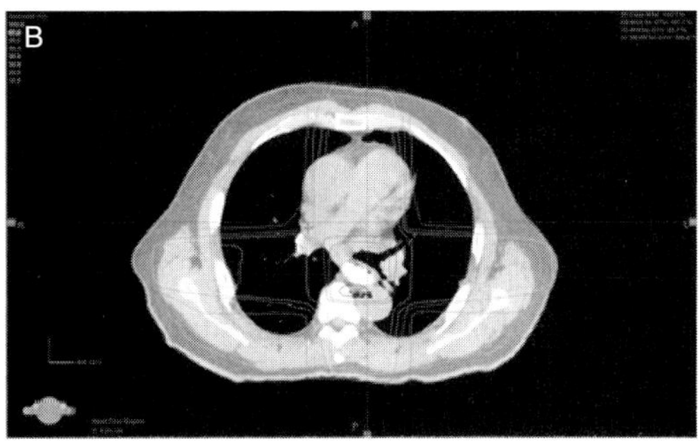

FIGURE 2 Acute pneumonitis and radiation plan. A 72-year-old man with multiple medical comorbidities and a history of tobacco and alcohol abuse presented with a T3N1M0 adenocarcinoma of the distal esophagus. He was treated with concurrent cisplatin, 5-FU, and 50.4 Gy with a four-field plan. Following treatment, he developed severe esophagitis and dehydration requiring hospitalization. An upper endoscopy showed ulceration consistent with radiation change, and multiple biopsies showed no evidence of tumor. He became progressively dyspneic, and a CT was obtained, (A) showing linear ground glass opacities in the lower lungs, corresponding to the radiation beams. (B) The infectious and metastatic workup was negative, and a diagnosis of radiation pneumonitis was made.

studied in a search for criteria that can quantify the risk of pneumonitis following thoracic radiotherapy. Graham et al. found that the volume of lung receiving at least 20 Gy (V20) was the only independent predictor of Grade 2 or higher pneumonitis in a cohort of 99 patients with non–small cell lung cancer treated with definitive radiation. The risk of grade 2 pneumonitis was 8% for a V20 of 22% to 31%.

Grade 3 pneumonitis first occurred at a V20 of over 32%, and there was a 23% incidence of grade 3 to 5 pneumonitis for a V20 of 40% (14). Mean lung dose (MLD) has also been evaluated in numerous series as a predictor of pneumonitis. Kwa et al. pooled 540 patients who had received thoracic radiotherapy at five institutions to show that the risk of grade 2 or higher pneumonitis was correlated with MLD. A MLD of 30 Gy was associated with a normal tissue complication probability of 13% to 24% (15).

Postoperative pulmonary complications are distinct from radiation pneumonitis and include respiratory events such as pneumonia or acute respiratory distress syndrome (ARDS) that occur in the postoperative period. Several groups have investigated the correlation between clinical and dosimetric factors in esophageal cancer patients and the likelihood of postoperative pulmonary complications. Reynolds et al. reported morbidity and mortality outcomes from a 200-patient Irish randomized trial of trimodality therapy versus surgery. Trimodality therapy was associated with significantly increased risk of postoperative respiratory failure and ARDS, but there was no difference in overall survival (16). Abou-Jawde et al. compared pre- and posttreatment pulmonary functions in 155 patients treated with three different neoadjuvant chemoradiation regimens. Chemoradiation decreased Dlco in a radiation-dose-dependent manner, and postoperative respiratory complications were more likely to occur in the 45 Gy group than in the 30 Gy group (17% vs 3%, $P = 0.025$). Patients who developed postoperative respiratory complications had a median survival of only 2.1 months (17). In a series of 35 patients treated with trimodality therapy, a forced respiratory volume in 1 second (FEV1) of less than 3 L was correlated with the development of respiratory complications after esophagectomy (18). Lee et al. reported on a group of 61 patients treated with neoadjuvant chemoradiation to a median dose of 45 Gy at the M.D. Anderson Cancer Center. Eleven patients (18%) had postoperative pulmonary complications, and two patients died of pneumonia. Pulmonary complications were more frequent when the lung volume receiving at least 10 Gy (V10) was over 40% (35% vs 8%, $P = 0.014$) (19). Wang et al. updated this series to include 110 patients treated with neoadjuvant chemoradiation and found that patients with a high volume of lung receiving at least 5 Gy (V5) were at increased risk of experiencing pneumonia or ARDS within 30 days of surgery (20).

Our understanding of the impact of dose–volume parameters on pulmonary function continues to evolve. Chemotherapy is almost always given concurrently with radiation for esophageal cancer and likely decreases pulmonary tolerance, although it is not clear to what extent. As an example, a recent report suggests that induction or concurrent therapy with taxanes increases the risk of radiation pneumonitis (21). Increasingly, it is becoming clear that even very low doses of radiation can be deleterious, if delivered to a large volume of lung (22). At the Yale Cancer Center, we use the following dose–volume guidelines when planning thoracic radiotherapy: V20 less than 30%, V10 less than 40%, V5 less than 60%, and an MLD of less than 15 Gy (Fig. 3). The planning tumor volume (PTV) is subtracted from the total lung volume when calculating the parameters. Uncertainties remain regarding the use of such parameters. For instance, there is the problem of which parameters to use, given that many of them, such as V20 and MLD, are highly correlated (14,23). Additionally, dose–volume histogram analysis inherently assumes that all parts of the lung are equal, when in fact the lower lobes of the lungs appear to be more sensitive to the development of radiation pneumonitis (24). Regarding postoperative respiratory complications, neoadjuvant chemoradiation appears to increase the rate of complications, but this may be balanced by improved oncologic outcomes in terms of overall survival. Careful treatment planning and selection of patients for trimodality therapy may help to improve outcomes and decrease postoperative morbidity.

■ DEFINING THE TREATMENT VOLUME WITH POSITRON-EMISSION TOMOGRAPHY

Compared to a conventional planning CT scan, PET-CT scans can highlight involved lymph nodes and previously undetected distant metastases (Fig. 4A and B). When coregistered or merged to a treatment planning CT, PET-CT scans may enable oncologists to delineate better the gross tumor volume (GTV) and distinguish tumor from normal esophagus and gastric cardia (Figs 5A and B). Leong et al. performed a prospective study in which 21 patients underwent radiation treatment planning with and without the aid of PET-CT. Four of the patients had previously unsuspected metastases diagnosed by PET-CT, and

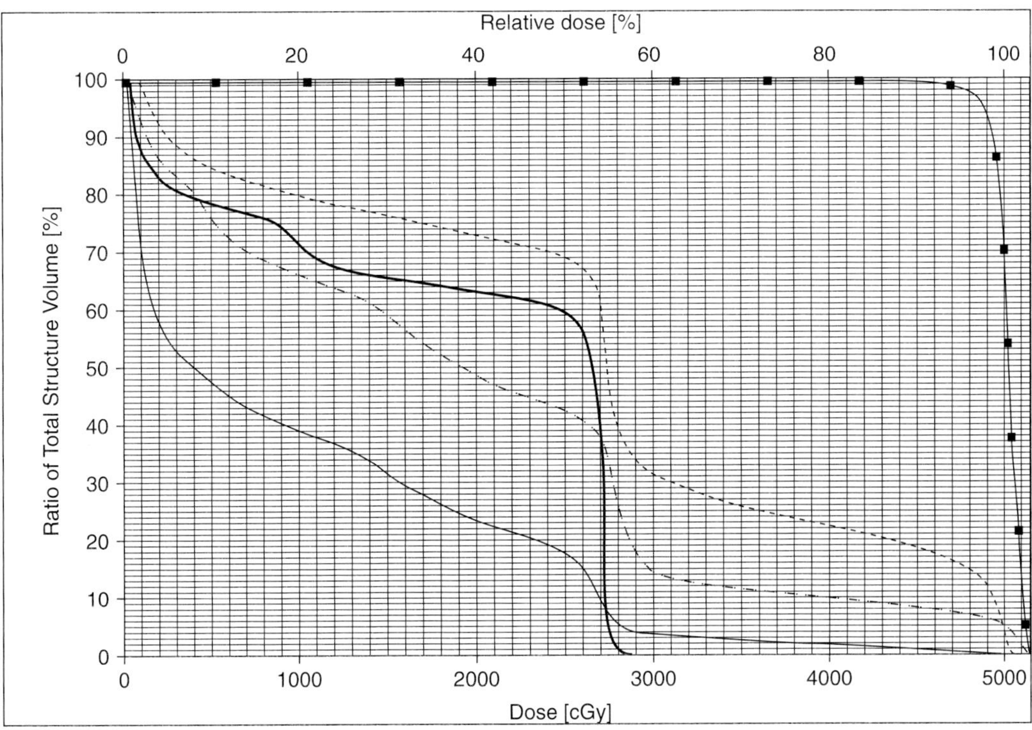

FIGURE 3 Dose–volume histograms for the patient in Figure 1. Histograms for (top to bottom) PTV, heart, spinal cord, liver, and lungs are displayed.

four additional patients had PET-avid nodal disease. Sixty-nine percent of patients had PET-avid GTV excluded from the GTV as planned by conventional CT, and 31% would have had a geographic miss of gross disease, with the PET-avid disease falling entirely outside of the margins of the conventionally planned PTV. PET-CT was felt to significantly improve the definition of the cranial and caudal borders of the esophageal GTV (25). Moreau-Zabutto et al. described their experience fusing PET-CT scans to treatment planning CT scans in 34 patients. Two patients were found to have metastatic disease and were excluded from definitive treatment. In 12 patients, the PET data led to a decrease in the GTV, whereas in 7 patients, the GTV had to be increased. In 18 of these patients, the changes were large enough that the PTV was affected (26). Konski and colleagues compared esophageal tumor length in 25 patients as measured by PET, CT, and endoscopy. Tumor length as measured by PET was significantly less than that measured by CT (5.4 vs 6.8 cm, $P = 0.0063$), and EUS was the best method

of the three for detecting periesophageal and celiac adenopathy (27). Gondi et al. analyzed treatment plans created with and without merged PET-CT data for 30 patients, including 16 esophageal cancer patients. The mean conformality index for the GTV (the ratio of the overlap of the two GTVs to the sum of the GTVs) was 0.46, and in 62.5% of the cases, the PET-defined GTV was smaller than the GTV defined by conventional planning CT (28).

While the use of PET-CT in treatment planning has been found to reduce interobserver variation in GTV definition (29), uncertainties remain about how to interpret PET-CTs for planning purposes. Hong et al. have demonstrated that GTV definition can vary significantly, depending on whether manual or semiautomated contouring is used (30). Recent clinicopathological correlation studies suggest that the threshold of standardized uptake value (SUV) used to characterize a PET-positive esophageal tumor can significantly affect the measurement of tumor length, and that a threshold of SUV 2.5 may correlate best with the actual pathological

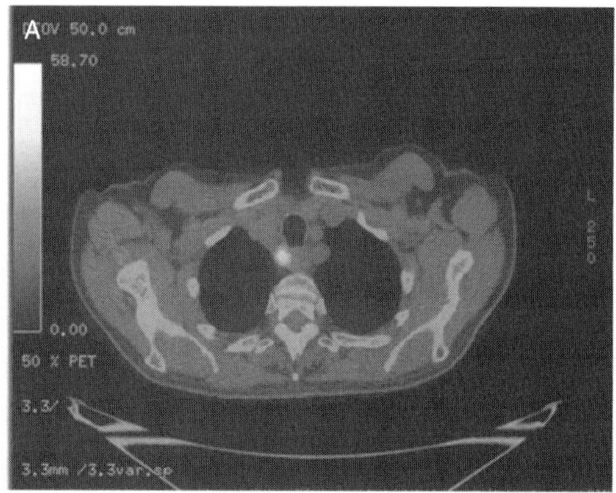

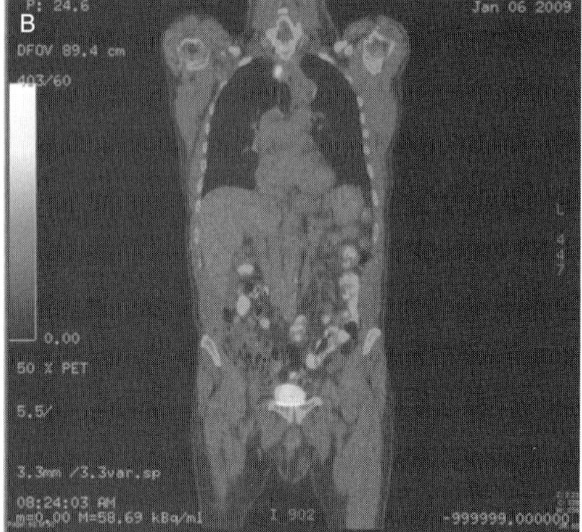

FIGURE 4 PET-CT of lymph nodes involved by esophageal cancer. (A) Axial and (B) coronal slices from a PET-CT scan in a patient with a clinical T3 tumor demonstrating a strong uptake in a paraesophageal lymph node.

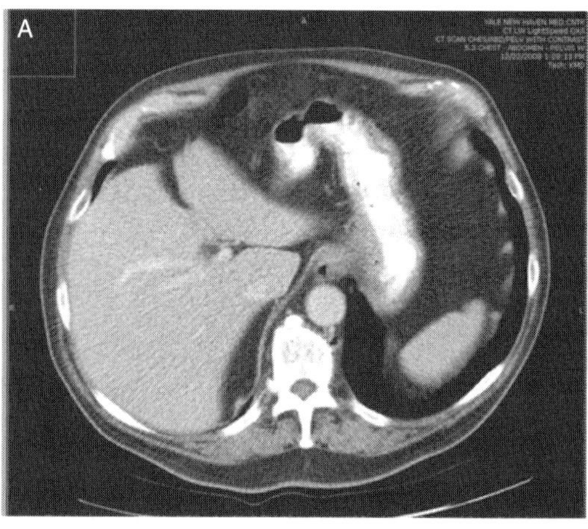

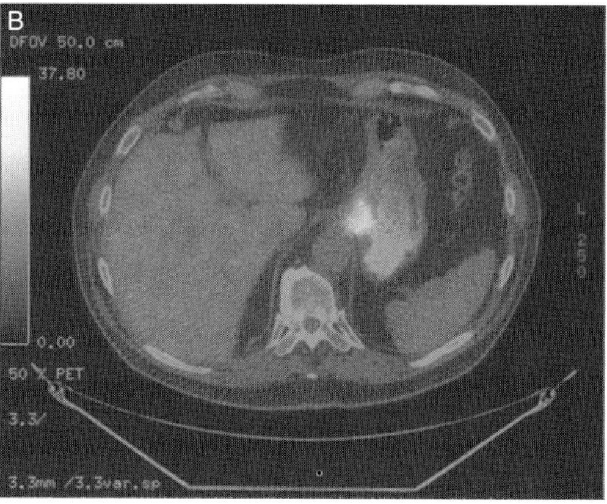

FIGURE 5 Tumor extension into the gastric cardia. (A) A slice from a PET-CT of a T3 gastroesophageal junction tumor. There is clear disease extension into the stomach that is not evident on a conventional CT (B).

tumor length in esophageal squamous cell carcinomas (31,32). It is unclear whether a standardized threshold method is superior to approaches that use an internal control (such as the liver) to determine a lower threshold for tumor involvement. Candidal infections and other nonmalignant lesions have also been reported to occasionally cause false-positive PET readings in esophageal cancer (33). Finally, PET-CT images are subject to respiratory and other sources of motion, as the images are acquired over an extended time period. While this could potentially be advantageous, it could also introduce error into SUV determination. Efforts are underway to correct for organ motion using respiratory-averaged PET-CT (34).

The National Comprehensive Cancer Network guidelines for the treatment of esophageal cancer now include a routine pretreatment PET-CT scan. It is not yet clear how to best integrate PET results into radiation treatment planning. A conservative approach would be to enlarge the GTV to include PET-positive disease not detected by other modalities, but not to reduce it in light of a negative PET if other information sources suggest there is disease present.

■ INTENSITY-MODULATED RADIATION THERAPY

Conventional 3D conformal radiation therapy (3DCRT) typically involves a small number of generous, dosimetrically homogeneous fields. In contrast, IMRT uses a larger number of fields that are divided into thousands of "pencil beams" of varying intensities, allowing for very sharp dose gradients and even treatment of concave target volumes. IMRT has been proposed as a method to improve tumor coverage and limit the volume of irradiated normal tissue. Clinical experience so far is limited to small series. Wang et al. reviewed the outcomes of seven patients with locally advanced cervical or upper thoracic esophageal squamous cell carcinoma who were treated with concurrent chemotherapy and IMRT to 64.8 Gy at the M.D. Anderson Cancer Center. Six evaluable patients had complete responses; two subsequently recurred and two developed metastases. There was one late tracheoesophageal fistula and two patients required frequent dilation of esophageal strictures (35). Koike et al. used IMRT as a boost in definitive treatment of 11 patients with cervical esophageal cancer. Conventional 3DCRT with cisplatin and 5-FU was given up to 36 to 40 Gy, and an IMRT boost was delivered to bring the total dose to 60 Gy. Median survival was 16.5 months, with a 2-year survival rate of 48%. One patient with a T4 tumor developed a fistula (36). Preliminary results of a series of 30 noncervical esophageal cancer have been reported by the group from Stanford. Patients were treated with chemoradiation to 50.4 Gy followed by surgery. Most patients had distal adenocarcinomas. Forty percent had grade 3 acute toxicity, and 10% needed a treatment break. One patient died from complications of feeding tube placement. Twenty-seven percent had late grade 3 toxicity (37).

Numerous dosimetric studies comparing conventional 3DCRT to IMRT in esophageal cancer have been published. Generally, these series have explored whether IMRT can reduce the amount of radiation delivered to the heart and lungs, with varying results. Chandra et al. found that IMRT with four, seven, or nine fields decreased lung V10, V20, and MLD compared to 3DCRT in distal esophageal cancers. The seven- and nine-field plans offered more conformal target coverage. IMRT did not improve heart or spinal cord sparing (38). Van

Liew and colleagues compared seven-field IMRT to four-field 3DCRT in mid- and distal esophageal cancers and found that IMRT decreased cardiac V40 and V50, but at the cost of increased pulmonary V10 (39). Nutting reported that four-field IMRT decreased MLD compared to 3DCRT, but that nine-field IMRT did not provide any further benefit (40).

Recognizing that using more fields for IMRT increases the amount of lung treated to low dose, some investigators have explored alternative modalities. Mayo et al. studied "hybrid" IMRT in 18 lung and esophageal patients. Two-thirds of the dose was delivered by two- or three-field 3DCRT and the remainder was given by IMRT. Compared to nine-field IMRT, the hybrid plans had lower V5 and V20, although nine-field IMRT delivered less cardiac dose. Compared to hybrid IMRT, four-field CRT had a lower V5 but higher V20 (41). Crowley et al. explored giving 36 Gy with 3DCRT followed by 14.4 Gy with IMRT, yielding improved sparing of the heart versus 3DCRT and improved sparing of the lungs compared to an all-IMRT approach. Dosimetry studies utilizing proton therapy, which has similar biological effects but superior dose-deposition characteristics compared to photon radiation, have also been published (42,43). At this point, the benefits conferred by these approaches remain theoretical. IMRT and in particular hybrid or combined plans require a substantial amount of extra work on the part of the physician and dosimetrist, and the extra cost is considerable. Likewise, proton radiotherapy is available at only a few select centers throughout the world and remains very costly. Prospective investigation with long-term follow-up and careful documentation of late toxicity will be needed to demonstrate the superiority of such techniques before they are widely implemented. Finally, while IMRT algorithms may be able to achieve the heart- and lung-sparing parameters entered by the planner, it is also worth repeating that these parameters continue to evolve and are still not completely understood.

■ 4D TREATMENT PLANNING

Yaremko and colleagues studied the motion of distal esophageal tumors in 31 patients using respiratory-gated 4D CT. Abdominal tumors moved by an average of 1.06 ± 0.04 cm, while thoracic tumors were less mobile, with an average of 0.81 ± 0.02 cm motion. A radial margin of 0.8 cm and an axial margin of 1.8 cm would have covered tumor motion in 95% of the cases (44). Patel et al. performed a similar study in 30 patients with mostly distal esophageal tumors, including 12 with involved celiac lymph nodes. Margins of 1.5 cm craniocaudal, 0.75 cm anteroposterior, and 0.75 laterally would have covered the esophageal tumor in 95% of the cases. Margins of 2.25 cm craniocaudal, 1.00 cm anteroposterior, and 0.75 laterally would have covered the celiac lymph nodes in 95% of the cases (45). Zhao et al. studied the motion of 25 distal esophageal tumors with 4D CT and recommended asymmetrical margins: 1.0 cm left (toward the stomach), 0.8 cm right, 1.1 cm anterior, 0.6 cm posterior, 1.0 cm superior (toward the distal esophagus), and 1.6 cm inferior (46). Tumor motion data from a 4D CT can be used to construct an internal target volume to decrease the likelihood of a geographic miss. It is also possible that abdominal compression or other methods to decreased respiratory motion could decrease tumor motion, allowing for reduction of margins.

■ CONCLUSIONS

Improvements in technology have led to a proliferation of techniques that have the potential to increase the therapeutic index of esophageal cancer radiotherapy. Validation of these technologies should be carried out in carefully designed prospective studies with long-term follow-up. At the same time, our understanding of normal tissue tolerances continues to grow and evolve, and this knowledge will play an integral role in the design of future trials. Eventually, it is conceivable that we will move away from standardized margins and beam arrangements toward individualized treatment plans that incorporate data from PET-CT and 4D scans and make use of fully optimized IMRT techniques to deliver radiation with maximum accuracy, precision, and safety.

■ REFERENCES

1. Akiyama H, Tsurumaru M, Kawamura T, Ono Y. Principles of surgical treatment for carcinoma of the esophagus: analysis of lymph node involvement. *Ann Surg* 1981;194(4):438.

2. Gao XS, Qiao X, Wu F, et al. Pathological analysis of clinical target volume margin for radiotherapy in patients with esophageal and gastroesophageal junction carcinoma. *Int J Radiat Oncol Biol Phys* 2007;67(2): 389–396.

3. Herskovic A, Martz K, al-Sarraf M, et al. Combined chemotherapy and radiotherapy compared with radiotherapy alone in patients with cancer of the esophagus. *N Engl J Med* 1992;326(24):1593–1598.

4. Minsky BD, Pajak TF, Ginsberg RJ, et al. INT 0123 (Radiation Therapy Oncology Group 94–05) phase III trial of combined-modality therapy for esophageal cancer: high-dose versus standard-dose radiation therapy. *J Clin Oncol* 2002;20(5):1167–1174.

5. Bosset JF, Gignoux M, Triboulet JP, et al. Chemoradiotherapy followed by surgery compared with surgery alone in squamous-cell cancer of the esophagus. *N Engl J Med* 1997;337(3):161–167.

6. Urba SG, Orringer MB, Turrisi A, Iannettoni M, Forastiere A, Strawderman M. Randomized trial of preoperative chemoradiation versus surgery alone in patients with locoregional esophageal carcinoma. *J Clin Oncol* 2001;19(2):305–313.

7. Walsh TN, Noonan N, Hollywood D, Kelly A, Keeling N, Hennessy TP. A comparison of multimodal therapy and surgery for esophageal adenocarcinoma. *N Engl J Med* 1996;335(7):462–467.

8. Button MR, Morgan CA, Croydon ES, Roberts SA, Crosby TD. Study to determine adequate margins in radiotherapy planning for esophageal carcinoma by detailing patterns of recurrence after definitive chemoradiotherapy. *Int J Radiat Oncol Biol Phys* 2009;73(3):818–823.

9. Emami B, Lyman J, Brown A, et al. Tolerance of normal tissue to therapeutic irradiation. *Int J Radiat Oncol Biol Phys* 1991;21(1):109–122.

10. MacAleer M, Smith GL, Smith BD, et al. Radiotherapy increases cardiac events in esophageal cancer patients: outcomes from the SEER-Medicare cohort with implications for improvement of tumor targeting and role of post-treatment pharmacomodulation. Proceedings of the American Radium Society 91st Annual meeting, Vancouver, BC; Canada. April 25–29, 2009, (abstract S042).

11. Hashimoto T, Asakura H, Zenda S, et al. Cardiac toxicities after concurrent chemoradiotherapy for esophageal cancer: dose volume histogram analysis. American Society for Clinical Oncology 2008 Gastrointestinal Cancers Symposium; (abstract 42).

12. Wei X, Liu HH, Tucker SL, et al. Risk factors for pericardial effusion in inoperable esophageal cancer patients treated with definitive chemoradiation therapy. *Int J Radiat Oncol Biol Phys* 2008;70(3):707–714.

13. Tripp P, Malhotra HK, Javle M, et al. Cardiac function after chemoradiation for esophageal cancer:

comparison of heart dose-volume histogram parameters to multiple gated acquisition scan changes. *Dis Esophagus* 2005;18(6):400–405.

14. Graham MV, Purdy JA, Emami B, et al. Clinical dose-volume histogram analysis for pneumonitis after 3D treatment for non-small cell lung cancer (NSCLC). *Int J Radiat Oncol Biol Phys* 1999;45(2):323–329.

15. Kwa SL, Theuws JC, Wagenaar A, et al. Evaluation of two dose-volume histogram reduction models for the prediction of radiation pneumonitis. *Radiother Oncol* 1998;48(1):61–69.

16. Reynolds JV, Ravi N, Hollywood D, et al. Neoadjuvant chemoradiation may increase the risk of respiratory complications and sepsis after transthoracic esophagectomy. *J Thorac Cardiovasc Surg* 2006;132(3):549–555.

17. Abou-Jawde RM, Mekhail T, Adelstein DJ, et al. Impact of induction concurrent chemoradiotherapy on pulmonary function and postoperative acute respiratory complications in esophageal cancer. *Chest* 2005;128(1):250–255.

18. Hsu F, Wu J, Lee Y, et al. Association of clinical and dosimetric factors with postoperative pulmonary complications in esophageal cancer patients receiving intensity modulated radiation therapy followed by esophagectomy [Abstract 1039]. *Int J Radiat Oncol Biol Phys* 2008;72(1, suppl): S130–S131.

19. Lee HK, Vaporciyan AA, Cox JD, et al. Postoperative pulmonary complications after preoperative chemoradiation for esophageal carcinoma: correlation with pulmonary dose-volume histogram parameters. *Int J Radiat Oncol Biol Phys* 2003;57(5):1317–1322.

20. Wang SL, Liao Z, Vaporciyan AA, et al. Investigation of clinical and dosimetric factors associated with postoperative pulmonary complications in esophageal cancer patients treated with concurrent chemoradiotherapy followed by surgery. *Int J Radiat Oncol Biol Phys* 2006;64(3):692–699.

21. McCurdy M, McAleer MF, Wei W, et al. Induction and Concurrent Taxanes Enhance both the Pulmonary Metabolic Radiation Response and the Radiation Pneumonitis Response in Patients with Esophagus Cancer. *Int J Radiat Oncol Biol Phys* 2009. In press.

22. Allen AM, Czerminska M, Jänne PA, et al. Fatal pneumonitis associated with intensity-modulated radiation therapy for mesothelioma. *Int J Radiat Oncol Biol Phys* 2006;65(3):640–645.

23. Kong FM, Hayman JA, Griffith KA, et al. Final toxicity results of a radiation-dose escalation study in patients with non-small-cell lung cancer (NSCLC): predictors for radiation pneumonitis and fibrosis. *Int J Radiat Oncol Biol Phys* 2006;65(4):1075–1086.

24. Bradley JD, Hope A, El Naqa I, et al. RTOG. A nomogram to predict radiation pneumonitis, derived from a combined analysis of RTOG 9311 and institutional data. *Int J Radiat Oncol Biol Phys* 2007;69(4): 985–992.

25. Leong T, Everitt C, Yuen K, et al. A prospective study to evaluate the impact of FDG-PET on CT-based radiotherapy treatment planning for oesophageal cancer. *Radiother Oncol* 2006;78(3):254–261.

26. Moureau-Zabotto L, Touboul E, Lerouge D, et al. Impact of CT and 18F-deoxyglucose positron emission tomography image fusion for conformal radiotherapy in esophageal carcinoma. *Int J Radiat Oncol Biol Phys* 2005;63(2):340–345.

27. Konski A, Doss M, Milestone B, et al. The integration of 18-fluoro-deoxy-glucose positron emission tomography and endoscopic ultrasound in the treatment-planning process for esophageal carcinoma. *Int J Radiat Oncol Biol Phys* 2005;61(4):1123–1128.

28. Gondi V, Bradley K, Mehta M, et al. Impact of hybrid fluorodeoxyglucose positron-emission tomography/computed tomography on radiotherapy planning in esophageal and non-small-cell lung cancer. *Int J Radiat Oncol Biol Phys* 2007;67(1):187–195.

29. Vesprini D, Ung Y, Kamra J, et al. The addition of 18-fluorodeoxyglucose positron emission tomography to CT based radiotherapy planning of carcinoma of the esophagus decreases both the intra- and interobserver variability of GTV definition [Abstract 2160]. *Int J Radiat Oncol Biol Phys* 2006; 66(3, Suppl): S299–S300.

30. Hong TS, Killoran JH, Mamede M, Mamon HJ. Impact of manual and automated interpretation of fused PET/CT data on esophageal target definitions in radiation planning. *Int J Radiat Oncol Biol Phys* 2008;72(5):1612–1618.

31. Fu X, Yu W, Zhang J, et al. A prospective evaluation of lymph node GTV delineation by 18-FDG PET/CT for patients with esophageal cancer [Abstract 2184]. *Int J Radiat Oncol Biol Phys* 2008;72(1 Suppl): S108–S109.

32. Zhong X, Yu J, Zhang B, et al. Using 18F-fluorodeoxyglucose positron emission tomography to estimate the length of gross tumor in patients with squamous cell carcinoma of the esophagus. *Int J Radiat Oncol Biol Phys* 2009;73(1): 136–141.

33. Shrikanthan S, Aydin A, Dhurairaj T, Alavi A, Zhuang H. Intense esophageal FDG activity caused by Candida infection obscured the concurrent primary esophageal cancer on PET imaging. *Clin Nucl Med* 2005;30(10):695–697.

34. Pan T, Luo D, Liu H, et al. Improving tumor localization and standard uptake value quantitation of non-small cell lung cancer and esophageal cancer patients by new respiration-averaged CT in PET/CT imaging [Abstract 2466]. *Int J Radiat Oncol Biol Phys* 2006; 66(3 Suppl): S468–S469.

35. Wang SL, Liao Z, Liu H, et al. Intensity-modulated radiation therapy with concurrent chemotherapy for locally advanced cervical and upper thoracic esophageal cancer. *World J Gastroenterol* 2006;12(34):5501–5508.

36. Koike R, Nishimura Y, Nakamatsu K, et al. Chemoradiotherapy using intensity-modulated radiation therapy for locally advanced cervical esophageal cancer [Abstract 2182]. *Int J Radiat Oncol Biol Phys* 2008;66(3): S310–S311.

37. La T, Minn A, Su Z, et al. Multi-modality treatment with intensity-modulated radiation therapy for esophageal cancer. American Society for Clinical Oncology 2009 Gastrointestinal Cancers Symposium; [Abstract 67].

38. Chandra A, Guerrero TM, Liu HH, et al. Feasibility of using intensity-modulated radiotherapy to improve lung sparing in treatment planning for distal esophageal cancer. *Radiother Oncol* 2005;77(3):247–253.

39. Van Liew S, Garofalo M, D'Souza D, et al. IMRT can effectively reduce cardiac dose over 3D-CRT in mid/distal esophageal cancer: 10 patient planning study. *Int J Radiat Oncol Biol Phys* 2006;66(3):S305–S306.

40. Nutting CM, Bedford JL, Cosgrove VP, Tait DM, Dearnaley DP, Webb S. A comparison of conformal and intensity-modulated techniques for oesophageal radiotherapy. *Radiother Oncol* 2001;61(2):157–163.

41. Mayo CS, Urie MM, Fitzgerald TJ, Ding L, Lo YC, Bogdanov M. Hybrid IMRT for treatment of cancers of the lung and esophagus. *Int J Radiat Oncol Biol Phys* 2008;71(5):1408–1418.

42. Zhang X, Zhao KL, Guerrero TM, et al. Four-dimensional computed tomography-based treatment planning for intensity-modulated radiation therapy and proton therapy for distal esophageal cancer. *Int J Radiat Oncol Biol Phys* 2008;72(1):278–287.

43. Crowley E, Kachinic L, Mamon H, et al. Optimizing the cardiac and pulmonary dose: a comparison of IMRT photon and 3-D proton treatment planning for distal esophageal cancer [Abstract 2829]. *Int J Radiat Oncol Biol Phys* 2008;72(1 Suppl): S539–S540.

44. Yaremko BP, Guerrero TM, McAleer MF, et al. Determination of respiratory motion for distal esophagus cancer using four-dimensional computed tomography. *Int J Radiat Oncol Biol Phys* 2008;70(1):145–153.

45. Patel AA, Wolfgang JA, Niemierko A, Hong TS, Yock T, Choi NC. Implications of respiratory motion as measured by four-dimensional computed tomography for radiation treatment planning of esophageal cancer. *Int J Radiat Oncol Biol Phys* 2009;74(1):290–296.

46. Zhao KL, Liao Z, Bucci MK, et al. Evaluation of respiratory-induced target motion for esophageal tumors at the gastroesophageal junction. *Radiother Oncol* 2007;84(3):283–289.

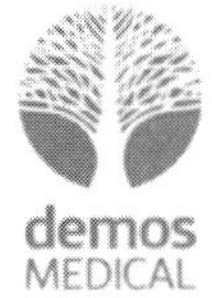

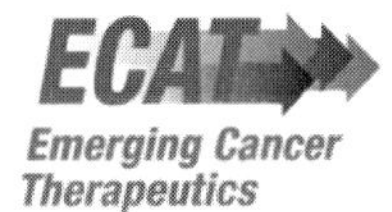

ECAT
**Emerging Cancer
Therapeutics**

Esophageal Cancer

Chemotherapy and Targeted Agents for Stage IV Cancer

M. Wasif Saif*

Yale Cancer Center, Yale University School of Medicine, New Haven, CT

■ ABSTRACT

Advanced esophageal carcinoma carries a poor prognosis with 5-year survival of less than 20%. This poor outcome is similar for patients with squamous cell carcinoma as well as adenocarcinoma. Surgical therapy, external radiation, and chemotherapy with curative intent are usually impossible because of the advanced disease. Advances have been achieved in the therapy of esophageal cancer, including new chemotherapeutic agents, such as oxaliplatin, docetaxel, capecitabine, and irinotecan. Encouraging results have been shown from recent preliminary data with biological and target-oriented agents in the treatment of esophageal cancer, in particular, epidermal growth factor receptor (EGFR) inhibitors. Limited experience is available with angiogenesis inhibitors, apoptosis inhibitors, and COX-2 inhibitors. Despite all the developments made in the treatment of esophageal cancer, it poses a continuous challenge to treat this highly virulent disease effectively. Future research should establish whether combinations of chemotherapy with targeted agents play a role in survival.

■ INTRODUCTION

Many agents are active in esophageal cancer. Objective response rates (RRs) of 30% to 60% and median survivals of less than 1 year are commonly reported with platinum-based combination regimens with fluorouracil, taxanes, topoisomerase inhibitors, hydroxyurea, or vinorelbine (1).

■ ROLE OF CYTOTOXIC AGENTS

Single Agents

Older single agents, including bleomycin, 5-fluorouracil (5-FU) given by bolus or continuous infusion, cisplatin, and mitomycin, have single-agent RRs ranging from 10% to 20% (1). Carboplatin, by contrast, has shown a lower single-agent RR in both squamous cell carcinoma (2–4) and adenocarcinoma (5), though carboplatin-based combination regimens appear similar to cisplatin combinations. Oxaliplatin, a new platinum analog, has not been evaluated as a single agent in esophageal cancer, but a combination of oxaliplatin with 5-FU and capecitabine has been evaluated in phase II and III trials. Oral 5-FU drugs,

---

*Corresponding author, Associate Professor of Medicine, Medical Oncology

Director, GI Cancers Program, Cancer Center, Yale University School of Medicine, New Haven, CT

E-mail address: Wasif.saif@yale.edu

Emerging Cancer Therapeutics 1 (2010) 69–76.

DOI: 10.5003/2151–4194.1.1.71

demosmedpub.com/ecat

capecitabine, S-1, and tegafururacil (UFT) have undergone evaluation in metastatic gastric (6,7) and gastroesophageal junction (GEJ) cancer. Capecitabine has been evaluated in Japanese and Korean trials, with reported RRs of 26% to 34% (8,9).

The alkaloids vindesine and vinorelbine have reported RRs ranging from 15% to 20% (10,11). Toxicity for vindesine included significant sensory neuropathy, while vinorelbine had significant hematologic toxicity, with grade 3 and 4 neutropenia seen in 59% of patients. Paclitaxel, another active single agent in esophageal cancer, has also been studied in combination chemotherapy trials. Phase II trials have evaluated a 24-hour, every 3-week schedule, and a weekly 1-hour schedule, with RRs ranging from 15% to 32% in combined adenocarcinoma and squamous cell carcinoma trials (12,13). Similar RRs were seen for both histologies with either infusion schedule, though the weekly 1-hour schedule had substantially less grade 3 and 4 neutropenia (5%) compared to the every 24-hour schedule administered every 3 weeks (86%), which also employed prophylactic granulocyte colony-stimulating factor (G-CSF). Docetaxel has been evaluated in esophageal squamous cell and adenocarcinoma at doses of 70 to 100 mg/m^2 every 3 weeks (14–16). RRs ranged from 20% to 25%. Hematologic toxicity was significant in these trials, with relatively high rates of grade 3 and 4 neutropenia (up to 88% of patients) and neutropenic fever (32%–45%).

The topoisomerase I inhibitor etoposide has been studied in both adenocarcinoma and squamous cell carcinoma, with RRs ranging from 0% to 19% (17,18). The topoisomerase II inhibitor irinotecan has been evaluated in two recent phase II trials in adenocarcinoma of the stomach and GEJ, with a RR of 15% observed (19,20).

Combination Chemotherapy

In recent years, combinations of these new agents have reported to result in at 50% or higher RR (Table 10).

Docetaxel, Cisplatin, and 5-FU (DCF)

A randomized international phase III study (V325) compared the combination of DCF (docetaxel 75 mg/m^2 on day 1, cisplatin 75 mg/m^2 on day 1, 5-FU 750 mg/m^2/day for 4 days in a 21-day cycle) to the conventional cisplatin and 5-FU (CF, cisplatin 100 mg/m^2 on day 1, 5-FU 1,000 mg/m^2/day for 4 days in a 28-day cycle) in metastatic gastric cancer population (21). A significant improvement in overall survival (OS; 9.2 vs 8.6 months, P = 0.0201), time to disease progression (TDP); 5.6 vs 3.7 months, P = 0.0004), and RR (36% vs 26%, P = 0.011) was demonstrated. However, increased toxicities were noticed in the DCF arm with grade 3/4 neutropenia 82% versus 57%, grade 3/4 diarrhea 20.4% versus 8%. Based on the results of the study, U.S. Food and Drug Administration (FDA) approved the regimen as a standard therapy for metastatic gastric cancer. However, dose modification is commonly needed and prophylactic G-CSF may be suggested in the practice.

EOX, EOF, ECX

A large randomized European phase III trial with a 2 × 2 factorial design evaluated the efficacy of capecitabine, an oral fluoropyrimidine, and oxaliplatin as alternatives to traditional infusion 5-FU and cisplatin in metastatic/advanced esophageal and gastric cancer (22). All the patients (N = 1,002) received triplet therapy with epirubicin (50 mg/m^2 on day 1) and cisplatin (60 mg/m^2 on day 1) plus either fluorouracil (200 mg/m^2/day continuous infusion) (ECF) or capecitabine (625 mg/m^2, orally twice a day) (ECX), or triplet therapy with epirubicin and oxaliplatin (130 mg/m^2 on day 1) plus either fluorouracil (EOF) or capecitabine (EOX) (every 3 weeks as a cycle for all 4 arms). The primary end point was no inferiority in OS for the triplet therapies containing capecitabine as compared with fluorouracil and for those containing oxaliplatin as compared with cisplatin. The toxic profiles of capecitabine and 5-FU were similar. As compared with cisplatin, there were lower incidences of grade 3/4 neutropenia, alopecia, renal toxicity, and thromboembolism, but with slightly higher incidences of grade 3 or 4 diarrhea and neuropathy in patients who received oxaliplatin. There was no significant difference in Progression free survival (PFS) and RRs among the regimens. Median survival times in the ECF, ECX, EOF, and EOX groups were 9.9, 9.9, 9.3, and 11.2 months, respectively. The OS was longer with EOX than with ECF (HR = 0.80 [95% CI 0.66–0.97]; P = 0.02).

Another randomized phase III study evaluated and confirmed the clinic benefits of the combinations

TABLE 10 Summary of combination chemotherapy regimens

Reference	RX	N	RR (%) (95% CI)	Median Survival (months)	P Value
ECF					
Ross (40)	ECF	289	42.4	9.4	NS
	MCF	285	44.1	8.7	
Webb (41)	ECF	121	46	8.7	$P < 0.01$
	FAMTX	116	21	6.1	
DCF					
Moiseyenko (42)	DCF	221	36.7	9.2	$P = 0.02$
	CF	224	25.4	8.6	
Irinotecan-based therapies					
Pooled results	Irinotecan/CDDP	105	48–58		
Pozzo (43)	Irinotecan/CDDP	56	32.1	6.9	$P = 0.002$
	Irinotecan/FU CI	59	42.4	10.7	
Dank (44)[a]	Irinotecan/FU CI	170	31.8	9.0	$P = 0.53$
	CF	165	25.8	8.7	

[a] Dank is a phase III study.

of 5-FU/leucovarinwith oxaliplatin versus cisplatin (23). Two hundred and twenty patients with untreated metastatic/advanced adenocarcinoma of the gastric or GEJ were randomly assigned to receive either 5-FU (2,600 mg/m^2 via 24-hour infusion), leucovorin (200 mg/m^2 on day 1), and oxaliplatin (85 mg/m^2 on day 1, every 2 weeks) (FLO) or 5-FU (2,000 mg/m^2 via 24-hour infusion), leucovorin (200 mg/m^2) weekly, and cisplatin (50 mg/m^2 every 2 weeks) (FLP). The combination with oxaliplatin was associated with significantly less toxicities except peripheral neuropathy. There was a trend toward improved median PFS with FLO versus FLP (5.8 vs 3.9 months; $P = 0.077$) and no significant difference in median overall survival (MOS; 10.7 vs 8.8 months). However, as compared with FLP, the combination of oxaliplatin (FLO) showed a significantly superior RR (41.3% vs 16.7%; $P = 0.012$), time-to-treatment failure (TTF) (5.4 vs 2.3 months; $P < 0.001$), PFS (6.0 vs 3.1 months; $P = 0.029$), and an improved OS (13.9 vs 7.2 months) in patients older than 65 years ($n = 94$).

All data suggest that the newer combination delivers equivalent benefits with less toxicity. More options are available for patients based on their tailored needs. However, the definitive role of anthrocyclines in the treatment of metastatic diseases is not clear.

S-1 in Combination Regimens

S-1, an oral fluoropyrimidine consisting of tegafur, CDHP (choro-2.4-dihydroxypyridine) and OXO (potassium oxonate) has been evaluated in phase III Japanese studies. Comparing S-1 (40 mg/m^2, bid, days 1–28, every 6 weeks) with continuous infusion 5-FU (800 mg/m^2/day, days 1–5, every 4 weeks) and irinotecan/cisplatin (irinotecan, 70 mg/m^2, days 1 and 15, cisplatin, 80 mg/m^2, day 1, every 4 weeks) for survival, RR, and toxicity, the three-arm randomized phase III study (JCOG 9912) concludes that S-1 is more favorable with overall profiles. S-1 is more effective as compared to 5-FU and not inferior to irinotecan/cisplatin combination (TTF 4.0 vs 2.3 vs 3.7 months, and OS of 11.4 vs 10.8 vs 12.3 months), but with much less toxicity (24).

The SPIRITS study tested the combination of cisplatin and S-1 versus S-1 alone in patients with advanced gastric cancer. In patients assigned to the combination arm (148 patients), S-1 was given orally (40–60 mg depending on the patient's body surface area [BSA]) twice daily for three consecutive weeks, and cisplatin (60 mg/m²) was administered intravenously on day 8, followed by a 2-week rest period, within a 5-week cycle. In patients assigned to the S-1–alone arm (150 patients), S-1 (40–60 mg) was administered twice daily for four consecutive weeks, followed by a 2-week rest period, within a 6-week cycle. MOS was significantly longer in the cisplatin and S-1 combination group (13.0 months [7.6–21.9]) than in S-1 alone (11.0 months [5.6–19.8]) (HR = 0.77; 95% CI 0.61–0.98; $P = 0.04$), and so was PFS (6.0 vs 4.0 months; $P < 0.0001$). There was 1 complete response (CR) and 46 partial responses (PRs) (RR 54% [43–65%]) in the combination arm and 1 CR and 32 PR (RR 31% [23–41]) in the S-1 alone arm. The combination of S-1 and cisplatin becomes a standard first-line treatment for patients with advanced gastric cancer in Japan (25).

A large randomized study testing the role of S-1 in the metastatic gastric cancer population in North America (5-FU with cisplatin vs S-1 with cisplatin) (FLAG) was completed, and the preliminary results suggest no survival difference between the two arms with less toxicity in the S-1/cisplatin arm (26).

■ ROLE OF TARGETED THERAPY

Esophageal cancer is an aggressive cancer constituting a major cause of cancer-related deaths worldwide. Recent advances in surgical techniques, incorporation of new therapeutic approaches—adjuvant/neoadjuvant chemoradiotherapy—and integration of new cytotoxic drugs, such as the taxanes and the camptothecin analogues, into the management of esophageal cancer have increased the RR to 40% to 50% with minor impact on OS. The 5-year survival rates after successful curative surgical resection have slightly improved from 4% to 14% while the relapse rate still remains high (1). The need for an efficacious therapy with minimal toxicity along with a better understanding of molecular pathways of esophageal carcinogenesis has led to the identification of

molecules (Table 11) whose action modification could inhibit the progress of esophageal cancer, and to the development of novel anticancer agents with targeted mechanisms of action. Success has been demonstrated in the treatment of colorectal, breast, lung, and renal cell carcinoma (RCC); similarly, preliminary data in esophageal and gastric cancer treatment from small studies are very encouraging (27–29). Epidermal growth factor receptors (EGFRs), HER-2/Neu, Ki-67, vascular endothelial growth factor (VEGF), VEGFR, p16, p21, cyclin D1, and p53 are potential targets for esophageal and gastric cancer treatment, and many of them are tested as predictive and prognostic factors for esophageal and gastric cancers. EGFR overexpression has been shown to predict poor prognosis in both esophageal squamous cell carcinoma and gastroesophageal adenocarcinoma. The expression of CXCR3, a chemokines receptor, is a strong and independent predictor of early relapse and poor prognosis in esophageal squamous cell carcinoma after neoadjuvant chemoradiotherapy (30). Mutations of p53 and KiRas have been implicated in chemoradiation resistance. A recent study suggests circulating anti-p53 antibodies as poor prognostic factor in esophageal squamous cell carcinoma patients treated with 5-FU and cisplatin-based chemoradiation (31).

EGFR Inhibitors

Available data of some of these biologic agents (with or without cytotoxic chemotherapy) in metastatic esophageal gastric cancer are encouraging (Table 12).

Cetuximab, an anti-EGFR monoclonal antibody, has been evaluated in esophageal and gastric cancer at locally advanced and metastatic setting. A combination of cetuximab with paclitaxel, carboplatin, and concurrent radiation was evaluated in patients with locally advanced esophageal/gastric cancer therapy (32). The study showed that 44 among 57 treated patients had surgical resection and 31 (69%) had their disease downstaged (with 22% pathological complete response). The combination was tolerable with limited toxicity. A phase II study tested the efficacy and safety of cetuximab combined with FOLFIRI as a first-line treatment of advanced gastric or GEJ adenocarcinoma (33). Thirty-eight patients were enrolled (13.2% locally advanced disease and 86.8% metastatic disease) and 34 patients were assessed for overall response rates (ORRs). The ORR was 44.1% (95% CI 27.5–60.9%). The median

TABLE 11   Molecular targets and their pathogenic role in esophageal carcinogenesis

Role	Molecular Targets
Cell-growth regulation	ErbB receptors family (EGFR, HER2/ new)
	EGFR or ErbB1
	HER2/new or ErbB2
Stimulation of angiogenesis	Vascular endothelial growth factor
Regulation of inflammatory response	Cyclooxygenase-2
Regulation of metastatic potential	Matrix metalloproteinases
Cell-cycle regulation	Cyclin-dependent kinases
	Histone deacetylases
Apoptosis regulation	Transcriptional nuclear factor kappa-b

TTP was 8 months (95% CI 7–9 months). At the median follow-up time of 11 months, 55.3% of patients were alive. There was one treatment-related death. The combination of cetuximab and FOLFOX was also tested. With a total of 40 patients treated as first-line therapy, the ORR was 50%, TTP 5.5 months (95% CI 4.8–6.2), and MOS 9.9 months.

The benefits of cetuximab as a second-line therapy in metastatic esophageal adenocarcinoma cancer were assessed via multicenter, open-label phase II Southwest Oncology Group (SWOG) study. Cetuximab was given (400 mg/m^2 IV on week 1, and 250 mg/m^2 IV weekly thereafter) and patients were evaluated for toxicity weekly and for response every 8 weeks. Twenty of 55 eligible and evaluable patients survived more than 6 months with MOS of 4 months (95% CI 3.2–5.9) and median PFS of 1.8 months (95% CI 1.7–1.9) (34). These data indicate that EGFR inhibitor(s) is effective in the esophageal gastric cancer treatment either as a single agent or in combination with conventional cytotoxic

chemotherapy or chemoradiation. A phase II study tested the EGFR tyrosine kinase inhibitor, erlotinib, in patients with GEJ and gastric adenocarcinoma as a single agent and first-line therapy. The study suggested an RR of 9% in GEJ patients (35).

VEGF Inhibitors

Meanwhile, the safety and efficacy of bevacizumab, an anti-VEGF monoclonal antibody was evaluated in esophageal gastric cancer. Thirty-four patients with measurable metastatic GEJ carcinoma were treated with a combination of bevacizumab (15 mg/kg on the day 1), irinotecan (65 mg/m^2, days 1 and 8), and cisplatin (30 mg/m^2, days 1 and 8 every 21 days) (36). The ORR was 65% (95% CI 46–80%). Median survival was 12.3 months (95% CI 11.3–17.2 months). There was no obvious increase in chemotherapy-related toxicity. Possible bevacizumab-related toxicities included a 28% incidence of grade 3 hypertension,

TABLE 12   Epidermal growth factor receptor (EGFR) tyrosine kinase inhibitors

Type of Inhibition	Agent
EGFR specific and reversible	ZD1839—Gefitinib
	OSI-774—Erlotinib
	PKI-166
EGFR specific and irreversible	EKB-569
Pan-HER reversible	GW-2016—Lapatinib
Pan-HER irreversible	CI-1033
Pan-HER and KDR reversible	AEE788

two cases of gastric perforation, one case of near perforation, and one case of myocardial infarction. However, 25 patients developed thromboembolic events during the study which was significantly higher than expected. Further investigation for thromboembolic events is needed before large phase III study with this bevacizumab could be conducted. Another phase II study evaluated the combination of bevacizumab docetaxel, cisplatin, and irinotecan (bevacizumab 10 mg/kg on day 1 every 3 weeks, docetaxel 30 mg/m², cisplatin 25 mg/m², irinotecan 50 mg/m² on days 1 and 8 of each 3-week cycle) in 26 patients with measurable, metastatic esophagogastric cancer. Among 22 evaluable patients, 15 (68%) had partial response and 4 (18%) had stable disease (37). These results suggest that bevacizumab is relatively safe and effective in the treatment of gastroesophageal cancer. However, patient selection may be crucial to maximize the benefits and minimize the toxicity especially when an antiangiogenic agent is used as part of perioperative therapy.

Several larger randomized studies are being done concurrently to test the efficacy of these biological agents (e.g., CALGB 80403 with comparison of cetuximab combining with ECF vs IC [irinotecan and cisplatin] vs FOLFOX [infusional 5-FU and oxaliplatin]).

Multitargeted Kinase Inhibitor

Other newer target-oriented agents have also been investigated in esophageal gastric cancer. Sunitinib malate is an oral, multitargeted tyrosine kinase inhibitor of VEGFRs, PDGFRs, KIT, RET, and FLT3, approved for the treatment of advanced RCC and imatinib-resistant or -intolerant gastrointestinal stromal tumor. A phase II study was performed to evaluate the efficacy and tolerability of sunitinib in previously treated metastatic gastric cancer (38). The preliminary findings suggested that sunitinib is generally well tolerated and may have single-agent antitumor activity in pretreated gastric cancer patients.

Ras/Raf Pathway

Alterations of the Ras/Raf pathway may contribute to the pathogenesis of esophageal and gastric cancer. Sorafenib is a potent inhibitor of Raf tyrosine kinase and of several receptor tyrosine kinases that are involved in tumor progression (e.g., VEGFR-2,

VEGFR-3, PDGFR-*b*). A phase II Eastern Cooperative Oncology Group study was conducted to evaluate the combination of sorafenib and docetaxel and cisplatin (sorafenib 400 mg orally twice a day, docetaxel 75 mg/m² on day 1, and cisplatin 75 mg/m² on day 1, every 21 days) (39). There were 44 patients with advanced and metastatic gastric and GEJ adenocarcinoma. The results were encouraging with an RR of 41%, median PFS of 5.8 months (90% CI 5.4–7.4), and a MOS of 13.6 months (90% CI 8.6–16.1). Grade 3 and 4 neutropenia was the main toxicity as expected. These newer agents hold promise and deserve further evaluation via large randomized studies.

Modest advances have been made in chemotherapy for esophageal cancer. A spectrum of single agents are active in esophageal cancer, including fluorinated pyrimidines, taxanes, platinum drugs, irinotecan, and mitomycin. Two-drug combinations modestly increase RRs, but translate into only a limited improvement in survival compared to single-agent therapy. The combination of 5-FU and cisplatin is widely used, and alternative two-drug regimens using either 5-FU or cisplatin as a backbone typically add either a taxane or irinotecan. Recent phase III trials, also treating patients with gastric cancer, indicate modest 10% to 15% improvements in response and 1–2 month improvements in median survival with the addition of a third agent to conventional infusional 5-FU/cisplatin—either epirubicin on the ECF regimen or docetaxel on the DCF regimen.

Cisplatin/5-FU-based chemotherapy is now a therapy standard in the preoperative treatment of esophageal and GEJ adenocarcinoma. Combined chemotherapy and radiation therapy are given preoperatively for esophageal adenocarcinoma and squamous cell carcinoma, and chemoradiotherapy without surgery is an accepted therapy standard for squamous cell cancer. Future research will focus on incorporating novel, molecularly targeted agents in the treatment of advanced disease and in the preoperative treatment of locally advanced disease.

■ REFERENCES

1. Enzinger PC, Ilson DH, Kelsen DP. Chemotherapy in esophageal cancer. *Semin Oncol* 1999;26(5 Suppl 15):12–20.
2. Mannell A, Winters Z. Carboplatin in the treatment of oesophageal cancer. *S Afr Med J* 1989;76(5):213–214.
3. Queisser W, Preusser P, Mross KB, et al. Phase II evaluation of carboplatin in advanced esophageal carcinoma.

A trial of the Phase I/II Study Group of the Association for Medical Oncology of the German Cancer Society. *Onkologie* 1990;13(3):190–193.

4. Sternberg C, Kelsen D, Dukeman M, Leichman L, Heelan R. Carboplatin: a new platinum analog in the treatment of epidermoid carcinoma of the esophagus. *Cancer Treat Rep* 1985;69(11):1305–1307.

5. Einzig A, Kelsen DP, Cheng E, et al. Phase II trial of carboplatin in patients with adenocarcinomas of the upper gastrointestinal tract. *Cancer Treat Rep* 1985;69(12):1453–1454.

6. Lee SJ, Cho SH, Yoon JY, et al. Phase II study of S-1 monotherapy in paclitaxel- and cisplatin-refractory gastric cancer. *Cancer Chemother Pharmacol* 2009;65(1):159–166.

7. Somali I, Meydan N, Tarhan MO, Oztop I, Alacacioglu A, Yilmaz U. Efficacy and toxicity of lower dose UFT without leucovorin in metastatic gastric cancer patients. *J BUON* 2009;14(3):429–433.

8. Kondo K, Takahashi Y, Ishikawa S, et al. Microscopic analysis of chromium accumulation in the bronchi and lung of chromate workers. *Cancer* 2003;98(11):2420–2429.

9. Hong YS, Song SY, Lee SI, et al. A phase II trial of capecitabine in previously untreated patients with advanced and/or metastatic gastric cancer. *Ann Oncol* 2004;15(9):1344–1347.

10. Kelsen DP, Bains M, Cvitkovic E, Golbey R. Vindesine in the treatment of esophageal carcinoma: a phase II study. *Cancer Treat Rep* 1979;63(11–12):2019–2021.

11. Conroy T, Etienne PL, Adenis A, et al. Phase II trial of vinorelbine in metastatic squamous cell esophageal carcinoma. European Organization for Research and Treatment of Cancer Gastrointestinal Treat Cancer Cooperative Group. *J Clin Oncol* 1996;14(1):164–170.

12. Ajani JA, Ilson DH, Daugherty K, Pazdur R, Lynch PM, Kelsen DP. Activity of taxol in patients with squamous cell carcinoma and adenocarcinoma of the esophagus. *J Natl Cancer Inst* 1994;86(14):1086–1091.

13. Ilson DH, Wadleigh RG, Leichman LP, Kelsen DP. Paclitaxel given by a weekly 1-h infusion in advanced esophageal cancer. *Ann Oncol* 2007;18(5):898–902.

14. Einzig AI, Neuberg D, Remick SC, et al. Phase II trial of docetaxel (Taxotere) in patients with adenocarcinoma of the upper gastrointestinal tract previously untreated with cytotoxic chemotherapy: the Eastern Cooperative Oncology Group (ECOG) results of protocol E1293. *Med Oncol* 1996;13(2):87–93.

15. Heath EI, Urba S, Marshall J, Piantadosi S, Forastiere AA. Phase II trial of docetaxel chemotherapy in patients with incurable adenocarcinoma of the esophagus. *Invest New Drugs* 2002;20(1):95–99.

16. Muro K, Hamaguchi T, Ohtsu A, et al. A phase II study of single-agent docetaxel in patients with metastatic esophageal cancer. *Ann Oncol* 2004;15(6):955–959.

17. Coonley CJ, Bains M, Heelan R, Dukeman M, Kelsen DP. Phase II study of etoposide in the treatment of esophageal carcinoma. *Cancer Treat Rep* 1983;67(4):397–398.

18. Kelsen DP, Magill GB, Cheng E, et al. Phase II trial of etoposide in adenocarcinomas of the upper gastrointestinal tract. *Cancer Treat Rep* 1983;67(5):509–510.

19. Harstrick A, Bokemeyer C, Preusser P, et al. Phase II study of single-agent etoposide in patients with metastatic squamous-cell carcinoma of the esophagus. *Cancer Chemother Pharmacol* 1992;29(4):321–322.

20. Enzinger PC, Ilson DH, Kelsen DP. Chemotherapy in esophageal cancer. *Semin Oncol* 1999;26(5 Suppl 15):12–20.

21. Van Cutsem E, Moiseyenko VM, Tjulandin S, et al., V325 Study Group. Phase III study of docetaxel and cisplatin plus fluorouracil compared with cisplatin and fluorouracil as first-line therapy for advanced gastric cancer: a report of the V325 Study Group. *J Clin Oncol* 2006;24(31):4991–4997.

22. Cunningham D, Starling N, Rao S, et al., Upper Gastrointestinal Clinical Studies Group of the National Cancer Research Institute of the United Kingdom. Capecitabine and oxaliplatin for advanced esophagogastric cancer. *N Engl J Med* 2008;358(1):36–46.

23. Al-Batran SE, Hartmann JT, Probst S, et al. Phase III trial in metastatic gastroesophageal adenocarcinoma with fluorouracil, leucovorin plus either oxaliplatin or cisplatin: a study of the Arbeitsgemeinschaft Internistische Onkologie. *J Clin Oncol* 2008, 26:1435–1442.

24. Boku N, Yamamoto S, Fujita S, Akasu T, Moriya Y. Impact of upward lymph node dissection on survival rates in advanced lower rectal carcinoma. *Dig Surg* 2007;24(5):375–381.

25. Koizumi W, Narahara H, Hara T, et al. S-1 plus cisplatin versus S-1 alone for first-line treatment of advanced gastric cancer (SPIRITS trial): a phase III trial. *Lancet Oncol* 2008;9(3):215–221.

26. Ajani JA, Rodriguez W, Bodoky G, et al. Multicenter phase III comparison of cisplatin/S-1 (CS) with cisplatin/ 5-FU (CF) as first-line therapy in patients with advanced gastric cancer (FLAGS). *Gastrointestional Cancers Symposium* 2009, abstract 8.

27. Syrigos KN, Zalonis A, Kotteas E, Saif MW. Targeted therapy for oesophageal cancer: an overview. *Cancer Metastasis Rev* 2008;27(2):273–288.

28. Tew WP, Shah M, Schwartz G, et al. Phase II trial of erlotinib for second-line treatment in advanced esophageal cancer. *Proc ASCO GI Can Symp* 2005, 85:abstract 5.

29. Shah A, Ramanathan RK, Ilson D, et al. Final results of a multicenter phase II study of irinotecn (CPT), cisplatin (CIS) and bevacizumab (BEV) in patients with metastatic gastric or gastroesophageal (GEJ) adenocarcinoma (NCI#6647). *J Clin Oncol* 2006, 24(N18)4020.

30. Suntharalingam M. The role of concurrent chemotherapy and radiation in the management of patients with squamous cell carcinomas of the head and neck. *Semin Oncol* 2003;30(4 Suppl 9):37–45.

31. Yoshikawa R, Koishi K, et al. Recurrence patterns and prognosis of esophageal cancer patients with persistent expression of chemokine receptor CXCR3 after neo-

adjuvant chemoradiotherapy. *Proc GI Can Symp* 2008, 1:abstract 98.

32. Blanchard P, Quero L, Schlageter MH, et al. Prognostic value of anti-p53 (p53 abs) and anti-Kiras (KiRas abs) circulating antibodies in esophageal carcinomas treated with chemoradiotherapy (CTRT). *Proc GI Can Symp* 2008, 1:abstract 24.

33. Safran H, Suntharalingam M, Dipetrillo T, et al. Cetuximab with concurrent chemoradiation for esophagogastric cancer: assessment of toxicity. *Int J Radiat Oncol Biol Phys* 2008;70(2):391–395.

34. Han SW, Kim HJ, Kim S, Ryu KH. Coronary ostial stenosis after aortic valvuloplasty (comprehensive aortic root and valve repair). *Eur J Cardiothorac Surg* 2009;35(6):1099–1101.

35. Gold PJ, Goldman B, Iqbal S, et al. Cetuximab as second-line therapy in patients with metastatic esophageal cancer: a phase II Southwest Oncology Group study [abstract 96]. *Proc GI Can Symp* 2008;1:39. Dragovich T, McCoy S, Fenoglio-Preiser CM. Phase II trial of erlotinib in gastroesophageal junction and gastric adenocarcinomas: SWOG 0127. *J Clin Oncol* 2006;24(30):4922–4927.

36. Shah MA, Ramanathan RK, Ilson DH, et al. Multicenter phase II study of irinotecan, cisplatin, and bevacizumab in patients with metastatic gastric or gastroesophageal junction adenocarcinoma. *J Clin Oncol* 2006;24(33):5201–5206.

37. Enzinger PC, Ryan DP, Regan EM, et al. Phase II trial of docetaxel, cisplatin, irinotecan, and bevacizumab in metastatic esophagogastric cancer. *Proc GI Can Symp* 2008, 1:abstract 97.

38. Bang Y, Kang YR, Seo MK, et al. Clinical Predictors of Incomplete ST-Segment Resolution in the Patients With Acute ST Segment Elevation Myocardial Infarction. *Korean Circ J* 2009;39(8):310–316.

39. Sun W, Chen H, Lei C, Lei X, Zhang Y. Genetic variation in eight Chinese cattle breeds based on the analysis of microsatellite markers. *Genet Sel Evol* 2008;40(6):681–692.

40. Ross P, Nicolson M, Cunningham D, et al. Prospective randomized trial comparing mitomycin, cisplatin, and protracted venous-infusion fluorouracil (PVI 5-FU) with epirubicin, cisplatin, and PVI 5-FU in advanced esophagogastric cancer. *J Clin Oncol.* 2002;20(8): 1996–2004.

41. Webb A, Cunningham D, Scarffe JH, et al. Randomized trial comparing epirubicin, cisplatin, and fluorouracil versus fluorouracil, doxorubicin, and methotrexate in advanced esophagogastric cancer. *J Clin Oncol* 1997;15(1):261–267.

42. Van Cutsem E, Moiseyenko VM, Tjulandin S, et al. Phase III study of docetaxel and cisplatin plus fluorouracil compared with cisplatin and fluorouracil as first-line therapy for advanced gastric cancer: a report of the V325 Study Group. *J Clin Oncol* 2006;24(31):4991–4997.

43. Pozzo C, Barone C, Szanto J, et al. Irinotecan in combination with 5-fluorouracil and folinic acid or with cisplatin in patients with advanced gastric or esophagealgastric junction adenocarcinoma: results of a randomized phase II study. *Ann Oncol* 2004;15(12):1773–1781.

44. Dank M, Zaluski J, Barone C, et al. Randomized phase III study comparing irinotecan combined with 5-fluorouracil and folinic acid to cisplatin combined with 5-fluorouracil in chemotherapy naive patients with advanced adenocarcinoma of the stomach or esophagogastric junction. *Ann Oncol* 2008;19(8):1450–1457.

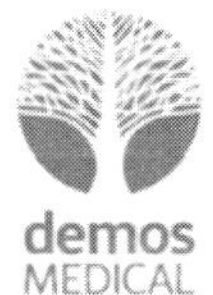

demos
MEDICAL

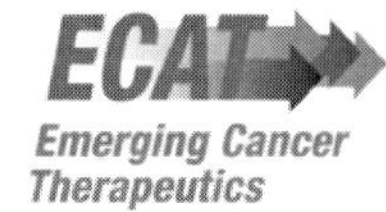

Gastric Cancer

Sobha Kurian[a]*, Susan Alsamarai[b], and M. Wasif Saif[b]

[a]*West Virginia University, Morgantown, WV*

[b]*Yale Cancer Center, Yale University School of Medicine, New Haven, CT*

■ ABSTRACT

Gastrointestinal malignancies are common, and despite recent advancements in treatment they still cause considerable morbidity and mortality worldwide. The development of new cytotoxic agents and targeted agents in the past decade has dramatically increased the number of treatment options available for these patients. These agents can have substantial benefit, often resulting in reduction of recurrences, increases in survival and improvements in quality of life. In addition, treatments may also be individualized to the specific patient based on the biology of the tumor and mechanism of the agent. We present in detail recent advances in the chemotherapeutic treatment of GI malignancies, and provide insight into many agents currently being investigated for these diseases.

■ INTRODUCTION

Despite a declining incidence worldwide, gastric cancer remains second to lung cancer as the leading cause of cancer deaths worldwide (1). It accounts for 9.9% of all new cancers. The world has seen a reduction in mortality from this disease, but it remains the fourth most common cancer. In the United States, in 2008, there were an estimated 21,500 new cases of gastric cancer with 10,800 resulting in death (2). In 2009, it is estimated that 21,130 Americans will be diagnosed with gastric cancer and 10,620 will die from it (3).

In the West, 5-year survival for all gastric cancer is approximately 10%, and in those surgically resected with curative intent, 5-year survival increases to about 20%.

In recent years, attention has been given to the anatomical location of the mass. Cancer of the gastric cardia and those of the more distal noncardia seem to be two epidemiologically different diseases. While gastric cancer decreases in incidence overall, cancers of the gastric cardia are increasing in incidence. Within the United States, Caucasians have higher rates of cancer involving the cardia than African Americans, whereas overall, African Americans have higher incidences. In males, gastric cardia cancer rates exceed female rates by greater than the 2:1 ratio overall (4).

*Corresponding author, West Virginia University, Morgantown, WV

E-mail address: skurian@hsc.wvu.edu

Emerging Cancer Therapeutics 1 (2010) 77–90.

DOI: 10.5003/2151–4194.1.1.79

demosmedpub.com/ecat

Age and gender differences exist in that most patients are diagnosed between the ages of 50 and 70, with a male-to-female ratio of 2:1 in those cases of noncardia location (5). In cases involving the gastric cardia, the gender difference is more striking with about a 6:1 male-to-female ratio (6).

Differences in geographic distribution are considerable. Some of the highest rates are seen in East Asia, South America, and Eastern Europe, with much lower incidences in North America and Western Europe. Yet, while some Asian countries such as Japan and Korea have high rates, other Asian countries such as India see much lower rates.

■ RISK FACTORS

H. pylori remains one of the most studied risk factors for gastric cancer since first reported in 1983. It is a major risk factor for the development of gastric cancer through chronic superficial gastritis that can progress to chronic atrophic gastritis and subsequently intestinal metaplasia and dysplasia (7). Cancers of the noncardia region have a strong association with *H. pylori* infection whereas cardia cancers have little or no association with *H. pylori* or in some cases even a negative association (8).

One recent cohort study using the Taiwan National Health Insurance Database looked at patients treated for *H. pylori* early (within 1 year of diagnosis) and late (greater than 1 year of diagnosis). No statistically significant difference existed between those patients treated early and the general populations, whereas the late treatment group was found to have an increased risk of gastric cancer with a standardized index ratio of 1.36. Other metaanalyses show a two- to threefold increase in gastric cancer in patients with chronic *H. pylori* infection (9).

The decline in gastric cancer overall is in parallel to the fall in *H. pylori* infection. In studies in the United States, the prevalence of *H. pylori* infection was found to be about 10% in those aged 18 to 29 and 47% in those aged 60 to 69 (10). Whereas in Japan, the prevalence is about 20.7% in those born after 1950 and increases to about 75% in those born prior to 1950 (11). The role of *H. pylori* in gastric cancer lies largely in the CagA virulence factor which is strongly associated with risk of adenocarcinoma, whereas a low risk is seen in its absence. In Japan, about 90% of the *H. pylori* strains are CagA positive, whereas the rate is closer to about 40% in the United States (12,13).

Cancers of the cardia overall do not show the same *H. pylori* association. Several studies show a negative association between *H. pylori* infection and esophageal adenocarcinoma. When looking at cancers involving the cardia, there seem to be two subtypes—one associated with *H. pylori* atrophic gastritis which is similar to noncardia cancer and another type with nonatrophic gastric mucosa that is more similar to esophageal adenocarcinoma. The possibility has been raised that this subgroup of gastric cancers of the cardia may have an etiology similar to esophageal adenocarcinoma and *H. pylori* may actually have a protective effect in those cases. The mechanism is hypothesized to be reduced acid production (8).

Socioeconomically, a lower status has consistently been shown to be associated with a higher risk overall. This association has been thought to be due to *H. pylori* infection among lower socioeconomic classes as when subdivided, the incidence of cardia cancer is largely seen in more professional classes (5).

Additionally, the socioeconomic difference can partially be explained by the negative relationship seen between a diet high in fruits and vegetables and risk of gastric cancer. One possible explanation for this finding is the antioxidant abilities of fruits and vegetables which are related to beta-carotene, alpha-tocopherol, and vitamin C content. *H. pylori* has been shown to substantially reduce the bioavailability of vitamin C. However, the role of diet also appears multifactor as one study in China did not show any change in risk of gastric cancer in patients receiving vitamin c supplementation whereas another study elsewhere showed regression of premalignant lesions when treating patients with a combination of vitamin C, beta-carotene, and eradication of *H. pylori* (5,4).

High salt intake has been reported to be a risk factor by two mechanisms: increasing the risk for *H. pylori* infection through mucosal damage that may increase the possibility of persistent infection as well as synergistic effect to promote gastric cancer by enhancing the carcinogenic effects of known gastric carcinogens such as N-methyl-N-nitro-N-nitrosoguanidine (MNNG) (14). Diets high in nitrite, as in preserved or cured meats, have been suggested to increase gastric cancer, but these are typically high salt foods so it is hard to separate the two, and the data for this is limited (5).

Similarly, alcohol consumption has been proposed as a risk factor, but the evidence is limited. In contrast, cigarette smoking has been shown to have an association with gastric cancer risk, with some studies showing a dose-dependent relationship (15).

Increased incidence has also been noted in conditions such as obesity (which predisposes to reflux esophagitis), blood group A, prior gastric resection, pernicious anemia, a family history of gastric cancer, hereditary nonpolyposis colon cancer, and Li-Fraumani syndrome.

■ SCREENING AND DIAGNOSIS

Screening methods are performed more routinely in countries with high incidences of gastric cancer—such as Japan where screening endoscopy starts at age 50. In the United States, by the time of diagnosis, about half the patients have disease extending beyond locoregional extension.

There is no specific tumor marker helpful in diagnosing or following gastric cancer. However, one recent study from Japan reported a novel fecal DNA methylation assay as a possible noninvasive screening test for colorectal and gastric cancers (16).

■ SIGNS AND SYMPTOMS

Most gastric cancers in the United States present at a later stage as surgically curable; early gastric cancers are generally not symptomatic and screening is not widely performed in the United States. Abdominal pain, which is generally vague and epigastric in location, and weight loss are common symptoms. Additionally, tumors arising at the proximal stomach or at the gastroesophageal junction (GEJ) often present with dysphagia. Nausea and early satiety can occur due to tumor mass or poor distensibility in the setting of linitis plastic. Advanced distal tumor can lead to gastric outlet obstruction.

Gastric cancer can spread regionally to the lesser and greater omentum, liver and diaphragm, spleen, pancreas, and transverse colon and can cause, for example, colonic obstruction. Lymphatic spread can be detected on physical exam with left supraclavicular adenopathy (Virchow's node), periumbilical node (Sister Mary Joseph's node), or left axillary lymphadenopathy (Irish node). Hematogenous metastases are generally to the liver, lungs, bone, or brain. Peritoneal spread can be apparent by development of ascites or a Krukenberg tumor of the ovary or mass in the cul-de-sac on rectal exam (Blumer's shelf). Paraneoplastic manifestations may also occur, such as diffuse seborrheic keratoses (sign of Leser-Trelat), acanthosis nigricans, microangiopathic hemolytic anemia, membranous nephropathy, hypercoagulable states, and polyarteritis nodosa.

■ PATHOLOGY

About 90% of gastric cancers are adenocarcinomas. The remaining 10% is comprised primarily of non-Hodgkin's lymphoma, leiomyosarcomas, and gastrointestinal (GI) stromal tumors. Rarely found are squamous cell carcinomas, small cell carcinomas, and carcinoid tumors. Occasionally, metastatic disease from tumors such as breast or melanoma can be found.

The adenocarcinomas are made up of intestinal or well-differentiated type and diffuse type.

Males and older age groups tend to present with well-differentiated tumors while younger groups tend to have diffuse carcinomas and the genders are more equivalent (5). Intestinal type is generally preceded by atrophic gastritis and metaplastic and dysplastic lesions as well as associated with H. pylori infection. In addition, polymorphisms in the IL-1β gene seem to lead to an increased risk of noncardia gastric cancer in the presence of H. pylori infection. Gastric expression of IL-1β was associated with gastric inflammation and subsequent neoplastic changes (17).

Diffuse-type gastric cancer can be subdivided into signet ring cell carcinoma and poorly differentiated carcinoma. Some suggest that signet ring cell can develop into poorly differentiated carcinoma. Downregulation of E-cadherin occurs early during the development of diffuse gastric cancer and is unique to this form.

Unlike intestinal-type gastric cancer, diffuse type has no clear association with H. pylori. Outcomes tend to be poorer due to more advanced stage at presentation.

■ STAGING AND PROGNOSIS

The importance of the preoperative evaluation is to divide patients into those with locoregional—stage I–III disease who are potentially curable and those with stage IV involvement who are treated in a palliative manner. Staging is done to rule out metastasis and to determine surgical resectability and the standard workup includes chest x-ray, chest CT scans, and abdominal imaging (Table 1). The role of endoscopic ultrasound (EUS) is less clear in gastric cancer compared to esophageal and GEJ cancers. Laproscopic staging may be needed in select patients.

■ GASTRIC CANCER TREATMENT

The standard treatment for patients with gastric cancer is surgical resection, unless the tumor is at an advanced, unresectable stage at diagnosis. The standard surgery in Asian countries like Japan includes meticulous resection of all regional lymph nodes (D2 resection), whereas in the United States, removal of only perigastric lymph nodes (D1 resection) is the standard. Data has suggested that the outcome of D2 resection may be better, but randomized trials have not clearly demonstrated a survival benefit. The disparity may be due to fundamental differences in the disease process itself rather than the surgical technique.

Early Stage Disease

Gastric Cancer–Adjuvant Treatment
Currently, the only chance for cure in gastric cancer is with surgical resection of the tumor and adjacent lymph nodes. However, only about 50% of patients have resectable disease on presentation (18). In the United States, unlike Japan where routine screening endoscopy starts at age 50, routine screening is not mainstream and gastric cancer symptoms remain vague overall. As distal cancers fall in number, more proximal tumors have risen in number and these convey a poorer prognosis. Despite resection, recurrence rates remain high with most patients dying of locoregional recurrence or distant metastasis. Five-year survival remains 30% at best in the United States. Adjuvant treatment has been shown to have a benefit in other GI malignancies and was subsequently studied in the setting of gastric cancer. An early metaanalysis by Herman et al. in 1993 failed to show a survival benefit with postoperative chemotherapy (19). A later analysis suggested a small survival benefit for patients treated adjuvantly—with a relative risk of 0.94 (95% CI 0.89–1.00). Subgroup analysis showed a greater effect in trials in which at least two-

thirds of the patients had nodal positive disease (20). When looking at adjuvant radiation alone, a decrease in locoregional failures was apparent (from 27% to 10.6%), but still no survival benefit overall.

A subsequent trial by MacDonald et al. combined the two treatment modalities and found a significant benefit in overall survival with postoperative chemoradiotherapy. Subsequent studies found a survival benefit with pre- and postoperative chemotherapy as well as the ability to downstage tumors from unresectable to resectable situations (21). Adjuvant therapy for nonmetastatic gastric cancer can be divided into three possibilities: (a) post-op chemoradiotherapy (MacDonald et al.) (22), (b) pre- and post-op (or perioperative) chemotherapy (MAGIC trial) (21), and (c) post-op chemotherapy (S-1, Japan) (23). All three treatment options confer significant survival benefit and the current standard of care in the United States is adjuvant therapy in all disease greater than stage 1. These three treatment approaches will be discussed in further detail.

Postoperative Chemoradiotherapy. Most patients develop locoregional or distant recurrence after curative resection for gastric cancer. A trial by Herskovic and Al-Sarraf indicated a benefit in disease-free survival for patients with esophageal cancer treated with radiation and chemotherapy (without a need for surgery) (24). Subsequently, a study was done by the SWOG 9008/INT 0116 group which paved the way for chemoradiotherapy as the standard of care for gastric cancer in the adjuvant setting. This study by MacDonald et al. randomized 556 patients with resected adenocarcinoma of the stomach or GEJ to surgery plus postoperative chemoradiotherapy versus surgery alone. The combination included chemotherapy for control of systemic micrometastatic disease as well as radiosensitization and radiation for local disease control. The patients ranged from stage 1B to IV (all nonmetastatic). Two hundred and eighty-one patients were randomized to the surgery plus chemoradiotherapy group and received fluorouracil 425 mg/m^2 of body surface area per day and leucovorin 20 mg/m^2 for 5 days. Chemoradiotherapy began 28 days after the initiation of chemotherapy and consisted of 4,500 cGy total of radiation, divided as 180 cGy/day for 5 days per week for 5 weeks with fluouracil (400 mg/m^2/day) and leucovorin (20 mg/m^2/day) on the first 4 and last 3 days of radiotherapy. One month following the completion of radiotherapy, two cycles of fluorouracil (425 mg/m^2/day), each 5 days in length, plus leucovorin (20 mg/m²/day) were given 1 month apart.

Of the chemoradiotherapy group, 68% had T3 or T4 disease and 85% node positive. Sixty-four percent completed treatment as planned, with 17% stopping treatment due to toxicities and 1% resulting in treatment-related deaths. The only surgical requirement was resection with curative intent and negative margins; however, critics have pointed out that only 54% of patients underwent D0 dissection (only partial removal of N1 nodes) and only 10% had D2 nodal dissections—which includes resection of all perigastric lymph nodes and some celiac, splenic or splenic-hilar, hepatic-artery, and cardial lymph nodes. However, this is comparable to general practice in North America.

After a 5-year median follow-up, median duration of survival was found to be 36 months in the chemoradiotherapy group compared to 27 months in the surgery only group (P = .005). Median disease-free survival was 30 months in the chemoradiotherapy group versus 19 months in the surgery only group (P < .0001) (22).

A study update in 2004 held up in terms of disease-free survival and overall survival, with 30-month median disease-free survival for chemoradiation and 19 months for surgery alone (P < .001). Overall survival was median 35 months in the chemoradiation group and 26 months in the group treated with surgery alone (P = .006) (25). A subsequent presentation at ASCO 2009 of 10-year follow-up of the phase III trial INT 0116 (SWOG 9008) continued to show a benefit in both disease-free and overall survival for the chemoradiation group (hazard ratio, HR = 1.32 with P =.004 for overall survival and HR = 1.51 with P < .001 for disease-free survival) with the additional finding that the subsets of women and patients with diffuse histology did not benefit. A multivariate analysis of gender and histology did not detect an effect once histology was included—women were significant more likely to have diffuse histology, and gender was not an independent risk factor. Additionally, there was no difference noted in late toxicities (26).

A follow-up to the MacDonald study is one by Fuchs et al. Intergroup Trial CALGB 80101 presented at ASCO 2006 is looking at a different and possibly more active regimen for chemoradiation—5-fluorouracil/leucovorin (5-FU/LV) was replaced with ECF. Patients are randomized either to the current standard of care of MacDonald regimen or to one cycle of ECF (epirubicin 50 mg/m² on day 1, cisplatin 60

mg/m² on day1, and 5-FU 200 mg/m²/day continuous infusion throughout radiation) followed by two cycles at a reduced dose (epirubicin 40 mg/m² on day 1, cisplatin 50 mg/m² on day 1, and 5-FU 200 mg/m²/day continuous infusion on days 1–21). The toxicity profile appears comparable, and since the study is ongoing the impacts this may make on practice are not yet clear (27). Another Dutch CRITICS study evaluates the addition of postoperative chemoradiation to preoperative ECX. Another ongoing study by a Swiss group randomizes patients to four cycles of DCF (docetaxel, cisplatin, and 5 FU) preoperatively versus postoperatively (28).

Pre- and Postoperative Chemotherapy. The MAGIC study published by Cunningham et al. in NEJM in 2006 (21) noted that a regimen of ECF—epirubicin, cisplatin, and infused 5-FU—has a survival benefit in patients with incurable locally advanced or metastatic gastric cancer and sought to see if this regimen could prove beneficial in the setting of surgically resectable and potentially curable gastric malignancies.

In this study, patients with resectable adenocarcinoma of the stomach (74%), GEJ (11%), or lower esophagus (15%) were randomized to either perioperative chemotherapy or surgery alone. Patients included were stage II or higher with no distant metastases, or had locally advanced inoperable disease. Two hundred and fifty patients were randomized to the chemotherapy group and they received three cycles of ECF (epirubicin 50 mg/m² iv bolus on day 1, cisplatin 60 mg/m² with hydration on day 1, and fluorouracil 200 mg/m² continuous iv infusion for 21 days) preoperatively and three cycles postoperatively. Surgery was scheduled 3 to 6 weeks after completion of the third cycle of chemotherapy and postoperative chemotherapy was to be initiated 6 to 12 weeks after surgery. Two hundred and fifty-three patients were randomized to surgery alone and this was scheduled to take place within 6 weeks after randomization. Of the patients assigned to receive perioperative chemotherapy, only 41.6% completed all six cycles, which is a limitation of the study. Patients did not complete the postoperative chemotherapy due to various reasons (37 patients due to early death or disease progression, 11 patients due to choice, 10 due to postoperative complications, 4 due to catheter problems, 3 due to prior toxicities, 2 due to lack of response to prior treatment, and 2 with worsened coexisting disease). The regimen was relatively well

TABLE 1 American Joint Committee on Cancer staging for gastric cancer

Tumor (T) Stage

TX	Primary tumor cannot be assessed
T0	No evidence of primary tumor
Tis	Carcinoma in situ: intraepithelial tumor without invasion of the lamina propria
T1	Tumor invades lamina propria or submucosa
T1a	Tumor invades lamina propria
T1b	Tumor invades submucosa
T2	Tumor invades muscularis propria
T3	Tumor invades subserosa without invasion of visceral peritoneum or adjacent structures
T4a	Tumor penetrates serosa (visceral peritoneum) without invasion of adjacent structures[a]
T4b	Tumor invades adjacent structures[a]

Nodal (N) Stage

NX	Regional lymph node(s) cannot be assessed
N0	No regional lymph node metastasis
N1	Metastasis in 1 to 2 regional lymph nodes
N2	Metastasis in 3 to 6 regional lymph nodes
N3	Metastasis in more than 6 regional lymph nodes
N3a	Metastasis in 7–15 regional lymph nodes
N3b	Metastasis in 16 or more regional lymph nodes

Metastasis (M) Stage

Mx	Presence of distant metastasis cannot be assessed
M0	No distant metastasis
M1	Distant metastasis

Anatomic Stage/Prognostic Groups

Stage 0	Tis	N0	M0
Stage 1A	T1	N0	M0
Stage 1B	T2	N0	M0
	T1	N1	M0
Stage IIA	T3	N0	M0
	T2	N1	M0
	T1	N2	M0
Stage IIB	T4a	N0	M0
	T3	N1	M0
	T2	N2	M0
	T1	N3	M0
Stage IIIA	T4a	N1	M0
	T3	N2	M0
	T2	N3	M0
Stage IIIB	T4b	N0–N1	M0
	T4a	N2	M0
Stage IIIc	T3	N3	M0
	T4b	N2–N3	M0
	T4a	N3	M0
Stage IV	Any T	Any N	M1

[a]The adjacent structures of the stomach include the spleen, transverse colon, liver, diaphragm, pancreas, abdominal wall, adrenal gland, kidney, small intestine, and retroperitoneum.

Source: AJCC Cancer Staging Manual, 7th edition. NewYork: Springer, 2010.

tolerated with the primary toxicities being hematologic with 24% grade ¾ granulocytopenia, 20% grade ¾ lymphocytopenia. Nonhematologic toxicities were primarily nausea (6.4% grade ¾) and vomiting (5.6% grade ¾).

This study made an important impact as it resulted in a significant survival benefit. Median follow-up was 49 months in the perioperative chemotherapy group and 47 months in the surgery group. Five-year survival rates were 36% in the perioperative chemotherapy group and 23% in the surgery group. Progression-free survival was significantly in favor of the perioperative chemotherapy group with HR for progression of 0.66 (95% CI 0.53–0.81, $P < .001$). Similar benefit was seen in terms of local and distant recurrence, with local recurrence identified in 14% of the perioperative chemotherapy group and 21% of the surgery group and distant metastases in 24% of the chemotherapy group and 37% of the surgery group.

An additional benefit was seen in the downstaging of patients after chemotherapy. The median maximum diameter of the resected tumor was smaller in the perioperative chemotherapy group than in the surgery group (3 vs 5 cm with $P < .001$). Additionally, 52% of the perioperative chemotherapy group were stage T1 or T2 at the time of surgery compared to 37% ($P = .002$) with less advanced (N0 or N1) nodal disease—84.4% compared to 70.5% ($P = .01$) favoring the perioperative chemotherapy group. Postoperative complications were equivalent between the two groups.

In comparison to the INT0116 trial, patient numbers and characteristics were similar. It is difficult to directly compare outcomes, but patients did better in the INT 0116 trial after surgery with 2-year survival of 52% compared to 2-year survival of 40% in the MAGIC trial and 2-year survival of 58% in INT 0116 compared to 48% in the MAGIC trial in looking at the treatment (chemoradiation/chemotherapy) arms.

From this trial comes the MAGIC-B trial which examines the addition of bevacizumab to perioperative chemotherapy. The chemotherapy regimen in this study is ECX rather than ECF due to findings of noninferiority of capecitabine in place of fluorouracil (29).

Postoperative Chemotherapy.   Rates of gastric cancer have generally been higher in Japan and in addition to epidemiological differences; there are also alternative chemotherapeutic options. One such drug used in Japan but not in the United States is the oral fluoropyrimidine S-1.

A trial of S-1 as adjuvant chemotherapy in patients with curatively resected gastric cancer was conducted in Japan by Sakuramoto et al. (23). S-1 is a combination of a prodrug flurouracil, gimeracil (which inhibits degradation of fluorouracil), and oteracil (which reduced the GI toxicities of fluorouracil by inhibiting its phosphorylation in the GI tract).

In this study, patients in Japan with stage II or III gastric cancer who underwent gastrectomy with extended (D2) lymph node dissection were randomized to surgery alone (standard of care at the time) or surgery followed by adjuvant therapy with S-1. Treatment was started within 6 weeks of surgery and continued for 1 year. The regimen was 40 mg/m² (but patients with body surface area of less than 1.25 m² were rounded up for a minimal dose of 80 mg) of S-1 for 4 weeks followed by 2 weeks off, making 6 week cycles. Sixty-six percent of patients completed 1 year of treatment.

Due to significance of overall survival in the chemotherapy group, the trial was stopped after the first interim analysis 1 year after enrollment was completed. Analysis of the data showed a 3-year survival rate overall of 80% in the S-1 group compared to 70% in the surgery only group, with relapse-free survival at 3 years of 72% in the S-1 group and 60% in patients treated with surgery alone. Chemotherapy was tolerated well overall with predominant side effects being anorexia in 6%, nausea in 3.7%, and diarrhea in 3.1% of patients.

One major difference of this study was the standard of D2 dissection in Japan, which is not routine in the West.

Locally Advanced Disease

For medically fit patients with apparent locoregional disease, laproscopic staging may be considered in addition to the standard staging scans and endoscopic ultrasound. Laproscopic staging is helpful to assess respectability, especially in GEJ tumors and those involving the whole stomach and helps to evaluate occult metastasis and peritoneal spread. If a lesion is deemed unresectable secondary to the extent of disease such as involvement of level 3 or 4 nodes or encasement of major vascular structures, either radiation therapy (RT) 45–50 Gy with concurrent 5-FU-based radiosensitizer dose or the alternate option of full dose systemic chemotherapy may be employed (30,31). However there are no trials directly comparing these two treatment options, and the current treatment practice is based on extrapolated data from the trials conducted in perioperative management of gastric cancer (see adjuvant section) (21,22).

External beam radiation as a single modality has minimal value in palliating locally unresectable gastric cancer. However, when used concurrently with 5-FU, external beam radiation improves survival (13 vs 9 months) compared to RT alone (32–34). Intensity-modulated radiation therapy (IMRT) has the potential to reduce radiation-related toxicity, but this modality still remains investigational in gastric cancer.

After completion of the primary treatment, medically fit patients with unresectable disease should undergo restaging studies (include pelvic imaging for women). If there is complete response, patients should be observed or they can undergo surgery if deemed appropriate based on extent of residual disease.

Metastatic Disease

Chemotherapy

The treatment of metastatic disease of the stomach is primarily palliative and confers only minimal effect on overall survival. A number of controlled trials and a metaanalysis provide evidence for the beneficial effect of palliative systemic chemotherapy as compared to supportive care alone for patients with advanced gastric cancer and have shown that patients undergoing combination chemotherapy survived for an average of 6 months longer than those receiving best supportive care (35).

When distal gastric adenocarcinomas were the most common stomach malignancy, most regimens for advanced gastric cancer were noncisplatin-containing regimens and were based upon 5-FU plus an anthracycline. More recently, cisplatin-based combinations were shown to be superior to 5-FU/ anthracycline-based and became the reference regimens for advanced gastric cancer.

Single Agents. Experience with older single agents like bleomycin, mitomycin-C, methotrexate, 5-FU,

etoposide, cisplatin, and doxorubicin were associated with only modest response rates of short duration of typically less than 6 months and infrequent complete responses. Newer agents that have been tested in gastric carcinomas include the taxanes (paclitaxel and docetaxel), irinotecan, capecitabine, S-1, and vinorelbine. In general, response rates are slightly higher than seen with older agents, but toxicity is prominent in many cases, and median survival durations have not exceeded 9 months. Table 4.2 summarizes response rates of single agents.

Combination Regimens. Higher response rates (up to 65%) are reported in phase II trials of combination therapy in patients with advanced gastric cancer, but in general the response rates have been lower in the setting of randomized trials. A metaanalysis of trials performed in patients with advanced gastric cancer predominantly using older combination regimens concluded that first-line combination therapy was associated with a modest but statistically significant survival benefit when compared to single agent therapy (35). The HR for death was 0.83 in favor of combination chemotherapy, but this translated into only a 1-month survival advantage. Newer triplet regimens using epirubicin or taxanes in combination with cisplatin and 5-FU (ECF, DCF) and irinotecan bases combinations may offer longer survival advantage, but these regimens have not been directly tested against single-agent therapy.

Anthracycline-based Regimens. ECF (epirubicin 50 mg/m^2 every 3 weeks, cisplatin 60 mg/m^2 every 3 weeks, plus infusional 5-FU 200 mg/m^2 daily) showed a response rate of 71% in a report involving 128 patients with advanced disease (36). In a subsequent randomized trial, 274 patients with advanced esophagogastric adenocarcinoma or undifferentiated cancer were randomly assigned to ECF or FAMTX (see below) (37). ECF was associated with a superior response rate (45% vs 21%) and median survival (8.9 vs 5.7 months). ECF caused more alopecia and nausea while FAMTX was associated with more hematologic toxicity and infections. Compared to patients treated with cisplatin and 5-FU alone, the addition of an anthracycline favorably impacted survival (HR for death = 0.77). This resulted in ECF regimen to be considered by many to be one of the reference regimens for first-line treatment of advanced upper GI cancer.

Due to the potential hazards and inconvenience of infusional therapy, efforts have been made to replace infusional 5-FU with orally administered fluoropyrimidine derivatives such as uracil-ftorafur (UFT) S-1, and capecitabine. At present, S-1 is not commercially available in the US and the dosing of S-1 may be different between the Western and Asian population due to differences in metabolism by CYP2A6.

The comparable efficacy of regimens substituting capecitabine for infusional 5-FU was studied in the REAL-2 trial, a randomized phase III study in which 1,002 patients with advanced gastric cancer were assigned, using a 2 × 2 factorial design, to 3-week cycles of epirubicin (50 mg/m^2) plus cisplatin (60 mg/m^2) and either capecitabine (625 mg/m^2 twice daily, ECX) or infusional 5-FU (200 mg/m^2 daily, ECF), or epirubicin (50 mg/m^2) plus oxaliplatin (130 mg/m^2) and either capecitabine (EOX) or infusional 5-FU (EOF) (29). The study was powered to demonstrate noninferiority. There were no significant differences among the groups in terms of objective response rate (41%, 42%, 46%, and 48% with ECF, EOF, ECX, and EOX, respectively) or progression-free survival. When outcomes of both capecitabine-containing arms were combined and compared to both 5-FU-containing arms (HR for death = 0.86, 95% CI 0.8–0.99), there was a statistically significant trend toward improved overall survival for capecitabine and toxic effects were similar. This trial also showed that outcomes were comparable when oxaliplatin was substituted for cisplatin in the ECF regimen. When the four groups were considered separately, median survival in patients treated with EOX was modestly longer when compared to ECF (median 11.2 vs 9.9 months, HR = 0.80, 95% CI 0.66–0.97).

Another randomized trial compared 21-day cycles of cisplatin (80 mg/m^2 day 1) given with either capecitabine (1,000 mg/m^2 twice daily for 14 days) or infusional 5-FU (800 mg/m^2/day days 1–5) in 316 patients with advanced gastric cancer and showed similar results (38). As with the REAL-2 study, this trial was also powered to demonstrate noninferiority. Median PFS (5.6 vs 5.0 months, respectively) and overall survival (10.5 vs 9.3 months, respectively) and the adverse effects were comparable in both groups. These studies suggest that the substitution of capecitabine for infusional 5-FU in these regimens provides similar efficacy.

S-1 in combination with cisplatin is highly active in Asian patients. A report from the SPIRITS trial supports a significant benefit for combined S-1 plus cisplatin over S-1 alone in terms of both response rate (54% vs 31%) and median survival (13 vs 11 months, P = 0.04) in Asian population (39). Trials done in the West with combination of S-1 plus cisplatin for advanced gastric cancer is limited but have shown some promising early results in phase II trials (40,41). The results from the phase II S-1 plus cisplatin trial led to the initiation of an international, prospective, randomized phase III trial, the First-Line Advanced Gastric Cancer Study (FLAGS) trial, which randomly assigned 1,053 patients to cisplatin plus either 5-FU or S-1. In a preliminary report from the 2009 ASCO Gastrointestinal Cancers Symposium, median overall survival (the primary end point) was not significantly better with cisplatin/S-1 as compared to cisplatin/5-FU (8.6 and 7.9 months, respectively) (42). The S-1 combination showed a more favorable side effect profile than cisplatin/5-FU, but lower cisplatin dose intensity was used in the cisplatin/S-1 arm (75 mg/m^2 on day 1 vs 100 mg/m^2 on day 1 in the cisplatin/5-FU arm) and this may have contributed to the difference noted in the survival and toxicity.

Older regimen include the combination of 5-FU plus an anthracycline (doxorubicin or epirubicin) studied in multiple phase II trials in conjunction with mitomycin (FAM/FEM) or methotrexate (FAMTX/FEMTX) in patients with advanced gastric adenocarcinoma. Initially encouraging results with 5-FU, doxorubicin, and mitomycin C (FAM) as well as high dose methotrexate, 5-FU plus doxorubicin (FAMTX) were not confirmed in subsequent trials and showed mainly partial responses only.

Taxane-based Combinations. Investigators have combined paclitaxel as well as docetaxel with cisplatin for the treatment of advanced gastric cancer using many different administration schedules.

The combination of low-dose cisplatin, etoposide, and paclitaxel is active in advanced upper GI cancer with an acceptable side effect profile and showed objective response rate of 70%, and median survival of 10 months (43).

The superiority of adding docetaxel to the combination of cisplatin and 5-FU (DCF regimen) compared to doublet of cisplatin and 5-FU alone was shown in a multinational TAX-325 trial which enrolled 457 patients with chemotherapy-naive advanced gastric cancer (44). Patients received either 21-day cycles of cisplatin (75 mg/m^2 on day 1) plus infusional 5-FU (750 mg/m^2 daily, days 1–5) and docetaxel (75 mg/m^2 on day 1) or 28-day cycles of cisplatin (100 mg/m^2 on day 1) plus infusional 5-FU (1,000 mg/m^2 per day days 1–5).

The docetaxel group showed higher response rates (37% vs 25%), time to tumor progression (TTP, 5.6 vs 3.7 months), and 2-year survival (18% vs 9%). DCF was also significantly superior to cisplatin/5-FU in time to definitive decline of performance status (median 6.1 vs 4.8 months) and in the duration of preserved quality of life (45,46). Based on these results, docetaxel was approved in the United States and Europe, in combination with cisplatin and 5-FU, in the treatment of advanced gastric cancer.

The contribution of cisplatin to the efficacy of this regimen is uncertain, as fairly similar results (overall response rate 38%, median survival 9.5 months) have been reported using docetaxel and infusional 5-FU without cisplatin (47). Combinations of docetaxel and capecitabine have also produced encouraging results (48). In published reports, response rates have ranged from 39% to 46% and the median TTP ranged between 4.2 and 6.1 months. Median and overall survival durations were between 8.4 and 15.8 months.

Irinotecan-containing Regimens. Irinotecan has been combined with cisplatin, docetaxel, and 5-FU showing encouraging results. However, there are no phase III trials supporting the use of an irinotecan-based combination instead of the current standard triplet regimen such as ECF, DCF, or EOX in the frontline therapy of advanced gastric cancer.

Weekly administration of irinotecan and cisplatin is active and fairly tolerated. In one phase II trial of 38 patients with untreated metastatic gastric cancer treated with irinotecan and cisplatin, both administered weekly for 4 of every 6 weeks showed complete responses in 10% and partial responses exceeding 40%, with a median time to progression of 24 weeks and median survival of 9 months (49).

The superiority of FOLFIRI (short-term infusional 5-FU plus leucovorin and irinotecan) over 5-FU/leucovorin with or without cisplatin was shown in a French randomized phase II trial involving 136 patients with advanced gastric cancer (50). Similar outcomes (response rate 44%, median survival 11 months) were obtained with irinotecan in combination with oral capecitabine in a nonrandomized phase II study (51).

A randomized phase III trial of irinotecan in gastric cancer compared 5-FU leucovorin irinotecan (FLI) (irinotecan 80 mg/m^2 on day 1, followed by leucovorin [folinic acid] 500 mg/m^2 over 2 hours, followed by 5-FU 2,000 mg/m^2 over 22 hours, weekly for 6 weeks) with cisplatin (100 mg/m^2 on day 1) followed by 5-FU (1,000 mg/m^2/day continuous infusion over 5 days) given every 4 weeks (52). There was no significant survival benefit of FLI over cisplatin/5-FU (median survival 9 and 8.7 months, respectively). However, this may be a viable noncisplatin-based regimen suited for second-line therapy and another phase III trial has shown better quality of life for this combination compared to cisplatin-based regimen (53).

Combinations of oxaliplatin with irinotecan are also effective and reasonably tolerated (54).

■ BIOLOGICAL AGENTS

HER2: Approximately 25% of advanced gastric cancers overexpress the type II epidermal growth factor receptor (EGFR) (HER2). The benefit of trastuzumab in advanced HER2-positive gastric cancer was evaluated in the phase III ToGA trial, which compared standard chemotherapy (six courses of infusional 5-FU/capecitabine plus cisplatin) with and without trastuzumab (8 mg/kg loading dose and 6 mg/kg every 3 weeks until disease progression) (55). The tumors of the enrolled patients (n = 594 of the 3,807 screened) were either 3+ for HER2 expression by immunohistochemistry or fluorescent in situ hybridization–positive.

In a preliminary report, the objective response rate was significantly higher with trastuzumab (47% vs 35%). At a median follow-up of 17.1 months, median overall survival (the primary end point) was significantly better with trastuzumab (13.8 vs 11.1 months). The toxicities in the two arms were comparable, except that a higher number of trastuzumab-treated patients had an asymptomatic decrease in left ventricular ejection fraction (5.9% vs 1.1%) and one patient developed grade 3 to 4 cardiac failure (vs two in the control group).

Lapatinib, an orally active small molecule inhibitor of both EGFR type I and II (HER2), is currently being studied in combination with weekly paclitaxel compared to paclitaxel alone in patients with previously treated advanced gastric cancer.

EGFR: Tumor overexpression of EGFR correlates with poor prognosis (56). The safety and efficacy of adding cetuximab to first-line chemotherapy

TABLE 2   Response rates of single agents

	Number of Patients	Objective Response Rate	Author (Ref.)
Paclitaxel (short infusion weekly)	26	14	Kii, T (61)
Paclitaxel (24-hour infusion)	18	23	Ajani, J (62)
Docetaxel	30	20	Mavroudis, D (63)
Irinotecan	40	20	Kohne, C (64)
5-FU	457	20	Earl, H (65)
Doxorubicin	180	17	Earl, H (65)
Mitomycin	189	29	Earl, H (65)
Cisplatin	20	22	Beer, M (66)
Methotrexate	28	11	Bruckner, H (67)

has been tested in multiple studies of advanced esophagogastric cancer (57). Studies suggest that this approach is safe and associated with objective response rates over 50% and median survival of 10 months. However, conclusions regarding the clinical use of cetuximab in patients with advanced esophagogastric cancer need confirmatory data from randomized phase III trials.

Vascular endothelial growth factor: Promising results were reported in a phase II study of bevacizumab (15 mg/kg on day 1) in combination with cisplatin (30 mg/m^2 days 1 and 8 of every 21-day cycle) and irinotecan (65 mg/m^2 on days 1 and 8) in 47 patients with advanced gastric or GEJ adenocarcinoma (58). The response rate was reported as 65% and median survival was 12.3 months. Promising results were also noted in another phase II trial of bevacizumab (5 mg/kg on days 1 and 15) plus docetaxel (35 mg/m^2 on days 1, 8, and 15 every 28 days) in 20 patients with metastatic esophagogastric cancer (59). An international phase III trial is currently underway to evaluate the benefit of adding bevacizumab to capecitabine plus cisplatin for first-line treatment of advanced gastric cancer.

■ PALLIATIVE PROCEDURES

Palliative gastrectomy may provide symptomatic relief of pain, nausea, bleeding, obstruction, and perforation. Gastric bypass with gastrojejunostomy to the proximal stomach is also often employed to palliate obstructive symptoms. Endoscopic placement of a stent provides a less-invasive alternative to surgery for symptom palliation and may possibly be more effective in symptom relief.

External beam RT has a well-defined role in the control of pain, bleeding, or obstruction in patients with localized but unresectable gastric cancer (60). Endoscopic laser treatment can effectively palliate dysphagia due to obstruction in patients with gastric cardia tumors.

■ REFERENCES

1. Parkin DM, Bray F, Ferlay J, Pisani P. Global cancer statistics, 2002. *CA Cancer J Clin* 2005;55(2):74–108.
2. Jemal A, Siegel R, Ward E, et al. Cancer Statistics. *CA Cancer J Clin* 2008; 58:71–96.
3. American Cancer Society. Cancer Facts and Figures 2009. Atlanta, GA: American Cancer Society, 2009.
4. Forman D, Burley VJ. Gastric cancer: global pattern of the disease and an overview of environmental risk factors. *Best Pract Res Clin Gastroenterol* 2006;20(4):633–649.
5. Kelley JR, Duggan JM. Gastric cancer epidemiology and risk factors. *J Clin Epidemiol* 2003;56(1):1–9.
6. Parkin DM, Whelan SL, Ferlay J, et al. Cancer incidence in five continents, vol. VII. Lyon: International Agency for Research on Cancer; 1997. pp. 922–924.
7. Correia M, Machado JC, Ristimäki A. Basic aspects of gastric cancer. *Helicobacter* 2009;14(Suppl 1):36–40.
8. Hansen S, Vollset SE, Derakhshan MH, et al. Two distinct aetiologies of cardia cancer; evidence from premorbid serological markers of gastric atrophy and Helicobacter pylori status. *Gut* 2007;56(7):918–925.
9. Eslick GD, Lim LL, Byles JE, Xia HH, Talley NJ. Association of Helicobacter pylori infection with gastric carcinoma: a meta-analysis. *Am J Gastroenterol* 1999;94(9):2373–2379.
10. Dooley CP, Cohen H, Fitzgibbons PL, et al. Prevalence of Helicobacter pylori infection and histologic

gastritis in asymptomatic persons. *NEJM* 1989;321: 1562–1566.

11. Sugiyama T, Nishikawa K, Komatsu Y, et al. Attributable risk of H. pylori in peptic ulcer disease: does declining prevalence of infection in general population explain increasing frequency of non-H. pylori ulcers? *Dig Dis Sci* 2001;46(2):307–310.

12. Maeda S, Ogura K, Yoshida H, et al. Major virulence factors, VacA and Cag A, are commonly positive in Helicobacter pylori isolates in Japan. *Gut* 1998;42:338–343.

13. Vicari JJ, Peek RM, Falk GW, et al. The seroprevalence of cagA-positive Helicobacter pylori strains in the spectrum of gastroesophageal reflux disease. *Gastroenterology* 1998;115(1):50–57.

14. Tsugane S. Salt, salted food intake, and risk of gastric cancer: epidemiologic evidence. *Cancer Sci* 2005;96(1):1–6.

15. Ji BT, Chow WH, Yang G, et al. The influence of cigarette smoking, alcohol, and green tea consumption on the risk of carcinoma of the cardia and distal stomach in Shanghai, China. *Cancer* 1996;77(12):2449–2457.

16. Nagasaka T, Tanaka N, Cullings HM, et al. Analysis of fecal DNA methylation to detect gastrointestinal neoplasia. *J Natl Cancer Inst* 2009;101(18):1244–1258.

17. McNamara D, El-Omar E. Helicobacter pylori infection and the pathogenesis of gastric cancer: a paradigm for host-bacterial interactions. *Dig Liver Dis* 2008;40(7):504–509.

18. Ng K, Meyerhardt JA, Fuchs CS. Adjuvant and neoadjuvant approaches in gastric cancer. *Cancer J* 2007;13(3):168–174.

19. Hermans J, Bonenkamp JJ, Boon MC, et al. Adjuvant therapy after curative resection for gastric cancer: meta-analysis of randomized trials. *J Clin Oncol* 1993;11(8):1441–1447.

20. Earle CC, Maroun JA. Adjuvant chemotherapy after curative resection for gastric cancer in non-Asian patients: revisiting a meta-analysis of randomised trials. *Eur J Cancer* 1999;35(7):1059–1064.

21. Cunningham D, Allum WH, Stenning SP, et al. Perioperative chemotherapy versus surgery alone for resectable gastroesophageal cancer. *N Engl J Med* 2006;355(1):11–20.

22. MacDonald JS, Smalley SR, Benedetti J, et al. Chemoradiotherapy after surgery compared with surgery alone for adenocarcinoma of the stomach or gastroesophageal junction. *N Engl J Med* 2001;345(10):725–730.

23. Sakuramoto S, Sasako M, Yamaguchi T, et al., ACTS-GC Group. Adjuvant chemotherapy for gastric cancer with S-1, an oral fluoropyrimidine. *N Engl J Med* 2007;357(18):1810–1820.

24. Herskovic A, Al-Sarraf M. Combination of 5-Fluorouracil and Radiation in Esophageal Cancer. *Semin Radiat Oncol* 1997;7(4):283–290.

25. MacDonald JS, Halleck MM. The toxicology of HMG-CoA reductase inhibitors: prediction of human risk. *Toxicol Pathol* 2004;32(Suppl 2):26–41.

26. Chemoradiation of resected gastric cancer: a 10-year follow-up of the phase III trial INT0116 (SWOG 9008). ASCO Annual Meeting; 2009.

27. Fuchs C, Tepper JE et al. Postoperative adjuvant chemoradiation for gastric or gastroesophageal adenocarcinoma using epirubicin, cisplatin, and infusional (CI) 5-FU (ECF) before and after CI 5-FU and radiotherapy (RT): *Interim toxicity results from Intergroup trial CALGB 80101.* Gastrointestinal Cancers Symposium 2006.

28. Swiss Group for Clinical Cancer Research. A phase III trial of preoperative vs. postoperative chemotherapy with taxotere-cisplatin-5FU (TCF) in patients with locally advanced operable gastric carcinoma. http://clinicaltrials.gov/ct2/show/NCT00005060

29. Cunningham D, Starling N, Rao S, et al. Upper Gastrointestinal Clinical Studies Group of the National Cancer Research Institute of the United Kingdom. Capecitabine and oxaliplatin for advanced esophagogastric cancer. *N Engl J Med* 2008;358(1):36–46.

30. Moertel CG, Childs DS, Reitemeier RJ, Colby MY, Holbrook MA. Combined 5-fluorouracil and supervoltage radiation therapy of locally unresectable gastrointestinal cancer. *Lancet* 1969;2(7626):865–867.

31. The Gastrointestinal Study Group: The concept of locally advanced gastric cancer: Effect of treatment on outcome. *Cancer* 1990;66:2324–2330.

32. Ajani JA, Mansfield PF, Crane CH, et al. Paclitaxel-based chemoradiotherapy in localized gastric carcinoma: degree of pathologic response and not clinical parameters dictated patient outcome. *J Clin Oncol* 2005;23(6):1237–1244.

33. Ajani JA, Mansfield PF, Janjan N, et al. Multi-institutional trial of preoperative chemoradiotherapy in patients with potentially resectable gastric carcinoma. *J Clin Oncol* 2004;22(14):2774–2780.

34. Ajani JA, Winter K, Okawara GS, et al. Phase II trial of preoperative chemoradiation in patients with localized gastric adenocarcinoma (RTOG 9904): quality of combined modality therapy and pathologic response. *J Clin Oncol* 2006;24(24):3953–3958.

35. Wagner AD, Grothe W, Haerting J, Kleber G, Grothey A, Fleig WE. Chemotherapy in advanced gastric cancer: a systematic review and meta-analysis based on aggregate data. *J Clin Oncol* 2006;24(18):2903–2909.

36. Findlay M, Cunningham D, Norman A, et al. A phase II study in advanced gastro-esophageal cancer using epirubicin and cisplatin in combination with continuous infusion 5-fluorouracil (ECF). *Ann Oncol* 1994;5(7):609–616.

37. Webb A, Cunningham D, Scarffe JH, et al. Randomized trial comparing epirubicin, cisplatin, and fluorouracil versus fluorouracil, doxorubicin, and methotrexate in advanced esophagogastric cancer. *J Clin Oncol* 1997;15(1):261–267.

38. Kang YK, Kang WK, Shin DB, et al. Capecitabine/cisplatin versus 5-fluorouracil/cisplatin as first-line therapy in patients with advanced gastric cancer: a randomised phase III noninferiority trial. *Ann Oncol* 2009;20(4):666–673.

39. Koizumi W, Narahara H, Hara T, et al. S-1 plus cisplatin versus S-1 alone for first-line treatment of advanced gastric cancer (SPIRITS trial): a phase III trial. *Lancet Oncol* 2008;9(3):215–221.

40. Ajani JA, Lee FC, Singh DA, et al. Multicenter phase II trial of S-1 plus cisplatin in patients with untreated advanced gastric or gastroesophageal junction adenocarcinoma. *J Clin Oncol* 2006;24(4):663–667.

41. Lenz HJ, Lee FC, Haller DG, et al. Extended safety and efficacy data on S-1 plus cisplatin in patients with untreated, advanced gastric carcinoma in a multicenter phase II study. *Cancer* 2007;109(1):33–40.

42. Ajani JA, Baker J, Pisters PW, Ho L, Feig B, Mansfield PF. Irinotecan plus cisplatin in advanced gastric or gastroesophageal junction carcinoma. *Oncology (Williston Park, NY)* 2001;15(3 Suppl 5):52–54.

43. Sharma A, Raina V, Lokeshwar N, Deo SV, Shukla NK, Mohanti BK. Phase II study of cisplatin, etoposide and paclitaxel in locally advanced or metastatic adenocarcinoma of gastric/gastroesophageal junction. *Indian J Cancer* 2006;43(1):16–19.

44. Van Cutsem E, Moiseyenko VM, Tjulandin S, et al., V325 Study Group. Phase III study of docetaxel and cisplatin plus fluorouracil compared with cisplatin and fluorouracil as first-line therapy for advanced gastric cancer: a report of the V325 Study Group. *J Clin Oncol* 2006;24(31):4991–4997.

45. Ajani JA, Moiseyenko VM, Tjulandin S, et al., V-325 Study Group. Clinical benefit with docetaxel plus fluorouracil and cisplatin compared with cisplatin and fluorouracil in a phase III trial of advanced gastric or gastroesophageal cancer adenocarcinoma: the V-325 Study Group. *J Clin Oncol* 2007;25(22):3205–3209.

46. Ajani JA, Moiseyenko VM, Tjulandin S, et al., V-325 Study Group. Quality of life with docetaxel plus cisplatin and fluorouracil compared with cisplatin and fluorouracil from a phase III trial for advanced gastric or gastroesophageal adenocarcinoma: the V-325 Study Group. *J Clin Oncol* 2007;25(22):3210–3216.

47. Thuss-Patience PC, Kretzschmar A, Repp M, et al. Docetaxel and continuous-infusion fluorouracil versus epirubicin, cisplatin, and fluorouracil for advanced gastric adenocarcinoma: a randomized phase II study. *J Clin Oncol* 2005;23(3):494–501.

48. Park YH, Ryoo BY, Choi SJ, Kim HT. A phase II study of capecitabine and docetaxel combination chemotherapy in patients with advanced gastric cancer. *Br J Cancer* 2004;90(7):1329–1333.

49. Ajani JA, Baker J, Pisters PW, et al. CPT-11 plus cisplatin in patients with advanced, untreated gastric or gastroesophageal junction carcinoma: results of a phase II study. *Cancer* 2002;94(3):641–646.

50. Bouché O, Raoul JL, Bonnetain F, et al., Fédération Francophone de Cancérologie Digestive Group. Randomized multicenter phase II trial of a biweekly regimen of fluorouracil and leucovorin (LV5FU2), LV5FU2 plus cisplatin, or LV5FU2 plus irinotecan in patients with previously untreated metastatic gastric cancer: a Federation Francophone de Cancerologie Digestive Group Study—FFCD 9803. *J Clin Oncol* 2004;22(21):4319–4328.

51. Oh SC, Sur HY, Sung HJ, et al. A phase II study of biweekly dose-intensified oral capecitabine plus irinote-can (bXELIRI) for patients with advanced or metastatic gastric cancer. *Br J Cancer* 2007;96(10):1514–1519.

52. Dank M, Zaluski J, Barone C, et al. Randomized phase III study comparing irinotecan combined with 5-fluorouracil and folinic acid to cisplatin combined with 5-fluorouracil in chemotherapy naive patients with advanced adenocarcinoma of the stomach or esophagogastric junction. *Ann Oncol* 2008;19(8):1450–1457.

53. Curran D, Pozzo C, Zaluski J, et al. Quality of life of palliative chemotherapy naive patients with advanced adenocarcinoma of the stomach or esophagogastric junction treated with irinotecan combined with 5-fluorouracil and folinic acid: results of a randomised phase III trial. *Qual Life Res* 2009;18(7):853–861.

54. Di Lauro L, Nunziata C, Arena MG, Foggi P, Sperduti I, Lopez M. Irinotecan, docetaxel and oxaliplatin combination in metastatic gastric or gastroesophageal junction adenocarcinoma. *Br J Cancer* 2007;97(5):593–597.

55. Van Cutsem E, Labianca R, Bodoky G, et al. Randomized phase III trial comparing biweekly infusional fluorouracil/leucovorin alone or with irinotecan in the adjuvant treatment of stage III colon cancer: PETACC-3. *J Clin Oncol* 2009;27(19):3117–3125.

56. Kopp R, Ruge M, Rothbauer E, et al. Impact of epidermal growth factor (EGF) radioreceptor analysis on long-term survival of gastric cancer patients. *Anticancer Res* 2002;22(2B):1161–1167.

57. Pinto C, Di Fabio F, Siena S, et al. Phase II study of cetuximab in combination with FOLFIRI in patients with untreated advanced gastric or gastroesophageal junction adenocarcinoma (FOLCETUX study). *Ann Oncol* 2007;18(3):510–517.

58. Shah MA, Ramanathan RK, Ilson DH, et al. Multicenter phase II study of irinotecan, cisplatin, and bevacizumab in patients with metastatic gastric or gastroesophageal junction adenocarcinoma. *J Clin Oncol* 2006;24(33):5201–5206.

59. Enzinger PC, Fidias P, Meyerhardt J, et al. Phase II study of bevacizumab and docetaxel in metastatic esophageal and gastric cancer (abstract). Data presented at the 2006 ASCO Gastrointestinal Cancers Symposium, San Francisco, CA; January 27, 2006.

60. Tey J, Back MF, Shakespeare TP, et al. The role of palliative radiation therapy in symptomatic locally advanced gastric cancer. *Int J Radiat Oncol Biol Phys* 2007;67(2):385–388.

61. Kil T, Takiuchi H, Gotoh M, et al. Weekly administration of Paclitaxel in patients with inoperable or recurrent gastric cancer, *Gan To Kagaku Ryoho* 2006;33:621.

62. Ajani JA, Fairweather J, Dumas P, et al. Phase II study of Taxol in patients with advanced gastric carcinoma cancer. *J Sci Am* 1998;4:269.

63. Mavroudis D, Kourousis C, Androulakis N, et al: Frontline treatment of advanced gastric cancer with docetaxel and G-CSF: a phase II trial. *Am J Clin Oncol* 2000;23:341.

64. Kohne CH, Catane R, Klein B, et al. Irinotecan is active in chemonaive patients with metastatic gastric cancer: a phase II multicentric trial. *Br J Cancer* 2003;89:997.

65. Earl HM, Coombes RC, Schein PS. Cytotoxic chemotheraphy for cancer of the stomach. *Clinics in Oncology* 1984;3:351.

66. Beer M, Cocconi G, Ceci G, et al. A phase II study of Cisplatin in advanced gastric cancer. *Eur J Cancer Clini Oncol* 1983;19:717.

67. Bruckner HW, Lokich JJ, Stablein DM. Studies of Baker's antifol, methotrexate and razoxane in advanced gastric cancer. A Gastrointestinal Tumor Study Group Report. *Cancer Treat Rep* 1982;66:1713.

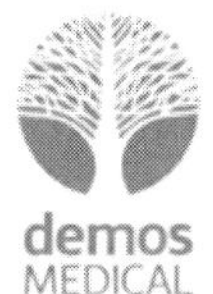

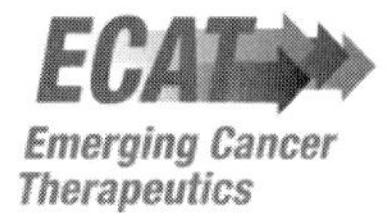

Hepatocellular Cancer

Yun Yen[a]*, Chiun Hsu[b], Ann-Lii Cheng[b], Antonio Arvelakis[c],
M. Wasif Saif[c], and Sukru Emre[d]

[a]*City of Hope Comprehensive Cancer Center, Duarte, CA*

[b]*National Taiwan University Hospital, Taipei, Taiwan*

[c]*Yale Cancer Center, Yale University School of Medicine, New Haven, CT,*

[d]*Yale New Haven Transplantation Center, New Haven, CT*

■ ABSTRACT

Hepatocellular carcinoma (HCC) is one of the major cancer deaths worldwide and is the most rapidly increased type of cancer in the United States and other developed countries. Although the etiologies of liver cancer are relatively well known, the mechanism and pathways leading to hepatocarcinogenesis is still elusive. A typical characteristic of HCC under different etiologies is its strong association with the chronic liver diseases of hepatitis and cirrhosis, in which hepatocyte regenerate continuously with higher proliferating rates. Recently, after SHARP trial data published, the sorafenib becomes the standard therapeutic agent for HCC. However, there are many agents still under investigation. The combination regimen contents sorafenib need to be studied as well. In this chapter, we discuss several targeted therapeutic agents and other modality such as Chinese herb medicine in HCC treatment. We would like to see the more treatment options in inhibiting HCC in the near future.

■ EPIDEMIOLOGY OF HCC AND THE SCOPE OF THE PROBLEM

Hepatocellular carcinoma (HCC) is one of the most common cancers, with increasing incidence. Today it is the fifth most common malignancy worldwide and the third most common cause of cancer-related death (1). It accounts for 84% of primary liver cancer. In the United States 95% of HCC cases develop in cirrhotic patients while this percentage is 80% worldwide. The risk of developing HCC in a cirrhotic patient is 3% a year, and the annual number of deaths in the United States due to this malignancy is over 20,000. The yearly fatality ratio of HCC is 1, which means that most of the new cases of HCC have less than 1-year survival (2).

HCC is the fastest growing cause of cancer-related death in men in the United States. Age-adjusted rates of HCC verified by histology or cytology increased from 1.3 per 100,000 in the period 1978 to 1980 to 3.3 per 100,000 in the period 1999 to 2001. The increase in HCC started in the mid-1980s, with the greatest proportional increases occurring during the 1990s. During recent years, as incidence rates have increased, the age distribution of HCC patients has shifted toward a relatively younger demographic, with the greatest proportional increases occurring between the ages of 45 and 60 (3).

---

*Corresponding author, Associate Cancer Center Director for Translational Research, City of Hope, Duarte, CA
E-mail address: yyen@coh.org

Emerging Cancer Therapeutics 1 (2010) 91–114.

DOI: 10.5003/2151–4194.1.1.93

The increasing number of persons living with cirrhosis is a likely explanation for the increasing incidence of HCC resulting from a combination of factors including: an increasing incidence of cirrhosis caused by hepatitis C virus (HCV), to a lesser extent, hepatitis B virus (HBV) infection, and a general improvement in survival among cirrhotic patients. It has been estimated that HCV began to infect large numbers of young adults in North America and South and Central Europe in the 1960s and the 1970s as a result of intravenous drug use. The virus then moved into national blood supplies and circulated until a screening test was developed in 1990, after which time rates of new infection decreased dramatically. Currently, it is estimated that HCV-related HCC will peak around 2010 (4).

The prevalence of HCV is not predicted to decrease or even plateau after that period though, due to the evolution of nonalcoholic steatohepatitis (NASH); HCC is part of the natural history of NASH. NASH-related cirrhosis carries a substantial risk of early HCC development. Patients who have obesity or diabetes are at risk for NASH and a variety of cancers. Given the epidemic of obesity and diabetes, the incidence of NASH-related HCC is expected to increase (5).

■ HISTORY OF TRANSPLANTATION FOR HCC

Currently, there are three treatment modalities for HCC: surgical resection, ablation, and orthotopic liver transplantation (OLT) (6). From these, it is widely acknowledged that transplantation is the only treatment with curative potential.

Since the underlying cirrhosis is the main predisposing factor for developing HCC, resection and ablation treat the cancer but leave the underlying disease behind.

Liver transplantation (LT) replaces the liver with a new healthy organ and thus it eliminates both the cancer and the predisposing cirrhotic factor.

The historical justifications of transplantation as a treatment for HCC have changed over the years (7). OLT for the definite treatment of HCC started in the late 1980s. Initially the approach mimicked the general surgical oncologic thinking of the time by removing all gross malignant disease for total cure or long-lasting control. Thus, LT was the logical, radical, surgical resection that would obviate

liver failure by removing advanced liver cancers with large vessel infiltration and even extrahepatic spread. During that period, high recurrence rates (32–54%) and poor outcomes (5-year survival rate, 20–40%) afflicted patients with adverse prognostic factors like macroscopic vascular invasion, lymph node involvement, and extrahepatic disease (8). Based on these poor early outcomes, most centers decided that HCC was a contraindication for LT, a perspective supported by the U.S. Department of Health and Human Services. However, in the years that followed several centers reported better results with transplantation for HCC; these centers had selected their transplant candidates more carefully. By the late 1990s, the enthusiasm for LT further increased as centers demonstrated that excellent results were possible through rigorous patient selection criteria. The general consensus gradually evolved and LT was deemed a treatment option only for patients who were not candidates for resection due to advanced liver cirrhosis (above child's A) but with tumors of a certain size and number. In 1996 Mazzaferro et al. showed excellent 5-year survival and low recurrence rates when LT for HCC was used for patients with a single tumor of 5 cm or less, or up to three tumors each no larger than 3 cm and without vascular, nodal or extrahepatic invasion. Their work established the well-known Milan criteria (9).

■ THE MILAN CRITERIA IN THE MELD ERA

In February 2002 a new liver allocation policy was implemented. The Model for End-Stage Liver Disease (MELD) allocation system based on measurable, objective parameters to evaluate the disease severity of the patient on the waiting list (10). The MELD score is calculated based on the patient's creatinine, total bilirubin, and INR and predicts the patient's mortality from liver disease within 3 months without LT.

It is recognized that the previous organ allocation policy in the United States discriminated the HCC patients on the waiting list which resulted in an increased number of dropouts. This problem was solved with the MELD allocation system. Based on this new system, the HCC patients with TNM stage 1 (1 lesion <2 cm) or stage 2 (1 lesion 2–5 cm or 2–3 nodules all <3 cm) were estimated to have respectively a 15% or 30% chance of exceeding the Milan criteria, corresponding to MELD scores of 24 and 29, respectively. Shortly after this policy was applied, it was clear that the HCC patients were favored over the non HCC cirrhotic patients in the waiting list. It took two subsequent adjustments in the attribution of MELD points for HCC patients (in April 2003 and January 2004) to reach the current policy; patients with stage 1 HCC do not receive any extra MELD points and patients with stage 2 HCC receive 22 points of exception and 3 points for every 3 months in the waiting list, provided that the tumor burden does not exceed the Milan criteria (11). It is our opinion that the current system is still not ideal and requires further adjustments. Authors propose that the patients with a single totally ablated tumor accruing MELD exception points and receiving transplant as a result of MELD exception with native MELD score <15 should not need priority. However, successfully downgraded patients above T2 criteria should be given priority if they are still in T2 criteria within 3 to 6 months after ablation therapy.

■ TREATMENT OF HCC PATIENTS WHILE ON THE WAITING LIST

LT is an established treatment for HCC, but the shortage of donors results in a significant dropout rate from the waiting list due to tumor progression beyond the Milan criteria (12). Long waiting times and high dropout rates have led most centers to adopt treatment modalities that delay or halt the progression of the tumor. The locoregional treatment options such as percutaneous ethanol injection (PEI), radiofrequency ablation (RFA), and transarterial chemoembolization (TACE) are the ones mostly used.

PEI was introduced in the late 1980s and has a long record of safety and efficacy in the treatment of small HCCs. RFA is a newer technique, and it uses radiowaves delivered by an electrode inserted directly into a tumor to create a zone of thermal necrosis. Two randomized studies compared RFA with PEI for the treatment of early-stage HCC and showed that the overall survival (OS) rates were superior in the RFA groups (13,14).

TACE is the administration of chemotherapeutic agents into the arterial branches that supply the tumor, followed by injection of occluding particles to induce ischemia. The combination of highly concentrated chemotherapy, including cisplatin or doxorubicin, and some degree of ischemia in the tumor

is synergistic in causing tumor necrosis. There is no standard approach in terms of drugs used, size and type of particles, or degree of selectivity with which the procedure is performed, making comparison of results among centers difficult.

Several studies have tried to evaluate these treatments on the basis of three criteria: (*a*) how much they reduce the number of HCC patients who drop out of the waiting list due to tumor growth beyond the Milan criteria, (*b*) how much they improve the posttransplant survival and tumor recurrence rate, and (*c*) whether they can downstage patients who are beyond Milan criteria, by decreasing the number and size of the tumors (15).

As for the impact of the locoregional treatments on the dropout rate, Lovet et al. were the first who showed that patients with HCC who are treated while on the waiting list have favorable results (16); the group used Marcov modeling to show that there is significant decrease in the dropout rate with the use of ablating techniques when the waiting time in the transplant list is more than 180 days. However, Yao et al. did not find a significant difference in their cohort of 58 patients (17), while Shah et al. from Toronto studied 79 nonrandomized patients and found statistically significant difference for waiting times more than 300 days (18).

The impact of the ablation techniques on the posttransplant survival is questionable. The two largest studies by Schwartz et al. (19) and Mazzaferro et al. (20) showed no increase in the posttransplant survival with the use of locoregional treatment in the waiting list. The use of ablation treatments for downstaging HCC patients who fall beyond the Milan criteria is not common and the reports are scarce. Graziadeli et al. reported 14 patients beyond Milan criteria who were downstaged with TACE and listed for LT; the 4-year survival after transplantation for those patients was 41% (21). Yao et al. reported 21 patients beyond Milan criteria who were downstaged and listed; their results were also poor (22).

Given the inconclusiveness of the aforementioned studies, it is clear that there are no constituent data points that give us level 1 evidence that waiting list HCC treatment is beneficial in all aspects (dropout rate, posttransplant survival, downstaging). More studies should be performed. However, it is well known that the tumor size and number are major risk factors for drop out and that the locoregional treatments have proven response rates on these factors. That makes the conduction of a randomized trial in which the control patients will be deprived of those treatments less acceptable.

■ LIVING DONOR LIVER TRANSPLANT FOR HCC

The severe disparity between the demand for liver transplants and the supply of organs from deceased donors (DDs) means that many HCC patients who would benefit from a transplant will die or drop out of the transplant list due to tumor progression before an organ becomes available (23). The use of Living Donor Liver Transplant (LDLT) significantly reduces the waiting time and thus minimizes the risk of tumor progression in the waiting list (24). Two decision analyses have supported the use of living donor transplants for the treatment of HCC, showing that LDLT is superior to deceased donor liver transplant (DDLT) for HCC patients who are within the Milan criteria and face waiting times of more than 6 months (25,26). However, LDLT has been proposed by many centers as an option for the patients who exceed the Milan criteria and do not have possibilities to receive a cadaveric organ (27,28).

Multiple studies have investigated the results of LDLT versus DDLT for HCC patients in regards to the posttransplant recurrence rate and survival. Interestingly enough the biggest and most reliable of them have shown controversial results. The three largest studies from Asia, where LDLT is much more common than in the United States, have shown that there is no difference in the recurrence rate and posttransplant survival between LDLT and DDLT (27,29,30). The largest U.S. study, conducted by the A2ALL consortium, showed that the LDLT recipients had higher recurrence rate within 3 years than DDLT recipients but there was no difference in mortality or the combined outcome of mortality or recurrence (31) (Table 1). The possible reasons for the differences

between these studies are unclear. The fact that in the United States the DDLT is much more common than in Asia and that the LDLT is usually offered to patients with tumors beyond the Milan criteria and low possibility to receive a cadaveric organ, may be an explanation.

Since the history of LDLT for HCC patients is fairly short, long-term results are still pending but the risk for the donors, although small, is real (32). However, the MELD system has significantly decreased the waiting times for HCC patients in most U.S. centers, making the demand for LDLT less prominent.

■ BEYOND MILAN CRITERIA

The 1996 study by Mazzaferro et al. (9), which established the Milan criteria, showed that LT can achieve excellent outcomes for HCC patients when restrictive criteria, based on preoperative imaging, are applied. These results have been validated by many studies (33). Since then, there has been a significant amount of debate in this area, with many investigators arguing that the Milan criteria are too restrictive. Many centers have suggested that a modest expansion of tumor size beyond the Milan criteria could achieve equally acceptable posttransplant survival rates (Table 2) (34–38). In order to critically analyze such suggestions one must review them with several key issues in mind: are the new criteria based on preoperative imaging/biopsy or postoperative pathology? How many patients are truly beyond the Milan criteria? How will these new criteria effect dropout rates and the intention-to-treat value of LT as a treatment option for HCC (39)?

TABLE 1 Survival of HCC patients after LDLT

Reference	*N*	Survival
Todo et al. (27)	137	80% 3 years
Hwang et al. (29)	151	91% 3 years
Takada et al. (30)	49	68% 3 years
A2ALL (31)	58	62% 4 years

TABLE 2 Beyond the Milan criteria used by different groups

Reference	Tumor Limits
Yao et al. (34) (UCSF criteria)	Solitary tumor ≤6.5 cm or up to 3 tumors with largest ≤4.5 cm and total tumor diameter ≤8 cm
Herrero et al. (35)	Solitary tumor ≤6 cm or up to 3 tumors with largest ≤5 cm
Roayaie et al. (36)	Solitary tumor ≤7 cm
Mazzaferro et al. (37)	Up to 7 rule

The largest study on this field was done by Mazzaferro et al. of the Metroticket study group (37). Unlike the previous studies, the investigators looked at the impact of the microvascular invasion of the tumor in the post-OLT survival, besides the number and size of tumors. They constructed a very interesting model that includes all these three parameters and suggested the up-to-seven rule; an HCC patient is a candidate for OLT if there is no microvascular invasion and the sum of the size of the largest tumor (in cm) and the number of tumors does not exceed seven.

At this time, whether acceptable outcomes using expanded criteria for patient selection can be achieved on a broader scale beyond a single center is quite controversial. The key to this debate may be what the transplant community would consider an acceptable threshold for patient survival using the expanded criteria; and whether a survival higher than the proposed 50% should be set to avoid causing harm to the non HCC transplant candidates (40).

■ NEW APPROACHES TO UNDERSTAND TUMOR BEHAVIOR AND IMPACT ON RECURRENCE AND SURVIVAL AFTER OLT

The evidence supports that vascular invasion is a major determinant of the outcome after LT for HCC (41,42); circulating cancer cells at the time of transplantation are responsible for tumor recurrence. Within the Milan criteria system (and the proposed expanded criteria) the factors that are recognized as the most important predictors of vascular invasion are the number and size of tumors. Novel approaches have emerged that evaluate the potential of vascular invasion using the biological behavior of the tumor rather than its size only (39). Those approaches use genomics and proteomics technologies (43), and tumor histology features (44,45).

Genomic study on HCC focuses on DNA sequence changes, chromosomal aberrations, and epigenetic abnormalities. According to the current understanding, most HCC patients contracted the disease from the accumulation of genetic abnormalities probably induced by exterior etiological factors especially HBV and HCV infections. These risk factors can induce mutations and damages in DNA sequences, such as p53 mutation induced by aflatoxin and DNA damages induced by the intrusion of the HBV genome.

Most proteomics studies on HCC are aimed at the discovery of new biomarkers. Proteomics is the large-scale study of total proteins, particularly their structures and functions at a given time and conditions in biological system. The 2D electrophoresis and mass spectrometry (MS) are the two major methods in proteomics. The use of the above methods as an additional tool to predict which HCC patients have higher potential of recurrence has been proposed by many centers including the well-known Pittsburg study (46).

The histological grade of differentiation in the HCC has also been shown to be an independent predictor of tumor recurrence and patient survival. Zavaglia et al. (44) showed in their study that the 5-year survival of patients with poorly differentiated (G3) HCC was significantly worse than that of patients with moderately (G2) or well-differentiated (G1) tumors. Cillo et al. (45) suggested routine prelisting biopsy, for tumor grading, and exclusion from transplantation of the patients with high grade (G3) tumors (Table 3).

■ SYSTEMIC TREATMENT

Chemotherapy Single and Combination

Introduction

The role of conventional cytotoxic chemotherapy is limited by its myelosuppressive toxicity, which is particularly threatening in patients with cirrhosis, hypersplenism, and cytopenia. Objective tumor response rate to single-agent cytotoxic therapies is usually less than 10%, and no survival benefit has been observed (Table 4) (54–56). Combination regimens can increase the objective response rate to approximately 20%, but at the expense of increased treatment-related toxicities. The most common grade 3–4 toxicity in these studies was myelosuppression. Therefore, cytotoxic chemotherapy can only be used with caution in selected patients with advanced HCC.

TABLE 3 Outcomes of transplantation for HCC

Author	Recurrence (%)	5-Year Survival
Mazzaferro et al. (9)	8	74% (4-year)
Bismuth et al. (8)	11	74%
Llovet et al. (16)	4	75%
Schlitt et al. (47)	16	71%

TABLE 4   Selected clinical trials of cytotoxic therapy for advanced hepatocellular carcinoma

Reference	Treatment	Patient No.	Objective Response	Median Survival (months)	
				OS	**TTP**
Yeo et al. (48)	Doxorubicin 60 mg/m² on day 1, every 3 weeks	94	RR: 10.5% (9 PR) SD: 39.4 %	6.8	NA
	Doxorubicin 40 mg/m² on day 1, every 3 weeks Cisplatin 20 mg/m² Interferon α–2b 5 MU/m² 5-FU 400 mg/m², days 1–4, every 3 weeks	94	RR: 20.9% (19 PR) SD: 37.2%	8.7	NA
Gish et al. (49)	Doxorubicin 60 mg/m² on day 1, every 3 weeks	222	RR: 2.7% (6 PR) SD: NA	7.4	2.3
	Nolatrexed 800 mg/m²/day, days 1–3, every 3 weeks	222	RR: 0.9% (1 PR) SD: NA	5.1	2.8
Patt et al. (50)	Capecitabine 2,000 mg/m²/day, days 1–14, every 3 weeks	37	RR: 11% (1 CR, 3 PR) SD: 11%	10.1	NA
Yen et al. (51)	Oxaliplatin 100 mg/m² every 2 weeks	36	RR: 2.8% (1 PR) SD: 47%	6	2
Yang et al. (52)	Gemcitabine 1,250 mg/m², days 1, 8, 15, every 4 weeks	28	RR: 17.8% (5PR) SD: 25%	4.3	2.8
Guan et al. (53)	Gemcitabine 1,250 mg/m², days 1, 8, every 3 weeks	48	RR: 2.1% (2 PR) SD: 43.9%	3.2	1.5

CR, complete response; NA, not available; OS, overall survival; PR, partial response; RR, response rate; SD, stable disease; TTP, time to tumor progression.

Doxorubicin

An earlier randomized trial comparing doxorubicin, 60 to 75 mg/m² every 3 weeks, with no treatment, indicated a borderline improvement in OS (10.6 vs 7.5 weeks) for patients who received doxorubicin (57). However, 25% of patients died of doxorubicin-related complications, including infection and cardiotoxicity. Doxorubicin was then used as the control treatment in several randomized clinical trials. Yeo et al. compared single-agent doxorubicin with the combination of doxorubicin, cisplatin, 5-fluorouracil (5-FU), and interferon-α-PIAF) (48). The PIAF regimen had higher objective response rate (20.9% vs 10.5%, p = 0.058) and longer OS (8.7 vs 6.8 months, P = 0.83) than single-agent doxorubicin. However, the PIAF regimen produced significantly more neutropenia, thrombocytopenia, and hypokalemia than single-agent doxorubicin. Gish et al. compared

single-agent doxorubicin with nolatrexed (49). Doxorubicin produced higher objective response rate (4.0% vs 1.4%) and longer OS (32.3 vs 22.3 weeks, P = 0.0068) than nolatrexed, and the toxicity, including stomatitis, diarrhea, and thrombocytopenia, was more severe in the nolatrexed group.

Liposomal doxorubicin was demonstrated to have a preferential localization into tumor tissues and decreased toxicity than conventional doxorubicin because of its pharmacokinetic features (58,59). Single-arm trials of liposomal doxorubicin have been reported for patients with advanced or metastatic HCC (60,61). Although the treatment was generally well tolerated, the efficacy of liposomal doxorubicin was not better than conventional doxorubicin.

We have tried to improve the antitumor effects of doxorubicin by adding high-dose tamoxifen as biochemical modulator. High-dose tamoxifen can enhance the cytotoxic effects of doxorubicin on HCC cells through, among other mechanisms, modulation of membrane translocation of protein kinase C and expression of the multidrug resistance (MDR) protein (62). Phase II trials for patients with advanced HCC indicated that the addition of tamoxifen, 160 mg/m^2/day for 7 days, can increase the objective response rate of doxorubicin to about 30% without significantly increasing the toxicity of doxorubicin (63,64).

Fluoropyrimidines

Oral and parenteral 5-FU has been tested extensively both as single-agent therapy and in various combinations. As single-agent therapy, 5-FU was well tolerated but no significant antitumor activity was found (65). Several approaches of biochemical modulation have been used to increase the antitumor efficacy of 5-FU. For example, leucovorin can enhance the binding of 5-FU to thymidylate synthase, and interferons and eniluracil can modulate 5-FU metabolism by inhibiting thymidylate phosphorylase and dihydropyrimidine dehydrogenase, respectively (66–70). Results from phase II trials indicated that addition of these biochemical modulators did not increase the treatment-related toxicity. Objective response rate of more than 20% was reported with the addition of leucovorin or interferon.

Several prodrugs of 5-FU are available. UFT is a combination of tegafur, a prodrug of 5-FU that is metabolized by liver microsonal enzymes to the active drug, and uracil, a competitive inhibitor of dihydropyrimidine dehydrogenase (DPD) (71). A small-scale randomized trial indicated that enteric-coated tegafur/uracil can prolong the survival time in patients with advanced HCC, although no objective responses were reported (72,73). Capecitabine is another 5-FU prodrug that is metabolized to the active drug by thymidylate phosphorylase. Thymidylate phosphorylase was found to be more abundant in tumor tissue and thus may preferentially activate capcitabine in the tumors than in surrounding normal tissue (74). A response rate of 11% was reported from a retrospective analysis of advanced HCC patients who were treated by single-agent capecitabine (50).

Platinum

Single-agent cisplatin produced an objective response rate of about 10% in selected patients with advanced HCC (75,76). Several cisplatin-containing combination regimens have been tested. The response rate improved to about 20% but was accompanied with increased incidence of myelosuppression, renal toxicity, and gastrointestinal toxicity (48,77). Oxaliplatin has a more favorable toxicity profile than cisplatin and is widely used for the treatment of gastrointestinal and pancreatic cancers. A phase II trial of single-agent oxaliplatin, 100 mg/m^2 every 2 weeks, reported a response rate of 2.8% and stable disease of 44.4% in 36 evaluable patients (51). The major adverse events included liver function abnormalities and fatigue. Myelosuppression was mild.

Gemcitabine

Gemcitabine is a nucleotide analogue of cytarabine that is phosphorylated in cells by deoxycytidine kinase to gemcitabine triphosphate, the active metabolite. Prolonged infusion of gemcitabine at a fixed dose rate of 10 mg/m^2/min was associated with a higher intracellular accumulation of gemcitabine triphosphate (78). Gemcitabine metabolites can inhibit ribonucleotide reductase and increase the cellular ratio of gemcitabine/deoxycytidine triphosphate, which favors incorporation of the former into DNA and further enhances its antitumor activity (79).

Yang et al. reported a single-arm study of gemcitabine, 1,250 mg/m^2/week for 3 weeks followed by 1-week rest, in patients with advanced HCC. The response rate was 17.8% (5 partial responses [PRs] in 28 patients) (52). Guan et al. compared the conventional 30-minute infusion with fixed dose-rate (10 mg/m^2/min) infusion of gemcitabine, 1,250 mg/m^2/week for 2 weeks followed by 1-week rest, in patients with unresectable HCC. The response rate was only 2.1% (1 PR in the conventional infusion group) (53).

Biological Agent Focus on Sorafenib and Other Tyrosine Kinase Studies

Recent advances in elucidating the molecular mechanisms of hepatocarcinogenesis have provided opportunities to develop molecular targeted therapy (MTT) for advanced HCC (80). Sorafenib, an oral multikinase inhibitor, has shown survival benefit in two randomized, placebo-controlled trials (81,82). Other MTT agents targeting different signaling pathways have also shown antitumor activity in patients with advanced HCC.

Sorafenib

Sorafenib inhibits the kinase activity of both wild-type B-raf (IC50 6 nM) and mutant Raf/v600E (IC50 38 nM). In addition, sorafenib inhibits vascular endothelial growth factor receptors (VEGFR), platelet-derived growth factor receptors (PDGFR), c-kit, Flt-3, and RET (IC50 <100 nM) (83). Therefore, both antiproliferative and antiangiogenic mechanisms may account for the antitumor effects of sorafenib.

The first randomized, placebo-controlled trial of sorafenib for the treatment of advanced HCC (the SHARP trial) was done primarily in Europe and the United States with the primary endpoint of OS (81). The second trial was designed originally as a bridging study to evaluate the overall efficacy and safety of sorafenib in the Asia-Pacific population (82). Patient eligibility of these two trials was almost identical (HCC patients whose tumors were not eligible for or had progressed after surgery or locoregional therapy, Child-Pugh liver function class A, and Eastern Cooperative Oncology Group [ECOG] performance score 2 or less). However, patients in the Asia-Pacific trial were younger and had more symptomatic disease (ECOG score 1 or 2) and extrahepatic metastases.

The treatment regimen was the same in the two trials (sorafenib 400 mg twice daily). Both trials were stopped early because per-protocol interim analysis indicated significant survival benefit of sorafenib over placebo. The hazard ratios of OS and time to progression were 0.69 and 0.58 in the SHARP trial and 0.68 and 0.57 in the Asia-Pacific trial. Exploratory subgroup analyses of the two trials indicated that sorafenib treatment prolonged survival regardless of patients' age, performance status, and tumor burden (vascular invasion or extrahepatic spread). Time to symptomatic progression was not significantly different between patients who received sorafenib and who received placebo in either trial. Sorafenib is generally well tolerated. The most common drug-related adverse events included diarrhea, fatigue, hand-foot skin reaction, and rash/desquamation. These events occurred in 20% to 40% of patients, most of which were grade 1 or 2. The most common causes of treatment interruption or dose reduction were hand-foot skin reaction, rash, and diarrhea.

Sorafenib has been approved for the treatment of advanced HCC by the European Medicines Agency and by the U.S. Food and Drug Administration (FDA). In the most recent practice guidelines recommended by the U.S. National Comprehensive Cancer Network, sorafenib is listed as a treatment option for HCC patients who are inoperable by performance status or comorbidity (local disease only) and who do not present with cancer-related symptoms (84). However, the efficacy and safety issues in patients with liver dysfunction need further clarification. A pharmacokinetic study suggested that patients with elevated bilirubin levels had lower tolerance to sorafenib treatment (85). In the phase II trial of sorafenib for HCC, stable disease for ≥4 months was noted in 49% of patients with Child-Pugh class A (n = 98) and 26% of patients with Child-Pugh class B (n = 38). Patients with Child-Pugh class B had higher rate of elevated bilirubin (18% vs 40%), encephalopathy (2% vs 11%), and worsening ascites (11% vs 18%) than patients with Child-Pugh class A, despite a similar incidence of all other adverse events and serious adverse events between these two groups of patients (86). There is no clinical data for patients with Child-Pugh class C.

Other Kinase Inhibitors

The results of early-phase clinical trials of selected MTT agents are summarized in Table 5.5. HCC is typically a hypervascular tumor, and the major mechanism of most of the MTT that have been tested is angiogenesis inhibition. The efficacy of these antiangiogenic MTT (bevacizumab (87), sunitinib (88,89), NGR-hTNF (90), pazopanib (91), brivanib (92), and ABT-869 (93)) appeared similar: an objective response rate of 5% to 10%, and the disease stabilization rate of 40% to 65%. In some trials, a decreased tumor perfusion after treatment was demonstrated by dynamic computed tomography or magnetic resonance imaging, suggesting that the angiogenesis inhibition is an important mechanism of antitumor activity. The most common toxicities included diarrhea, hypertension, skin rashes, and fatigue. An uncommon but potentially life-threatening toxicity is gastrointestinal bleeding. A careful evaluation of bleeding risks such as esophageal and gastric varices is recommended before the use of antiangiogenic MTT for HCC.

EGFR Inhibitors

Several data indicate the potential involvement of epidermal growth factor receptor (EGFR) signaling pathway in hepatocarcinogenesis (102). Hepatitis viral proteins can induce the expression of transforming growth factor-α, an EGFR ligand, and may

TABLE 5 Early-phase clinical trials of molecular targeted therapy for advanced hepatocellular carcinoma

Reference	Treatment	Major Targets	Phase	Patient No.	Objective Response	Overall Survival (months)	TTP (months)
Siegel et al. (87)	Bevacizumab 5–10 mg/kg every 2 weeks	Anti-VEGF antibody	II	46	RR : 13% (1 CR and 5 PR) SD : 65% (progression-free at 6 months)	12.4	6.9 (PFS)
Zhu et al. (88)	Sunitinib 37.5 mg qd for 4 weeks, followed by 2-week rest	VEGFR, PDGFR, stem-cell factor receptor, CSF-1, RET, Flt-3	II	34	RR : 2.9% (1 PR) SD : 47%	9.9	4.0
Faivre et al. (89)	Sunitinib 50 mg qd for 4 weeks, followed by 2-week rest		II	37	RR : 2.7% (1 PR) SD : 35.1%	10.3	4.8
Santoro et al. (90)	NGR-hTNF 0.8 µg/m^2 1-hour infusion every 3 weeks	Vascular disrupting agent	II	27	RR : 7.4 % (1 CR, 1 PR)	NA	2.39 (PFS)
Yau et al. (91)	Pazopanib 200–800 mg daily p.o.	VEGFR	I	28	RR : 7.1% (1 PR at 800 mg, 1 PR at 600 mg) MTD: 600 mg/day	NA	4.2 (PFS)
Raoul et al. (92)	Brivanib 800 mg daily p.o.	VEGFR, FGFR	II	101	First-line: RR: 6 (4 PR, 2 unconfirmed PR) SD: 47.2% Second-line: RR: 2.7% (1PR) SD: 43.2%	10 (first line) 9.8 (second line)	2.8 (first line) 1.4 (second line)
Toh et al. (93)	ABT-869 0.25 mg/kg daily (for Child A) or every 2 days (for Child B)	VEGFR, PDGFR	II	44	RR: 6.8% (3 PR)	9.3	5.4
Philip et al. (94)	Erlotinib 150 mg qd	EGFR	II	38	RR : 9% (3 PR in 34 evaluable patients) SD : 50%	13	3.2
Thomas et al. (95)	Erlotinib 150 mg qd	EGFR	II	40	RR : 0 SD : 42.5%	10.8	6.5
O'Dwyer et al. (96)	Gefitinib 250 mg qd	EGFR	II	31	RR: 3.2% (1 PR) SD: 22.6%	6.5	2.8 (PFS)
Zhu et al. (97)	Cetuximab 400 mg/m^2 loading, then 250 mg/m^2/week.	EGFR	II	30	RR: 0 SD: 16.7%	9.6	1.4 (PFS)

continued

TABLE 5   Early-phase clinical trials of molecular targeted therapy for advanced hepatocellular carcinoma (continued)

Treatment		Major Targets	Phase	Patient No.	Objective Response	Overall Survival (months)	TTP (months)
Decaens et al. (98)	Sirolimus 30 mg weekly	mTOR	II	14	RR: 40% (1 CR and 5 PR)	NA	NA
Chen et al. (99)	Everolimus Daily dosing: 2.5, 5.0, 7.5, 10 mg/kg p.o Weekly dosing: 20, 30, 50, 70 mg/kg p.o.	mTOR	I	39 (21, daily; 18, weekly)	RR: 2.6% (1 PR, at 50 mg/week) MTD: 7.5 mg/day 70 mg/week	NA	NA
Hsu et al. (100)	Thalidomide 100 mg bid	Antiangiogenesis	II	63	RR : 6.3 % (1 CR, 3 PR in 63 evaluable patients)	4.3	NA
Patt et al. (101)	Thalidomide 400 mg qd	Antiangiogenesis	II	32	RR 3.2 % (1 PR in 32 evaluable patients) SD : 31%	6.8	NA

CR, complete response; EGFR, epidermal growth factor receptor; FGFR, fibroblast growth factor receptor; MTD, maximum tolerated dose; mTOR, mammalian target of rapamycin; NA, not available; OS, overall survival; PDGFR, platelet-derived growth factor receptor; PFS, progression-free survival; PR, partial response; RR, response rate; SD, stable disease; TTP, time to tumor progression; VEGF, vascular endothelial growth factor; VEGFR, vascular endothelial growth factor receptor.

act synergistically with viral infection in hepatocarcinogenesis (103–105). The EGFR expression pattern amongst HCC tumor tissues studied mainly via immunohistochemistry (IHC) gave varying results (106), and the activating mutation of EGFR, that is, the major determinant of efficacy of EGFR inhibitors in lung cancer (107), was rarely observed in HCC tumor tissue (108). Nevertheless, as the hepatocarcinogenesis is a multistep process involving multiple molecular pathways, the growth factor receptor activation and angiogenesis may play a significant role (109). The overexpression of EGFR2 (Her2/neu) is rarely observed in HCC (110), but it may play an important role in predicting the response to EGFR targeting agents (111).

Two phase II studies were conducted to test the efficacy of the oral EGFR inhibitor erlotinib in patients with advanced HCC. Philip et al. evaluated erlotinib in 38 patients. Through IHC, the overexpression of EGFR was detected in 88% of specimens (94). Erlotinib was well tolerated and a radiological PR was seen in three patients (8%) with the median OS of 13 months. Thomas et al. evaluated it in 40 patients with HCC; no objective responses were

reported and the median survival of patients was 10.8 months (95). Gefitinib and cetuximab did not show significant antitumor efficacy in HCC (96,97).

Lapatinib, an oral dual kinase inhibitor of EGFR and Her-2/neu, was tested in patients with biliary tree and HCC. This was based on the hints of activity from the erlotinib clinical trials and the preclinical observation that inhibiting the dual EGF family members has a greater inhibitory effect on downstream signaling pathways than inhibiting either receptor alone as reported by Ramanathan et al. through California Cancer Consortium (112). In this study, 17 patients with biliary tract cancer (BTC) and 40 with HCC were evaluated. In both BTC and HCC subjects, the treatment was well tolerated. Hematological toxicities were uncommon though grade 3/4 anemia and thrombocytopenia were observed in 4% and 2% of patients, respectively. Elevated liver function tests were seen though mostly of grade 1 or 2. A grade 1/2 skin rash was observed in 19 patients (35%), one patient developed a grade 3 rash, and no changes in LVEF occurred following the treatment. The most common grade 3/4 toxicities were diarrhea (7%), fatigue (6%), and elevations of liver transaminases (9%), while common grade 1–2 toxicities were diarrhea (46%), nausea (32%), and fatigue (46%).

In patients with HCC, 13 stable diseases (35%) and 2 objective responses (5%) were reported. PRs were observed in a patient with no prior therapy and in another following TACE. The median OS for BTC and HCC patients were 5.2 months (95% CI 3.3–∞) and 6.2 months (95% CI 5.1–∞), respectively. The median PFS for patients with BTC and HCC were 1.8 months (95 % CI 1.7–5.2) and 2.3 months (95% CI 1.7–5.6), respectively. The onset of rash tightly correlates with prolonged PFS (increased from 2.0 to 5.0 months, $P = 0.03$) and OS (increased from 5.0 to 10.0 months, $P = 0.004$).

Of interests to this chapter is the overexpression of EGFR observed in 7 of 12 (58%) of specimens that had sufficient archival tumor material for analysis. A total of 5 out of 10 HCC patient samples showed staining for EGFR in 30% to 100% of tumor cells analyzed. The wild-type KRAS was detected and mutations were absent in all these samples. Out of 40 (70%) HCC patients 28 were genotyped. To assess the relevance of the number of (CA)n repeats on the clinical outcome, patients were segregated into two subgroups: 8 patients (29%) had (CA)n repeats <20 and 20 patients (71%) had any (CA)n repeats ≥ 20. Patients with (CA)n repeats < 20 showed lower PFS compared to those with (CA)n repeats < 20 ($P = 0.016$, log-rank test). No statistically significant association was observed between the EGFR (CA) n repeats and the clinical response or OS. No significant associations occurred between other tested genes from the EGFR pathway ($n = 8$) and response, PFS, or OS.

Skin rash was observed in approximately one-third of the patients associated with improved PFS and survival, suggesting an effect on the ERB1 pathway. The correlation of skin rash to the clinical outcome previously observed for colon and pancreatic cancer patients who were treated with cetuximab and erlotinib (113) was not previously reported for HCC (94). In a randomized study of breast cancer patients treated with capecitabine or the combination of capecitabine and lapatinib, skin rash was infrequent and its onset did not correlate with the outcome (114). Lapatinib has shown dual inhibitory activity on ERB1 and ERB2 in preclinical models, but its predominant inhibitory action may be on the ERB2 pathway. In HCC, the frequency of ERB2 overexpression and activating mutations are low, which may

account for the disappointing outcome for our study. Resistance to EGFR therapy may be dependent on the KRAS status as resistance occurred in KRAS-mutant tumors (115). In HCC, KRAS appears mutated in approximately 30% of the tumors, which may associate with the exposure to vinyl chloride (116). In our study, KRAS mutations were absent in all 12 samples examined.

As the collection of tumor and genomic biomarker was optional, its assessment and correlation to efficacy was limited by the number of samples and the limited scrutiny. We focused on EGFR genotyping based on the following: the overexpression of EGFR mRNA and protein was associated with the aggressiveness of tumor and the poor clinical outcome in a variety of epithelial malignancies including HCC (117,118). A highly polymorphic region within the intron 1 of the EGFR gene shows association with the transcription level of EGFR in vitro and in vivo (119,120). The length of this (CA) n dinucleotide polymorphism shows an inverse correlation with its transcriptional activity. In vitro, the EGFR transcription in cells containing a prolonged polymorphic region (>20 CA repeats) was markedly attenuated when compared to cells with a shorter allele (121). These findings were recaptured in human breast cancer samples. A constant decline in the intratumoral EGFR protein expression associated with an increase in the allele length. Furthermore, hemizygous tumors showed a higher EGFR expression if the longer allele was lacking when compared to tumors that retained the longer allele (117). To date, EGFR polymorphisms have not been causatively linked to the clinical outcome in HCC patients. In our study, short repeat alleles of EGFR (CA)n, which code for an increased EGFR gene expression, showed a significant association with PFS ($P = 0.016$, log-rank test).

The response rate of 5% observed for HCC patients in our study is similar to the published studies employing single-agent therapy with erlotinib and cetuximab (94,95,97). Baseline characteristics of the etiology or viral titers in HCC patients were not collected, but our patient population can be expected to be similar to other studies. However, the median survival of 6.2 months (95% CI 5.1–∞) is lower than other studies, whereas the OS of 8 to 13 months was reported. The low median survival in our study may be due to the smaller sample size, but it appears also likely that lapatinib may not register a significant activity in HCC.

mTOR Inhibitors

The mammalian target of rapamycin (mTOR) signaling pathway plays a pivotal role in the control of protein synthesis, cell growth, and survival (122). An increased mTOR signaling activity has been demonstrated in human HCC (123,124). In xenograft models of HCC, the mTOR inhibitor everolimus demonstrated promising growth-inhibitory effects (125). Early-phase clinical trials of sirolimus and everolimus have also shown disease-stabilizing effects (98,126). The most common drug-related toxicities included mucositis, diarrhea, and elevation of liver transaminases.

Thalidomide

Thalidomide was found to have antiangiogenic properties in the early 1990s and has been tested for the treatment of various cancers (99,127). Several phase II studies have explored the efficacy of thalidomide as a treatment for advanced HCC (100,101,128,129). Objective response, defined as complete response (CR) and PR, occurred in approximately 5% of the patients. In addition, about 10% to 30% of patients had disease stabilization for more than 2 to 4 months after thalidomide treatment. Disease stabilization after thalidomide treatment was associated with decreased tumor vascularity (130) and blood perfusion (131), suggesting that the antitumor effect of thalidomide is in part due to antiangiogenesis. The most common drug-related toxicities in all the series were somnolence, constipation, dizziness, and skin rash albeit generally manageable.

■ COMBINATION OF CHEMOTHERAPEUTIC AGENTS AND TYROSINE KINASE INHIBITORS

A combination therapy with MTT has been investigated. A randomized phase II trial of sorafenib plus doxorubicin versus doxorubicin alone reported a superior median OS (13.7 vs 6.5 months) and time to progression (8.6 vs 4.8 months) for patients receiving the former (132). These results should be interpreted with caution because a sorafenib-alone arm was not included and high incidence of adverse events related to doxorubicin was noted. Many small-scale trials of combining MTT with cytotoxic chemotherapy have been reported (133–136). However, the efficacy in terms of tumor response and patient survivability were similar to those reported for the cytotoxic regimens alone (Table 6) (48,137,138).

A second approach is to combine antiangiogenic MTT with chemotherapy given in small doses on a frequent (daily, several times a week, or weekly) and uninterrupted basis for prolonged periods. The latter is usually referred to as "metronomic chemotherapy" (139). The cumulative doses of metronomic chemotherapy are generally lower than when the same agents are given in the maximum-tolerated-dose approach and the treatment-related toxicity is significantly lower (140). Preclinical studies suggested that metronomic chemotherapy can even be effective in cancers that have developed resistance to the same chemotherapeutic agents administered in the conventional way, suggesting distinct mechanisms of antitumor action (141). Antiangiogenesis has been the most frequently cited mechanism of metronomic chemotherapy (142), and synergistic antitumor effects may exist between metronomic chemotherapy and antiangiogenic therapy (143,144). We have tested several combination regimens, including bevacizumab/capecitabine (145), sorafenib/tegafur-uracil (146), and thalidomide/tegafur-uracil (147). These regimens are generally safe and can be easily administered on an outpatient basis. Disease stabilization was achieved in about 40% of patients with advanced HCC.

A third approach is to combine MTT targeting different molecular pathways. A phase II trial done in the United States combining bevacizumab (10 mg/kg every 2 weeks) with erlotinib (150 mg daily) for advanced HCC patients showed a response rate of 28% (14 PR in 57 patients) and a median time to tumor progression of 7.9 months (148). However, a second trial in Asia combining a lower dose of bevacizumab (5 mg/kg every 2 weeks) with erlotinib reported a much lower response rate (5.9%, 3 PR in 51 patients) (149). It is not known whether the difference resulted from the difference in bevacizumab dosage or from the difference in the baseline characteristics of HCC patients from different geographic areas. Larger studies are needed to clarify the clinical potential of this combination regimen.

Chinese Herbal Medicine

The use of traditional Chinese medicine (TCM) is based on the interaction of multiple components acting synergistically and multifactorially on the body.

TABLE 6 Selected clinical trials of cytotoxic therapy or cytotoxic therapy plus MTT for advanced hepatocellular carcinoma

Cytotoxic Therapy				Cytotoxic Therapy Plus MTT			
Author	Regimen	Objective Response	Overall Survival (months)	Author	Regimen	Objective Response	Overall Survival (months)
Yeo et al. (48)	Doxorubicin	RR: 10.5% (9 PR) SD: 39.4 %	6.8	Abou-Alfa et al. (132)	Sorafenib + Doxorubicin	RR: 2% (4 PR) SD: 77%	13.7
					Doxorubicin	RR: 1% (2 PR) SD: 55%	6.5
Louafi et al. (137)	GEMOX (gemcitabine + oxaliplatin)	RR: 18% (6 PR) SD: 58%	11.5	Zhu et al. (133)	Bevacizumab + GEMOX	RR : 20% (6 PR in 30 evaluable patients) SD : 27%	9.6
				Asnacios et al. (134)	Cetuximab + GEMOX	RR: 20% (9 PR) SD: 40%	9.5
Boige et al. (138)	XELOX (capecitabine + oxaliplatin)	RR: 6% (3 PR) SD: 58%	9.3	Sun et al. (135)	Bevacizumab + XELOX	RR: 13.3% (4 PR in 30 evaluable patients) SD: 76.6%	10.3
				O'Neil et al. (136)	Cetuximab + XELOX	RR: 10% (2 PR in 23 evaluable patients) SD: 65%	4.5

CR, complete response; GEMOX, gemcitabine/oxaliplatin; MTT, molecular targeted therapy; NA, not available; OS, overall survival; PR, partial response; RR, response rate; SD, stable disease; TTP, time to tumor progression; XELOX, capecitabine/oxaliplatin.

The multiple components in a Chinese herbal formulation serve various functions; some provide efficacy while others decrease toxicity or increase absorption (150). Using a mixture of plant extracts, instead of an isolated compound, for the management of diseases is gaining greater acceptance in Western countries and is at the core of Chinese herbal medicine (151,152). Chinese herbal formulas are derived from empirical observations, complex TCM theory, and over 2,000 years of human use (153,154). Often, multiple therapeutic claims are made for Chinese herbal medicine. It is common that one Chinese medicine formula, perhaps consisting of multiple herbs and certainly multiple compounds, may relieve more than one side effect associated with the use of cancer chemotherapeutic agents. We have performed a literature search of Chinese medicine formulae that have been used for the treatment of gastrointestinal symptoms similar to those observed in the use of chemotherapeutic agents. Among the many formulae examined, we focused on those that (*a*) were well established, used for hundreds of years to successfully treat a variety of ailments including diarrhea, abdominal spasms, fever, headache, vomiting, nausea, and loss of appetite (152–154), (*b*) had documented prior human use which would permit, under recently FDA-established guidelines for botanical drugs, fast-tracking during clinical trials (154), and (*c*) had a well-defined botanical composition of individual herbs that have been well documented and can be manufactured under Good Manufacturing Practice (GMP) conditions. Of the several candidates selected and studied, PHY906 was found to be the most superior in preliminary animal studies, both in protecting against toxicity-induced weight loss, mortality, and in slowing tumor growth.

PHY906

PHY906 has been described in the Chinese Pharmacopeia for over 1,800 years (154). The four individual herbs of PHY906 (*Scutellaria baicalensis* Georgi, *Glycyrrhiza uralensis* Fisch, *Paeonia lactiflora* Pall., and the fruit of *Ziziphus jujuba* Mill.) reportedly have a variety of pharmacological activities including antiviral activity, immunological stimulation, analgesic activity, vasodilatation, liver protection, nausea reduction, diarrhea treatment, antioxidation, and appetite improvement (154). Many of these are similar to the gastrointestinal side effect profile associated with many cancer chemotoxic agents, and our preliminary studies of PHY906 indicated a reduction in GI-induced toxicity, and surprisingly, a therapeutic synergism with Western chemotherapeutics. PHY906 has been evaluated in two clinical trials. In the first study entitled "A Phase I, Multicenter, Double-Blind, Randomized, Placebo-Controlled, Crossover, Dose Escalation, Safety and Phase II Open-Label Efficacy Study of PHY906 + CPT-11 in Advanced Colorectal Cancer Patients Refractory to First-line Chemotherapeutics," PHY906 at the dose of 800 mg, TID (i.e., 2,400 mg/day) was determined to be safe in patients with colorectal cancer. The second, currently ongoing PHY906 HCC study, entitled "A Phase I/II, Multicenter, Open-Label, Dose-Escalation, Safety, and Efficacy Study of PHY906 plus Capecitabine in Patients with Unresectable Hepatocellular Carcinoma," has also demonstrated that PHY906 at dose level of 800 mg, BID (i.e.1,600 mg/day) in combination with capecitabine at dose level 750 mg/m^2, BID, is safe. PHY 906 has been shown to have a synergistic effect on a broad spectrum of chemotherapeutic agents in vitro and in animal models. Previous human liver cancer and colon cancer trials reported its safety and tolerability. Thus, by utilizing PHY 906 + gemcitabine combination chemotherapy for advanced pancreatic cancer, we hope to improve quality of life and survival.

PHY906 Drug Substance and Drug Product

The production of PHY906 involves the extraction of a mixture of the root of *Scutellaria baicalensis* Georgi (33.3%), *Glycyrrhiza uralensis* Fisch (22.2%), *Paeonia lactiflora* Pall. (22.2%), and the fruit of *Ziziphus jujuba* Mill. (22.2%) with water at elevated temperature followed by filtration. The decoctions are concentrated by evaporation under reduced pressure to yield concentrated extract. After an appropriate amount of corn starch is added into the concentrated extract, the resulting mixture is then spray-dried to yield a powdered extract that can be formulated into the desired dosage form.

PHY906 powdered extract is formulated as a capsule by Sage Pharmaceuticals, Inc., of Shreveport, LA, a company that has formulated prior batches of PHY906 powdered extract into capsules for previous PHY906 U.S. clinical trials. This formulation is done under FDA current Good Manufacturing Practice (cGMP) regulations and the facility has passed FDA inspection. Dark green #0 gelatin capsules are used to contain the PHY906. The following color agents are used in the manufacture of these capsules: Glob. Yellow iron oxide (FD/E172), sicomet-85 black iron oxide (FDA/E172) and titanium dioxide (E171). Each PHY906 capsule will contain 200 mg of PHY906 powdered extract and excipients of starch, sodium starch glycolate, and magnesium stearate.

PHY906 in HCC Clinical Phase I/II Trial

This study was a multicenter, open-label, dose escalation phase I/II safety and efficacy trial.

From preclinical studies, PHY906 combined with capecitabine (Xeloda™) in HepG2 xenografted NCr athymic nude mice was found to enhance the antitumor activity of capecitabine. Capecitabine had been used off-label for the treatment of patients with HCC prior to the FDA approval of the first drug, sorafenib (Nexavar®), for the treatment of HCC in November 2007. The first clinical study conducted with PHY906/capecitabine combination by Yen et al. was a multicenter, open-label, dose escalation phase I/II safety and efficacy clinical trial of PHY906 given concomitantly with capecitabine to patients with advanced HCC (155). Phase I was designed to determine a safe and tolerable dosing regimen of PHY906 plus capecitabine, and phase II was designed to determine whether PHY906 enhanced the response rate of capecitabine, time to tumor progression (TTP), and OS time. The QoL of patients undergoing treatment was monitored. The study was conducted at the City of Hope National Medical Center (Duarte, CA), Stanford University School of Medicine (Stanford, CA), Yale Cancer Center (New Haven, CT), and the VA Healthcare System (West Haven, CT).

Forty-two patients with HCC were enrolled: 18 patients in phase I and 24 patients in phase II (155). Twenty-five patients (59.5%) were classified Child-Pugh class A and 17 (40.5%) Child-Pugh class B. All patients were eligible for safety evaluation; 2 who received the cohort 1 treatment regimen and 27 who received the cohort 2 or cohort 3 regimen were evaluable for efficacy. Of the 42 patients, 7 (16.7%) had received no prior treatment, 18 (43%) received prior chemoembolization, 9 (21.4%) received other pretreatment, and the pretreatment statuses of 8 patients were unavailable. Among 27 efficacy-evaluable patients, 13 (48%) received prior chemoembolization, 4 (15%) other prior treatments, and previous treatment information was unavailable for 4 (15%). Three cohorts were involved in this study: (a) capecitabine 1,000 mg/m^2 BID and PHY906 1,000 mg BID; (b) capecitabine 750 mg/m^2 BID and PHY906 600 mg BID; and (c) capecitabine 750 mg/m^2 BID and PHY906 800 mg BID.

Of the first three patients recruited into cohort 1, two developed drug-related grade 3 dose-limiting toxicity: one with colitis, hyperbilirubinemia, and stomatitis, and one with hand-foot skin reaction. Enrollment of further patients into this cohort was therefore terminated and both capecitabine and PHY906 doses were adjusted downward. The combination of PHY906 (600 or 800 mg BID) and capecitabine (750 mg/m^2 BID) was well tolerated (N = 39). Of 39 patients, 28 (71.8%) reported adverse events (AEs). The most common grade 1 drug-related AEs were diarrhea (28.2%), fatigue (23.0%), abdominal pain (10.3%), pruritus (10.3%), and nausea (10.3%). The most frequently experienced grade 2 drug-related AEs were leukopenia (7.7%), fatigue (7.7%), and hyperbilirubinemia (7.7%). The most frequently experienced grade 3 drug-related AEs were mucositis/stomatis (7.7%), dehydration (5.1%), neutropenia (2.6%), hyperbilirubinemia (2.6%), and hand-foot skin reaction (2.6%). No patient experienced drug-related grade 4 or 5 toxicities. Among 27 efficacy-evaluable patients, 5 patients each had one drug-related grade 3 toxicity: neutropenia, dehydration, ALP elevation, hyperglycemia, or hand-foot skin reaction. One patient experienced two drug-related grade 3 toxicities (poor appetite and AST elevation). Among 20 efficacy-evaluable Child-Pugh class A patients, 4

patients each experienced one drug-related grade 3 toxicity: neutropenia, dehydration, ALP elevation, or hyperglycemia. No correlation was observed between grade-3 drug-related toxicity and ethnicity, Child-Pugh status, hepatitis, or previous treatment.

Among four patients treated with capecitabine 750 mg/m^2/PHY906 600 mg, two patients had minor response (MR, tumor reduced 33.5% and 34%, respectively), one had SD, and one had PD after two cycles of treatment. At the capecitabine 750 mg/m^2/PHY906 800 mg dose level (N = 23), no CR or PR were seen; 8.7% (N = 2) had an MR (39.7% and 44% tumor reduction, respectively), 56.5% (N = 13) exhibited SD, and 34.8% (N = 8) had PD. Median time to progression was 3.4 months and median OS was 9.2 months. The 12-month survival rate was 44.5%. Seventy-four percent (N = 20) of the 27 efficacy-evaluable patients were classified as Child-Pugh class A. Median OS values for Child-Pugh class A and Child-Pugh class B patients were 10.9 and 6.5 months, respectively. No difference in the 6-month survival rate was observed between Child-Pugh class A and Child-Pugh class B patients. However, the 12-month survival rate for was 51% for Child-Pugh class A patients and 29% for Child-Pugh class B patients.

Median OS values for Asian and non-Asian subgroups were 16.5 and 6.2 months, respectively (P = 0.03, Fig. 5.1). Median OS values for Asian and non-Asian Child-Pugh class A patients were 16.5 and 6.7 months, respectively (P = 0.05, Fig. 5.2). No significant correlation was observed for either nuclear grade or degree of differentiation of tumor. The results suggest that the PHY906/capecitabine combination provides a survival benefit and a tolerable safety profile in advanced HCC patients and that the combination has promise as a treatment for this disease. Use of the PHY906/capecitabine combination may prove to be particularly efficacious for Asian Child-Pugh class A HCC patients. In light of the very poor prognosis of HCC patients and the 100% tumor progression rate seen with sorafenib therapy, the PHY906/capecitabine combination provides an additional opportunity to stabilize the disease for relatively longer periods of time.

The data illustrate that a widely used TCM formulation, PHY906, can be used in combination with a widely used Western cancer chemotherapeutic agent, capecitabine, to successfully treat patients with advanced HCC (155). The results with Asian patients are particularly noteworthy. A follow-up

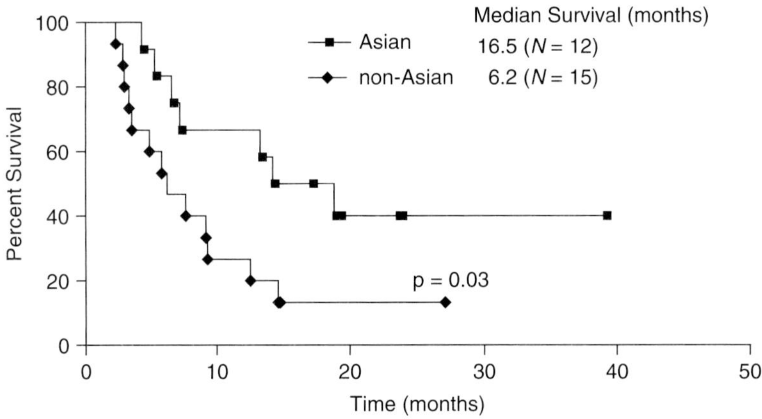

FIGURE 1 Survival curve of Asian versus non-Asian patients treated with PHY906 (600 or 800 mg) + capecitabine (750 mg/m²).

phase II study is currently conducted in Taiwan. An additional large size, randomized, double-blind, controlled study of capecitabine/PHY906 in HCC patients is required to validate these findings.

The mechanisms of PHY906 drug action are multifactorial. In preclinical studies, PHY906 has been shown to have inhibitory activity on MDR protein and CYP450; the presence of these inhibitions can facilitate the oral uptake of chemotherapeutic agents (156). Examination of the tumor tissues and compounds involved suggest that the integrity of blood vessels and the pathways of HIF-∝ and Fos/Juk transcription are affected by PHY906. In vitro studies also reveal that PHY906 has inhibitory

activities against NF-κB and matrix metalloproteases (MMPs), which are possible contributors to the enhancement of the antitumor action of chemotherapeutic agents. Possible mechanisms of action for the reduction of gastrointestinal toxicity by PHY906 are the inhibition of Tachykinin NK-1, and/or opiate δ receptors, and may be acetylcholinesterase-based. The structures for 64 bioactive compounds, including flavonoids, triterpene saponins, and monoterpene glycosides, were proposed based on the LC/MS analysis (155).

Summary of PHY906 in HCC Clinical Trial

From many previous trials, including those with capecitabine, it is evident that HCC is resistant to chemotherapy (156,157). Capecitabine, as a monotherapy, has been used off-label in HCC, yielding response rates of up to 15% (155,156). Myelosuppression and skin toxicity are the most common side effects seen with capecitabine-containing combinations, with severe GI toxicity being the most limiting side effect. Sorafenib in HCC patients also exhibits drug toxicities; these include fatigue, weight loss, rash or superficial skin shedding, hand or foot skin reaction, hair loss, diarrhea, anorexia, nausea, and abdominal pain (138,142,152,157–159). Diarrhea was reported in 55% of patients who received sorafenib (160,161). Agents that reduce the toxicities of these chemotherapeutics without compromising their antitumor activities would provide an added benefit to the patients.

PHY906, a TCM formulation, has been in continuous use for a variety of gastrointestinal ailments since AD 300. In preclinical studies, PHY906

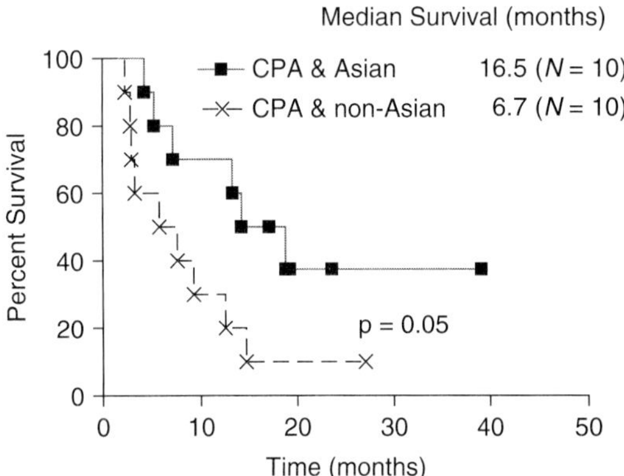

FIGURE 2 Kaplan-Meier survival curve of Asian versus non-Asian patients (both Child-Pugh class A) treated with PHY906 (600 or 800 mg) plus capecitabine (750 mg/m²).

did not appear to have toxicities that overlap with those of other agents used for HCC chemotherapy (155,156,162). More significantly, in a double-blind, randomized, placebo-controlled, cross-over phase I/II clinical trial with a two-step dose escalation of PHY906 in colon carcinoma patients treated concomitantly with irinotecan/5-FU/leucovorin, PHY906 decreased the incidence of vomiting, nausea, and grade 3/4 diarrhea (163). The mechanisms of PHY906 drug action are multifactorial. PHY906 has inhibitory activity on MDR protein and CYP450. The presence of these inhibitions facilitated the oral uptake of chemotherapeutic agents. Examination of the tumor tissues and compounds involved suggest that the integrity of the blood vessel and the pathways of HIF-α and Fos/Juk transcription were affected.

In vitro studies also reveal that PHY906 has inhibitory activities against NF-κB and MMPs, which are possible contributors to the enhancement of the antitumor action of chemotherapeutic agents (164).

For the current phase I/II study, the PHY906/capecitabine combination resulted in only a few grade 3 drug-related toxicities and no grade 4 or 5 drug-related toxicities; the combination was generally well tolerated. The nausea and emesis rates seen with PHY906/capecitabine are lower than would be expected using capecitabine alone. Moreover, fewer patients discontinued treatment in the current combination trial as a consequence of adverse effects (9.5%) than were reported in trials using capecitabine or sorafenib monotherapy (29%) (155,156,165,166).

Based on the results of SHARP and Asian phase III studies, sorafenib has been approved for HCC treatment. Ninety-five percent of patients enrolled in these studies were classified Child-Pugh class A and had no prior treatment. The median OS of patients enrolled in the SHARP and Asian studies were 10.7 and 6.5 months, respectively, while that of placebo was 7.9 and 4.2 months, respectively (81,82). The patients enrolled in the current study would generally be expected to have a poorer prognosis, as 26% of the patients were classified Child-Pugh class B and >64% had previous treatments. However, the median OS in our study was 9.2 months with fewer grade 3 or 4 drug-related toxicities than seen with sorafenib (81). Moreover, the median OS among Child-Pugh class A (n = 20) patients was 10.9 months with no grade 3 or 4 sorafenib-type toxicities. In our study, Asian Child-Pugh class A patients had a median OS of 16.5 months—a marked increase over that seen with sorafenib in the same cadre of patients.

Our results suggest that the PHY906/capecitabine combination provides a survival benefit and a tolerable safety profile in advanced HCC patients and that the combination has promise as a treatment for this disease. Use of the PHY906/capecitabine combination may prove to be particularly efficacious for Asian Child-Pugh class A HCC patients. In light of the very poor prognosis of HCC patients and the 100% tumor progression rate seen with sorafenib therapy, the PHY906/capecitabine combination provides an additional opportunity to stabilize the disease for relatively longer periods of time.

Use of the PHY906/capecitabine combination may not be limited to HCC. A phase II clinical trial in patients with advanced and recurrent pancreatic cancer refractory to gemcitabine is currently ongoing, and preliminary reports indicate that the combination is safe and well tolerated (124). The data provided in this report illustrate that a widely used TCM formulation, PHY906, can be used in combination with a widely used Western cancer chemotherapeutic agent, capecitabine, to successfully treat patients with advanced HCC. The results with Asian patients are particularly noteworthy.

■ REFERENCES

1. Bosch F, Ribes J, Díaz M, Cléries R. Primary liver cancer: worldwide incidence and trends. *Gastroenterology* 2004;127(5 Suppl 1):S5–S16.
2. Barbara L, Benzi G, Gaiani S, et al. Natural history of small untreated hepatocellular carcinoma in cirrhosis: a multivariate analysis of prognostic factors of tumor growth rate and patient survival. *Hepatology* 1992;16(1):132–137.
3. El-Serag H, Davila J, Petersen N, McGlynn K. The continuing increase in the incidence of hepatocellular carcinoma in the United States: an update. *Ann Intern Med* 2003;139(10):817–823.
4. Wong J, McQuillan G, McHutchison J, Poynard T. Estimating future hepatitis C morbidity, mortality, and costs in the United States. *Am J Public Health* 2000;90(10):1562–1569.
5. Bugianesi E. Non-alcoholic steatohepatitis and cancer. *Clin Liver Dis* 2007;11(1):191–207, x–xi.
6. Roayaie K, Feng S. Allocation policy for hepatocellular carcinoma in the MELD era: room for improvement? *Liver Transpl* 2007;13(11 Suppl 2):S36–S43.
7. Yoo H, Patt C, Geschwind JF, Thuluvath P. The outcome of liver transplantation in patients with hepatocellular carcinoma in the United States between 1988 and 2001: 5-year survival has improved significantly with time. *J Clin Oncol* 2003;21(23):4329–4335.
8. Bismuth H, Chiche L, Adam R, Castaing D, Diamond T, Dennison A. Liver resection versus transplantation for

hepatocellular carcinoma in cirrhotic patients. *Ann Surg* 1993;218(2):145–151.

9. Mazzaferro V, Regalia E, Doci R, et al. Liver transplantation for the treatment of small hepatocellular carcinomas in patients with cirrhosis. *N Engl J Med* 1996;334(11):693–699.

10. Kamath P, Wiesner R, Malinchoc M, et al. A model to predict survival in patients with end-stage liver disease. *Hepatology* 2001;33(2):464–470.

11. UNOS. United Network for Organ Sharing. Policy 3.6 Organ Distribution: Allocation of Livers. Revised December 14, 2006. http://www.unos.org/policiesandb-ylaws/policies.asp?resources=true. Accessed: 19 October, 2007.

12. Ishizaki Y, Kawasaki S. The evolution of liver transplantation for hepatocellular carcinoma (past, present, and future). *J Gastroenterol* 2008;43(1):18–26.

13. Lin S, Lin C, Lin C, Hsu C, Chen Y. Randomised controlled trial comparing percutaneous radiofrequency thermal ablation, percutaneous ethanol injection, and percutaneous acetic acid injection to treat hepatocellular carcinoma of 3 cm or less. *Gut* 2005;54(8):1151–1156.

14. Lencioni R, Allgaier H, Cioni D, et al. Small hepatocellular carcinoma in cirrhosis: randomized comparison of radio-frequency thermal ablation versus percutaneous ethanol injection. *Radiology* 2003;228(1):235–240.

15. Belghiti J, Carr B, Greig P, Lencioni R, Poon R. Treatment before liver transplantation for HCC. *Ann Surg Oncol* 2008;15(4):993–1000.

16. Llovet J, Mas X, Aponte J, et al. Cost effectiveness of adjuvant therapy for hepatocellular carcinoma during the waiting list for liver transplantation. *Gut* 2002;50(1):123–128.

17. Yao F, Bass N, Nikolai B, et al. A follow-up analysis of the pattern and predictors of dropout from the waiting list for liver transplantation in patients with hepatocellular carcinoma: implications for the current organ allocation policy. *Liver Transpl* 2003;9(7):684–692.

18. Shah S, Cleary S, Tan J, et al. An analysis of resection vs transplantation for early hepatocellular carcinoma: defining the optimal therapy at a single institution. *Ann Surg Oncol* 2007;14(9):2608–2614.

19. Schwartz J, Schwartz M, Mandeli J, Sung M. Neoadjuvant and adjuvant therapy for resectable hepatocellular carcinoma: review of the randomised clinical trials. *Lancet Oncol* 2002;3(10):593–603.

20. Mazzaferro V, Battiston C, Perrone S, et al. Radiofrequency ablation of small hepatocellular carcinoma in cirrhotic patients awaiting liver transplantation: a prospective study. *Ann Surg* 2004;240(5):900–909.

21. Graziadei I, Sandmueller H, Waldenberger P, et al. Chemoembolization followed by liver transplantation for hepatocellular carcinoma impedes tumor progression while on the waiting list and leads to excellent outcome. *Liver Transpl* 2003;9(6):557–563.

22. Yao F, Roberts J. Applying expanded criteria to liver transplantation for hepatocellular carcinoma: too much too soon, or is now the time? *Liver Transpl* 2004;10(7):919–921.

23. Yao F, Bass N, Nikolai B, et al. Liver transplantation for hepatocellular carcinoma: analysis of survival according to the intention-to-treat principle and dropout from the waiting list. *Liver Transpl* Oct 2002;8(10):873–883.

24. Brown RJ, Russo M, Lai M, et al. A survey of liver transplantation from living adult donors in the United States. *Engl J Med*. Feb 2003;348(9):818–825.

25. Cheng S, Pratt D, Freeman RJ, Kaplan M, Wong J. Living-donor versus cadaveric liver transplantation for non-resectable small hepatocellular carcinoma and compensated cirrhosis: a decision analysis. *Transplantation* Sep 2001;72(5):861–868.

26. Sarasin F, Majno P, Llovet J, Bruix J, Mentha G, Hadengue A. Living donor liver transplantation for early hepatocellular carcinoma: A life-expectancy and cost-effectiveness perspective. *Hepatology* May 2001;33(5):1073–1079.

27. Todo S, Furukawa H; Japanese Study Group on Organ Transplantation. Living donor liver transplantation for adult patients with hepatocellular carcinoma: experience in Japan. *Ann Surg* 2004;240(3):451–459; discussion 459–461.

28. Volk M, Marrero J, Lok A, Ubel P. Who decides? Living donor liver transplantation for advanced hepatocellular carcinoma. *Transplantation* 2006;82(9):1136–1139.

29. Hwang S, Lee S, Lee Y, et al. Donor selection for procurement of right posterior segment graft in living donor liver transplantation. *Liver Transpl* 2004;10(9):1150–1155.

30. Takada Y, Tanaka K. Living related liver transplantation. *Transplant Proc* 2004;36(2Suppl):271S–273S.

31. Fisher R, Kulik L, Freise C, et al. A2ALL Study Group. Hepatocellular carcinoma recurrence and death following living and deceased donor liver transplantation. *Am J Transplant* 2007;7(6):1601–1608.

32. Trotter J, Adam R, Lo C, Kenison J. Documented deaths of hepatic lobe donors for living donor liver transplantation. *Liver Transpl* 2006;12(10):1485–1488.

33. Befeler A, Hayashi P, Di Bisceglie A. Liver transplantation for hepatocellular carcinoma. *Gastroenterology* 2005;128(6):1752–1764.

34. Yao F, Ferrell L, Bass N, et al. Liver transplantation for hepatocellular carcinoma: expansion of the tumor size limits does not adversely impact survival. *Hepatology* 2001;33(6):1394–1403.

35. Herrero J, Sangro B, Quiroga J, et al. Influence of tumor characteristics on the outcome of liver transplantation among patients with liver cirrhosis and hepatocellular carcinoma. *Liver Transpl* 2001;7(7):631–636.

36. Roayaie S, Frischer J, Emre S, et al. Long-term results with multimodal adjuvant therapy and liver transplantation for the treatment of hepatocellular carcinomas larger than 5 centimeters. *Ann Surg* 2002;235(4):533–539.

37. Mazzaferro V, Llovet J, Miceli R, et al. Metroticket Investigator Study Group. Predicting survival after liver transplantation in patients with hepatocellular carcinoma beyond the Milan criteria: a retrospective, exploratory analysis. *Lancet Oncol* 2009;10(1):35–43.

38. Duffy J, Vardanian A, Benjamin E, et al. Liver transplantation criteria for hepatocellular carcinoma should be expanded: a 22-year experience with 467 patients

at UCLA. *Ann Surg* 2007;246(3):502–509; discussion 509–511.

39. Roayaie S, Schwartz M. Expansion of criteria for transplanting patients with hepatocellular carcinoma. *Liver Transpl* 2008;14(8):1071–1072.

40. Volk M, Vijan S, Marrero J. A novel model measuring the harm of transplanting hepatocellular carcinoma exceeding Milan criteria. *Am J Transplant* 2008;8(4):839–846.

41. Iwatsuki S, Dvorchik I, Marsh J, et al. Liver transplantation for hepatocellular carcinoma: a proposal of a prognostic scoring system. *J Am Coll Surg* 2000;191(4):389–394.

42. Hemming A, Cattral M, Reed A, Van Der Werf W, Greig P, Howard R. Liver transplantation for hepatocellular carcinoma. *Ann Surg* 2001;233(5):652–659.

43. Pei Y, Zhang T, Renault V, Zhang X. An overview of hepatocellular carcinoma study by omics-based methods. *Acta Biochim Biophys Sin (Shanghai)* 2009;41(1):1–15.

44. Zavaglia C, De Carlis L, Alberti A, et al. Predictors of long-term survival after liver transplantation for hepatocellular carcinoma. *Am J Gastroenterol* 2005;100(12):2708–2716.

45. Cillo U, Vitale A, Bassanello M, et al. Liver transplantation for the treatment of moderately or well-differentiated hepatocellular carcinoma. *Ann Surg* 2004;239(2):150–159.

46. Marsh J, Dvorchik I. Should we biopsy each liver mass suspicious for hepatocellular carcinoma before liver transplantation?—yes. *J Hepatol* 2005;43(4):558–562.

47. Schlitt HJ, Neipp M, Neimann A, et al. Recurrence patterns of hepatocellular and fibrolamellar carcinoma after liver transplantation. *J Clin Oncol* 1999;17(1):326–331.

48. Yeo W, Mok TS, Zee B, et al. A randomized phase III study of doxorubicin versus cisplatin/interferon alpha-2b/doxorubicin/fluorouracil (PIAF) combination chemotherapy for unresectable hepatocellular carcinoma. *J Natl Cancer Inst* 2005;97(20):1532–1538.

49. Gish RG, Porta C, Lazar L, et al. Phase III randomized controlled trial comparing the survival of patients with unresectable hepatocellular carcinoma treated with nolatrexed or doxorubicin. *J Clin Oncol* 2007;25(21):3069–3075.

50. Patt YZ, Hassan MM, Aguayo A, et al. Oral capecitabine for the treatment of hepatocellular carcinoma, cholangiocarcinoma, and gallbladder carcinoma. *Cancer* 2004;104:578–586.

51. Yen Y, Lim DW, Chung V, et al. Phase II study of oxaliplatin in patients with unresectable, metastatic, or recurrent hepatocellular cancer: a California Cancer Consortium Trial. *Am J Clin Oncol* 2008;31(4):317–322.

52. Yang TS, Lin YC, Chen JS, Wang HM, Wang CH. Phase II study of gemcitabine in patients with advanced hepatocellular carcinoma. *Cancer* 2000;89(4):750–756.

53. Guan Z, Wang Y, Maoleekoonpairoj S, et al. Prospective randomised phase II study of gemcitabine at standard or fixed dose rate schedule in unresectable hepatocellular carcinoma. *Br J Cancer* 2003;89(10):1865–1869.

54. Hsu C, Cheng JC, Cheng AL. Recent advances in non-surgical treatment for advanced hepatocellular carcinoma. *J Formos Med Assoc* 2004;103(7):483–495.

55. Zhu AX. Systemic therapy of advanced hepatocellular carcinoma: how hopeful should we be? *Oncologist* 2006;11(7):790–800.

56. Lopez PM, Villanueva A, Llovet JM. Systematic review: evidence-based management of hepatocellular carcinoma—an updated analysis of randomized controlled trials. *Aliment Pharmacol Ther* 2006;23(11):1535–1547.

57. Lai CL, Wu PC, Chan GC, Lok AS, Lin HJ. Doxorubicin versus no antitumor therapy in inoperable hepatocellular carcinoma. A prospective randomized trial. *Cancer* 1988;62(3):479–483.

58. Gabizon A, Martin F. Polyethylene glycol-coated (pegylated) liposomal doxorubicin. Rationale for use in solid tumours. *Drugs* 1997;(54 Suppl 4):15–21.

59. Hong RL, Tseng YL. Phase I and pharmacokinetic study of a stable, polyethylene-glycolated liposomal doxorubicin in patients with solid tumors: the relation between pharmacokinetic property and toxicity. *Cancer* 2001;91(9):1826–1833.

60. Halm U, Etzrodt G, Schiefke I, et al. A phase II study of pegylated liposomal doxorubicin for treatment of advanced hepatocellular carcinoma. *Ann Oncol* 2000;11(1):113–114.

61. Hong RL, Tseng YL. A phase II and pharmacokinetic study of pegylated liposomal doxorubicin in patients with advanced hepatocellular carcinoma. *Cancer Chemother Pharmacol* 2003;51(5):433–438.

62. Cheng AL, Chuang SE, Fine RL, et al. Inhibition of the membrane translocation and activation of protein kinase C, and potentiation of doxorubicin-induced apoptosis of hepatocellular carcinoma cells by tamoxifen. *Biochem Pharmacol* 1998;55(4):523–531.

63. Cheng AL, Yeh KH, Fine RL, et al. Biochemical modulation of doxorubicin by high-dose tamoxifen in the treatment of advanced hepatocellular carcinoma. *Hepatogastroenterology* 1998;45(24):1955–1960.

64. Lu YS, Hsu C, Li CC, et al. Phase II study of combination doxorubicin, interferon-alpha, and high-dose tamoxifen treatment for advanced hepatocellular carcinoma. *Hepatogastroenterology* 2004;51(57):815–819.

65. Falkson G, Moertel CG, Lavin P, Pretorius FJ, Carbone PP. Chemotherapy studies in primary liver cancer: a prospective randomized clinical trial. *Cancer* 1978;42(5):2149–2156.

66. Tetef M, Doroshow J, Akman S, et al. 5-Fluorouracil and high-dose calcium leucovorin for hepatocellular carcinoma: a phase II trial. *Cancer Invest* 1995;13(5):460–463.

67. Porta C, Moroni M, Nastasi G, Arcangeli G. 5-Fluorouracil and d,l-leucovorin calcium are active to treat unresectable hepatocellular carcinoma patients: preliminary results of a phase II study. *Oncology* 1995;52(6):487–491.

68. Patt YZ, Hassan MM, Lozano RD, et al. Phase II trial of systemic continuous fluorouracil and subcutaneous

recombinant interferon Alfa-2b for treatment of hepatocellular carcinoma. *J Clin Oncol* 2003;21(3):421–427.

69. Benson AB, Mitchell E, Abramson N, et al. Oral eniluracil/5-fluorouracil in patients with inoperable hepatocellular carcinoma. *Ann Oncol* 2002;13(4):576–581.

70. Llovet JM, Ruff P, Tassopoulos N, et al. A phase II trial of oral eniluracil/5-fluorouracil in patients with inoperable hepatocellular carcinoma. *Eur J Cancer* 2001;37(11):1352–1358.

71. Hoff PM, Pazdur R, Benner SE, et al. UFT and leucovorin: a review of its clinical development and therapeutic potential in the oral treatment of cancer. *Anticancer Drugs* 1998;9(6):479–490.

72. Ishikawa T, Ichida T, Sugitani S, et al. Improved survival with oral administration of enteric-coated tegafur/uracil for advanced stage IV-A hepatocellular carcinoma. *J Gastroenterol Hepatol* 2001;16(4):452–459.

73. Mani S, Schiano T, Garcia JC, et al. Phase II trial of uracil/tegafur (UFT) plus leucovorin in patients with advanced hepatocellular carcinoma. *Invest New Drug* 1998–1999;16:279–283.

74. Schüller J, Cassidy J, Dumont E, et al. Preferential activation of capecitabine in tumor following oral administration to colorectal cancer patients. *Cancer Chemother Pharmacol* 2000;45(4):291–297.

75. Falkson G, Ryan LM, Johnson LA, et al. A random phase II study of mitoxantrone and cisplatin in patients with hepatocellular carcinoma. An ECOG study. *Cancer* 1987;60(9):2141–2145.

76. Okada S, Okazaki N, Nose H, Shimada Y, Yoshimori M, Aoki K. A phase 2 study of cisplatin in patients with hepatocellular carcinoma. *Oncology* 1993;50(1):22–26.

77. Boucher E, Corbinais S, Brissot P, Boudjema K, Raoul JL. Treatment of hepatocellular carcinoma (HCC) with systemic chemotherapy combining epirubicin, cisplatinum and infusional 5-fluorouracil (ECF regimen). *Cancer Chemother Pharmacol* 2002;50(4):305–308.

78. Tempero M, Plunkett W, Ruiz Van Haperen V, et al. Randomized phase II comparison of dose-intense gemcitabine: thirty-minute infusion and fixed dose rate infusion in patients with pancreatic adenocarcinoma. *J Clin Oncol* 2003;21(18):3402–3408.

79. Plunkett W, Huang P, Searcy CE, Gandhi V. Gemcitabine: preclinical pharmacology and mechanisms of action. *Semin Oncol* 1996;23(5 Suppl 10):3–15.

80. Llovet JM, Bruix J. Molecular targeted therapies in hepatocellular carcinoma. *Hepatology* 2008;48(4):1312–1327.

81. Llovet J, Ricci S, Mazzaferro V, et al. SHARP Investigators Study Group. Sorafenib in advanced hepatocellular carcinoma. *N Engl J Med* 2008;359(4):378–390.

82. Cheng AL, Kang YK, Chen Z, et al. Efficacy and safety of sorafenib in patients in the Asia-Pacific region with advanced hepatocellular carcinoma: a phase III randomised, double-blind, placebo-controlled trial. *Lancet Oncol* 2009;10(1):25–34.

83. Wilhelm S, Carter C, Lynch M, et al. Discovery and development of sorafenib: a multikinase inhibitor for treating cancer. *Nat Rev Drug Discov* 2006;5(10):835–844.

84. National Comprehensive Cancer Network: Practice guidelines in oncology, v.2.2008—hepatobiliary cancers. Available at URL: http://www.nccn.org; Accessed Nov 6, 2008.

85. Miller AA, Murry DJ, Owzar K, et al. Phase I and pharmacokinetic study of sorafenib in patients with hepatic or renal dysfunction: CALGB 60301. *J Clin Oncol* 2009;27(11):1800–1805.

86. Abou-Alfa GK, Amadori D, Santoro A, et al. Is sorafenib (S) safe and effective in patients (pts) with hepatocellular carcinoma (HCC) and Child-Pugh B (CPB) cirrhosis? [Abstract 4518]. *J Clin Oncol* 26:2008 (May 20 Suppl).

87. Siegel AB, Cohen EI, Ocean A, et al. Phase II trial evaluating the clinical and biologic effects of bevacizumab in unresectable hepatocellular carcinoma. *J Clin Oncol* 2008;26(18):2992–2998.

88. Zhu AX, Sahani DV, Duda DG, et al. Efficacy, safety, and potential biomarkers of sunitinib monotherapy in advanced hepatocellular carcinoma: a phase II study. *J Clin Oncol* 2009;27(18):3027–3035.

89. Faivre S, Raymond E, Boucher E, et al. Safety and efficacy of sunitinib in patients with advanced hepatocellular carcinoma: an open-label, multicentre, phase II study. *Lancet Oncol* 2009;10(8):794–800.

90. Santoro A, Citterio G, Pressiani T, et al. Phase II study of NGR-hTNF, a selective vascular targeting agent (VTA), in previously treated patients with hepatocellular carcinoma (HCC) [Abstract e15500]. *J Clin Oncol* 2009:27.

91. Yau CC, Chen PJ, Curtis CM, et al. A phase I study of pazopanib in patients with advanced hepatocellular carcinoma [Abstract 3561]. *J Clin Oncol* 2009;27:15s.

92. Raoul JL, Finn RS, Kang YK, et al. An open-label phase II study of first- and second-line treatment with brivanib in patients with hepatocellular carcinoma (HCC) [Abstract 4577]. *J Clin Oncol* 2009;27:15s.

93 Toh H, Chen PJ, Carr BI, et al. A phase II study of ABT-869 in hepatocellular carcinoma (HCC): Interim analysis [Abstract 4581]. *J Clin Oncol* 2009;27:15s.

94. Philip PA, Mahoney MR, Allmer C, et al. Phase II study of Erlotinib (OSI-774) in patients with advanced hepatocellular cancer. *J Clin Oncol* 2005;23(27):6657–6663.

95. Thomas MB, Chadha R, Glover K, et al. Phase 2 study of erlotinib in patients with unresectable hepatocellular carcinoma. *Cancer* 2007;110(5):1059–1067.

96. O'Dwyer PJ, Giantonio BJ, Levy DE, Kauh JS, Fitzgerald DB, Benson AB. Gefitinib in advanced unresectable hepatocellular carcinoma: Results from the Eastern Cooperative Oncology Group's Study E1203. *J Clin Oncol* 2006 ASCO Annual Meeting Proceedings Part I. Vol 24, No. 18S (June 20 Suppl), 2006; 4143.

97. Zhu AX, Stuart K, Blaszkowsky LS, et al. Phase 2 study of cetuximab in patients with advanced hepatocellular carcinoma. *Cancer* 2007;110(3):581–589.

98. Chen LT, Shiah HS, Chen CY, et al. Randomized, phase I, and pharmacokinetic (PK) study of RAD001, an mTOR inhibitor, in patients (pts) with advanced hepatocellular carcinoma (HCC) [Abstract 4587]. *J Clin Oncol* 2009;27:15s.

99. D'Amato RJ, Loughnan MS, Flynn E, et al. Thalidomide is an inhibitor of angiogenesis. *Proc Natl Acad Sci USA* 1994;91(9):4082–4085.

100. Hsu C, Chen CN, Chen LT, et al. Low-dose thalidomide treatment for advanced hepatocellular carcinoma. *Oncology* 2003;65(3):242–249.

101. Patt YZ, Hassan MM, Lozano RD, et al. Thalidomide in the treatment of patients with hepatocellular carcinoma: a phase II trial. *Cancer* 2005;103(4):749–755.

102. Breuhahn K, Longerich T, Schirmacher P. Dysregulation of growth factor signaling in human hepatocellular carcinoma. *Oncogene* 2006;25(27):3787–3800.

103. Ono M, Morisawa K, Nie J, et al. Transactivation of transforming growth factor alpha gene by hepatitis B virus preS1. *Cancer Res* 1998;58(9):1813–1816.

104. Sato Y, Kato J, Takimoto R, et al. Hepatitis C virus core protein promotes proliferation of human hepatoma cells through enhancement of transforming growth factor alpha expression via activation of nuclear factor-kappaB. *Gut* 2006;55(12):1801–1808.

105. Jakubczak JL, Chisari FV, Merlino G. Synergy between transforming growth factor alpha and hepatitis B virus surface antigen in hepatocellular proliferation and carcinogenesis. *Cancer Res* 1997;57(16):3606–3611.

106. Kiss A, Wang NJ, Xie JP, Thorgeirsson SS. Analysis of transforming growth factor (TGF)-alpha/epidermal growth factor receptor, hepatocyte growth Factor/c-met,TGF-beta receptor type II, and p53 expression in human hepatocellular carcinomas. *Clin Cancer Res* 1997;3(7):1059–1066.

107. Yang CH. EGFR tyrosine kinase inhibitors for the treatment of NSCLC in East Asia: present and future. *Lung Cancer* 2008;(60Suppl 2):S23–S30.

108. Su MC, Lien HC, Jeng YM. Absence of epidermal growth factor receptor exon 18–21 mutation in hepatocellular carcinoma. *Cancer Lett* 2005;224(1):117–121.

109. Berasain C, Castillo J, Prieto J, et al. New molecular targets for hepatocellular carcinoma: the ErbB1 signaling system. *Liver Int* 2007;27(2):174–185.

110. Hsu C, Huang CL, Hsu HC, Lee PH, Wang SJ, Cheng AL. HER-2/neu overexpression is rare in hepatocellular carcinoma and not predictive of anti-HER-2/neu regulation of cell growth and chemosensitivity. *Cancer* 2002;94(2):415–420.

111. Bekaii-Saab T, Williams N, Plass C, et al. A novel mutation in the tyrosine kinase domain of ERBB2 in hepatocellular carcinoma. *BMC Cancer* 2006;6:278.

112. Ramanathan RK, Belani CP, Singh D, et al. Phase II Study of Lapatinib in patients with Advanced Biliary tree and hepatocellular cancer. *Cancer Chemo Phar.* 2009. In press.

113. Peréz-Soler R, Saltz L. Cutaneous adverse effects with HER1/EGFR-targeted agents: is there a silver lining? *J Clin Oncol* 2005;23(22):5235–5246.

114. Geyer CE, Forster J, Lindquist D, et al. Lapatinib plus capecitabine for HER2-positive advanced breast cancer. *N Engl J Med* 2006;355(26):2733–2743.

115. Van Cutsem E, Lang I, D'haens G, et al. KRAS status and efficacy in the first-line treatment of patients with metastatic colorectal cancer (mCRC) treated with FOLFIRI with or without cetuximab: the CRYSTAL experience [Abstract 2]. *J Clin Oncol* 2008; 26: (May 20 Suppl).

116. Weihrauch M, Benicke M, Lehnert G, Wittekind C, Wrbitzky R, Tannapfel A. Frequent k-ras -2 mutations and p16(INK4A)methylation in hepatocellular carcinomas in workers exposed to vinyl chloride. *Br J Cancer* 2001;84(7):982–989.

117. Mayoral R, Fernández-Martínez A, Boscá L, Martín-Sanz P. Prostaglandin E2 promotes migration and adhesion in hepatocellular carcinoma cells. *Carcinogenesis* 2005;26(4):753–761.

118. Mitchell C, Nivison M, Jackson LF, et al. Heparin-binding epidermal growth factor-like growth factor links hepatocyte priming with cell cycle progression during liver regeneration. *J Biol Chem* 2005;280(4):2562–2568.

119. Buerger H, Gebhardt F, Schmidt H, et al. Length and loss of heterozygosity of an intron 1 polymorphic sequence of egfr is related to cytogenetic alterations and epithelial growth factor receptor expression. *Cancer Res* 2000;60(4):854–857.

120. Gebhardt F, Zänker KS, Brandt B. Modulation of epidermal growth factor receptor gene transcription by a polymorphic dinucleotide repeat in intron 1. *J Biol Chem* 1999;274(19):13176–13180.

121. Schiffer E, Housset C, Cacheux W, et al. Gefitinib, an EGFR inhibitor, prevents hepatocellular carcinoma development in the rat liver with cirrhosis. *Hepatology* 2005;41(2):307–314.

122. Bjornsti MA, Houghton PJ. The TOR pathway: a target for cancer therapy. *Nat Rev Cancer* 2004;4(5):335–348.

123. Sieghart W, Fuereder T, Schmid K, et al. Mammalian target of rapamycin pathway activity in hepatocellular carcinomas of patients undergoing liver transplantation. *Transplantation* 2007;83(4):425–432.

124. Sahin F, Kannangai R, Adegbola O, Wang J, Su G, Torbenson M. mTOR and P70 S6 kinase expression in primary liver neoplasms. *Clin Cancer Res* 2004;10(24):8421–8425.

125. Huynh H, Chow KH, Soo KC, et al. RAD001 (everolimus) inhibits tumour growth in xenograft models of human hepatocellular carcinoma. *J Cell Mol Med* 2009;13(7):1371–1380.

126. Decaens T, Luciani A, Itti E, et al. Pilot study of sirolimus in cirrhotic patients with advanced hepatocellular carcinoma. ASCO Gastrointestinal Cancers Symposium 2009 [Abstract 244].

127. Kruse FE, Joussen AM, Rohrschneider K, et al. Thalidomide inhibits corneal angiogenesis induced by vascular endothelial growth factor. *Graefes Arch Clin Exp Ophthalmol* 1998;236(6):461–466.

128. Lin AY, Brophy N, Fisher GA, et al. Phase II study of thalidomide in patients with unresectable hepatocellular carcinoma. *Cancer* 2005;103(1):119–125.

129. Chiou HE, Wang TE, Wang YY, et al. Efficacy and safety of thalidomide in patients with hepatocellular carcinoma. *World J Gastroenterol* 2006;12(43):6955–6960.

130. Hsu C, Chen CN, Chen LT, et al. Effect of thalidomide in hepatocellular carcinoma: assessment with power doppler US and analysis of circulating angiogenic factors. *Radiology* 2005;235(2):509–516.

131. Wang J, Chen LT, Tsang YM, et al. Dynamic contrast-enhanced MRI analysis of perfusion changes in advanced hepatocellular carcinoma treated with an antiangiogenic agent: a preliminary study. *AJR Am J Roentgenol* 2004;183(3):713–719.

132. Abou-Alfa GK, Johnson P, Knox J, et al. Preliminary results from a phase II, randomized, double-blind study of sorafenib plus doxorubicin versus placebo plus doxorubicin in patients with advanced hepatocellular carcinoma . In: Proceedings of the 14th European Cancer Conference of the European Cancer Organisation (ECCO); [Abstract 3500] September 23–27, 2007; Barcelona, Spain.

133. Zhu AX, Blaszkowsky LS, Ryan DP, et al. Phase II study of gemcitabine and oxaliplatin in combination with bevacizumab in patients with advanced hepatocellular carcinoma. *J Clin Oncol* 2006;24(12):1898–1903.

134. Asnacios A, Fartoux L, Romano O, et al. Gemcitabine plus oxaliplatin (GEMOX) combined with cetuximab in patients with progressive advanced stage hepatocellular carcinoma: results of a multicenter phase 2 study. *Cancer* 2008;112(12):2733–2739.

135. Sun W, Haller DG, Mykulowycz K, et al. Combination of capecitabine, oxaliplatin with bevacizumab in treatment of advanced hepatocellular carcinoma (HCC): A phase II study. *J Clin Oncol 2007* ASCO Annual Meeting Proceedings Part I. 2007. Vol 25, No. 18S (June 20 Supplement):4574.

136. O'Neil BH, Bernard SA, Goldberg RM, et al. Phase II study of oxaliplatin, capecitabine, and cetuximab in advanced hepatocellular carcinoma [Abstract 4604]. *J Clin Oncol* 2008;26(May 20 Suppl).

137. Louafi S, Boige V, Ducreux M, et al. Gemcitabine plus oxaliplatin (GEMOX) in patients with advanced hepatocellular carcinoma (HCC): results of a phase II study. *Cancer* 2007;109(7):1384–1390.

138. Boige V, Raoul JL, Pignon JP, et al. Multicentre phase II trial of capecitabine plus oxaliplatin (XELOX) in patients with advanced hepatocellular carcinoma: FFCD 03–03 trial. *Br J Cancer* 2007;97(7):862–867.

139. Hanahan D, Bergers G, Bergsland E. Less is more, regularly: metronomic dosing of cytotoxic drugs can target tumor angiogenesis in mice. *J Clin Invest* 2000;105(8):1045–1047.

140. Emmenegger U, Man S, Shaked Y, et al. A comparative analysis of low-dose metronomic cyclophosphamide reveals absent or low-grade toxicity on tissues highly sensitive to the toxic effects of maximum tolerated dose regimens. *Cancer Res* 2004;64(11):3994–4000.

141. Klement G, Huang P, Mayer B, et al. Differences in therapeutic indexes of combination metronomic chemotherapy and an anti-VEGFR-2 antibody in multidrug-resistant human breast cancer xenografts. *Clin Cancer Res* 2002;8(1):221–232.

142. Kerbel RS, Kamen BA. The anti-angiogenic basis of metronomic chemotherapy. *Nat Rev Cancer* 2004;4(6):423–436.

143. Klement G, Baruchel S, Rak J, et al. Continuous low-dose therapy with vinblastine and VEGF receptor-2 antibody induces sustained tumor regression without overt toxicity. *J Clin Invest* 2000;105(8):R15–R24.

144. Man S, Bocci G, Francia G, et al. Antitumor effects in mice of low-dose (metronomic) cyclophosphamide administered continuously through the drinking water. *Cancer Res* 2002;62(10):2731–2735.

145. Hsu CH , Yang TS, Hsu C, et al. Phase II study of bevacizumab (A) plus capecitabine (X) in patients (pts) with advanced/metastatic hepatocellular carcinoma (HCC): final report [Abstract 4603]. *J Clin Oncol* 2008;26(May 20 Suppl).

146. Shen YC, Hsu CH, Hsu C, et al. A phase II study of sorafenib in combination with tegafur/uracil (UFT) for Asian patients with advanced hepatocellular carcinoma (HCC) [Abstract 4589]. *J Clin Oncol* 2009;27:15s.

147. Hsu CY, Lin ZZ, Lee KT, et al. A phase II trial of thalidomide plus tegafur/uracil for patients with advanced/metastatic hepatocellular carcinoma (HCC): Final report [Abstract e15533]. *J Clin Oncol* 2009;27.

148. Kaseb AO, Iwasaki M, Javle M, et al. Biological activity of bevacizumab and erlotinib in patients with advanced hepatocellular carcinoma (HCC) [Abstract 4522]. *J Clin Oncol* 2009;27:15s.

149. Hsu CH, Kang Y, Yang T, et al. A phase II study of bevacizumab (B) and erlotinib (E) in combination for Asian patients (pts) with advanced/metastatic hepatocellular carcinoma (HCC): An interim safety report [Abstract 4585]. *J Clin Oncol* 2009;27:15s.

150. *Chinese Botany*, vol. 7, 1st ed. Shanghai, China: Shanghai Science and Technology Publishing Company, 1999.

151. Tang W, Eisenbrand G. Chinese *Drugs of Plant Origin: Chemistry, Pharmacology and Use in Traditional and Modern Medicine, 1st ed*. New York: Springer-Verlag; 1992.

152. Hsu HY, Hsu CS. *Commonly Used Chinese Herb Formulas With Illustrations*. Los Angeles, CA: Oriental Healing Art Institute; 1980.

153. Yuko T, Yukio K, Masako U, et al. Investigation of 5-FU disposition after oral administration of capecitabine, a triple-prodrug of 5-FU, using a physiologically based pharmacokinetic model in a human cancer xenograft model: comparison of the simulated 5-FU exposures in the tumor tissue between human xenograft model. *Biopharm Drug Dispos.* 2001(22): 1–14.

154. *Guidance for Industry: Botanical Drug Products.* US Food and Drug Administration; 2004.

155. Yen Y, Chu E, et al. PHY906 and capecitabin in liver cancer treatment. *Anti-Cancer Research.* 2009. In press.

156. von Delius S, Lersch C, Mayr M, et al. Capecitabine for treatment of advanced hepatocellular carcinoma. *Hepatogastroenterology* 2007;54(80):2310–2314.

157. Shin D, Lee J, Park J, et al. Systemic chemotherapy with capecitabine, doxorubicin and cisplatin for metastatic hepatocellular carcinoma [Abstract 4177]. *J Clin Oncol* 2005;23:16s.

158. Liu SH, Jiang Z, Cheng YC. A Chinese medicine formulation, PHY-906, can enhance the therapeutic index of CPT-11 and other anticancer drugs against cancer in mice [Abstract 458]. *Proc Am Assoc Cancer Res* 2001;42.

159. Liu SH, Jiang Z, Gao W. PHY906, a Chinese herbal formulation enhances the therapeutic effect of cancer chemotherapy in human colorectal and liver cancer [Abstract 864]. *Proc Am Soc Clin Oncol* 2003; 22:864.

160. Liu SH, Foo A, Jiang Z, et al. PHY906 as a broad-spectrum enhancer in therapy: clinical and preclinical results in hepatocellular carcinoma [Abstract 2142]. *Proc Am Assoc Cancer Res* 2006;47.

161. Liu SH, Jiang Z, Su TM, et al. Developing PHY906 as a broad-spectrum modulator of chemotherapeutic agents in cancer therapy [Abstract 557]. *Proc Am Assoc Cancer Res* 2004;45.

162. O'Neil BH, Venook AP. Hepatocellular carcinoma: the role of the North American GI Steering Committee Hepatobiliary Task Force and the advent of effective drug therapy. Oncologist 2007;12:1425–1432.

163. Abou-Alfa GK, Venook AP. The impact of new data in the treatment of advanced hepatocellular carcinoma. *Curr Oncol Rep* 2008;10(3):199–205.

164. Farrell MP, Kummar S. Phase I/IIA randomized study of PHY906, a novel herbal agent, as a modulator of chemotherapy in patients with advanced colorectal cancer. *Clin Colorectal Cancer* 2003;2(4):253–256.

165. Liu SH, Jiang Z, Foo A, et al. PHY906 in hepatocellular carcinoma [Abstract 1841]. *Proc Am Assoc Cancer Res* 2007; 48.

166. Hoimes CJ, Lamb L, Ruta S, et al. A phase I/II study of PHY906 plus capecitabine (CAP) in patients (pts) with advanced pancreatic cancer [Abstract 15538]. *J Clin Oncol 2008*; 26(May 20 Suppl).

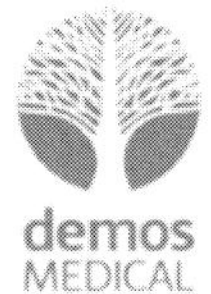

demos
MEDICAL

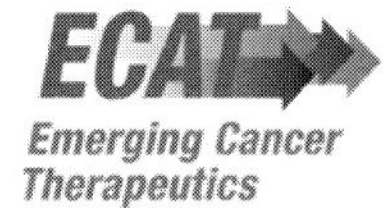

Emerging Cancer
Therapeutics

Colorectal Cancer

Robert Diasio* and M. Wasif Saif

Mayo Clinic, Rochester, MN

Yale Cancer Center, Yale University School of Medicine, New Haven, CT

■ ABSTRACT

Colorectal cancer is the third most common malignancy in the United States, with an estimated 150,000 new cases diagnosed each year, and it is the second leading cause of cancer-related deaths. Approximately 20% of new cases present with metastatic disease. Of the patients who present with localized disease, up to 20% will subsequently relapse with distant metastases. Over the last decade, the options for systemic therapy for patients with colorectal cancer have progressed significantly, from single agent 5-fluorouracil (5-FU) alone in 1957 to an armamentarium of seven chemotherapy and three biological agents. Along with these choices, however, comes complexity in terms of the optimal selection, timing, sequencing, and interval cessation of therapy. However, the availability of new strategies allows the medical oncologist to offer a number of different treatment options with the intent to both maximize therapeutic impact and tailor the toxicity profile to each individual patient following an informed discussion between the patient and the treating oncologist. Metastatic colorectal cancer remains a significant burden on patients, their families, and the oncology community in general. We present in detail these recent advances and provide some insight into several promising future strategies.

■ INTRODUCTION

Colorectal cancer (CRC) is the third most common malignancy in the United States, with an estimated 150,000 new cases diagnosed each year, and it is the second leading cause of cancer-related deaths (1). Among these patients, 19% present at stage IV, 37.2% present at stage III, 27.9% at stage II, and 11% at stage I (2). In locoregionally advanced CRC, surgery is the primary treatment modality and has a curative intent. However, as many as 40% to 50% of the patients will relapse and require additional treatment

of their disease. Clinical failure following resection of CRC is predominantly secondary to the clinical progression of previously undetected distant metastatic disease (3). Except for the patients who are candidates for resection of liver metastasis, the approach in treating metastatic colorectal cancer (mCRC) patients is palliative systemic chemotherapy.

Over little more than a decade, the options for systemic therapy have progressed significantly, from 5-fluorouracil (5-FU) alone to an armamentarium of seven chemotherapy and biological agents (4,5). Along with these choices, however, comes complexity in terms of the optimal selection, timing, sequencing, and interval cessation of therapy. Because these therapies may impact quality of life (QoL) within the context of anticipated outcome as well as the financial burden, it is important that one must consider

____

*Corresponding author, Mayo Clinic Cancer Center, Mayo Clinic, Rochester, MN
E-mail address: Diasio.Robert@mayo.edu

Emerging Cancer Therapeutics 1 (2010) 115–136.

DOI: 10.5003/2151–4194.1.1.117

and discuss the potential impact of any therapy on the patient and assess what is meaningful to an individual patient.

■ STAGES OF COLON CANCER

The stage of CRC at the time of diagnosis plays a significant role in determining the course of treatment. Treatment decisions should be made with reference to the tumor–node–metastasis (TNM) classification rather than to the older Dukes' or the Modified Astler-Coller classification schema (Table 1) (6). The American Joint Committee on Cancer and a National Cancer Institute–sponsored panel recommended that at least 12 lymph nodes be examined in patients with colon and rectal cancer to confirm the absence of nodal involvement by tumor (7). This recommendation takes into consideration that the number of lymph nodes examined is a reflection of the aggressiveness of lymphovascular mesenteric dissection at the time of surgical resection and the pathologic identification of nodes in the specimen.

■ ADJUVANT TREATMENT OF CRC

5-FU

Studies from the National Surgical Adjuvant Breast and Bowel Project (NSABP) and other cooperative groups have clearly demonstrated that adjuvant chemotherapy has resulted in improvement in disease-free survival (DFS) and overall survival (OS) (8–18). These adjuvant regimens included 5-FU + levamisole (LEV) and 5-FU + leucovorin (LV) (5-FU/LV). The Intergroup 0035 study using 5-FU and LEV for 1 year, the Intergroup study using 6 months of 5-FU/LV, and the IMPACT study using 5-FU/LV for 6 months demonstrated similar improvements in DFS and survival rates (11–13). These encouraging results led to direct comparison of these regimens. Intergroup study (INT-0089) randomly assigned 3,759 patients (20% with high-risk Dukes' stage B2 disease) to receive standard 5-FU + LEV for 12 months, 5-FU + high-dose LV, 5-FU + low-dose LV, or 5-FU + low-dose LV + LEV (14). The latter three regimens were administered for approximately 6 months. The results affirmed that 6 months of therapy with 5-FU/LV should represent standard adjuvant treatment for patients with resected high-risk colon cancer. The results of NSABP C-04, in which 2,152 patients (41% Dukes' B) were randomized, were similar. The 5-year DFS was 74% for 5-FU/LV, 70% for 5-FU + LEV, and 73% for 5-FU + LV + LEV; therefore, LEV did not appear to add to the survival advantage associated with 5-FU/LV. Duration of therapy was approximately 1 year for all groups. No significant differences in toxicity were noticed. Based on data from these trials, adjuvant chemotherapy using 6 months of 5-FU/LV became a current standard of care in the United States.

FOLFOX and FLOX

The superior efficacy of oxaliplatin and 5-FU regimens in the treatment of advanced CRC provided the rationale for trials assessing oxaliplatin-based combination regimens in the adjuvant setting. A large trial conducted in Europe used an oxaliplatin + 5-FU/LV regimen as adjuvant therapy for stages II and III CRC.

The MOSAIC trial randomized 2,246 patients with stage II and stage III CRC to receive either 6 months of LV5-FU2 (bolus plus infusional 5-FU/LV) or FOLFOX4 (folinic acid + 5-FU + oxaliplatin) (19). FOLFOX4 was found to be superior to LV5-FU2 in terms of 3-year DFS, a parameter that is highly predictive of 5-year OS. A combined analysis for stage II and stage III patients demonstrated a 23% risk reduction for 3-year recurrence (hazard ratio [HR] 0.77, 95% CI 0.65–0.91, $P = .002$). DFS after 3 years was 78.2% in the FOLFOX4 arm and 72.9% in the LV5-FU2 arm. After a median follow-up of 81.9 months, FOLFOX4 was associated with a 16% reduction in the risk for death compared with LV5-FU2 alone (95% CI, 0.71–1.00). The main prognostic factor of OS was disease stage (HR = 1.85; 95% CI, 1.47–2.34). Therefore, the researchers conducted additional independent OS analyses for patients with stage II and III tumors; however, there was no statistical significance for the relationship between disease stage and treatment. Fewer deaths occurred in the FOLFOX4 group compared with LV5-FU2 (21.8% vs 25.2%); most deaths occurred as a result of relapse or recurrence, but adverse events (AEs) accounted for six deaths in each group. At 6 years, FOLFOX4 was associated with a 20% reduction in the risk for death among patients with stage III disease. Similarly, FOLFOX4 was associated with a 20% reduction in the risk for relapse in all patients. Grade 3 peripheral sensory neuropathy occurred

TABLE 1   Stages of colon cancer: TNM definitions

Primary tumor (T)

TX: Primary tumor cannot be assessed

T0: No evidence of primary tumor

Tis: Carcinoma *in situ*: intraepithelial or invasion of the lamina propria[a]

T1: Tumor invades submucosa

T2: Tumor invades muscularis propria

T3: Tumor invades through the muscularis propria into the subserosa or into nonperitonealized pericolic or perirectal tissues

T4: Tumor directly invades other organs or structures and/or perforates visceral peritoneum[b]

Regional lymph nodes (N)c

NX: Regional nodes cannot be assessed

N0: No regional lymph node metastasis

N1: Metastasis in one to three regional lymph nodes

N2: Metastasis in four or more regional lymph nodes

Distant metastasis (M)

MX: Distant metastasis cannot be assessed

M0: No distant metastasis

M1: Distant metastasis

AJCC stage groupings

Stage 0

Tis, N0, M0

Stage I

T1, N0, M0

T2, N0, M0

Stage IIA

T3, N0, M0

Stage IIB

T4, N0, M0

Stage IIIA

T1, N1, M0

T2, N1, M0

Stage IIIB

T3, N1, M0

T4, N1, M0

Stage IIIC

Any T, N2, M0

Stage IV

Any T, any N, M1

---

[a]This includes cancer cells confined within the glandular basement membrane (intraepithelial) or lamina propria (intramucosal) with no extension through the muscularis mucosae into the submucosa.

[b]Direct invasion in T4 includes invasion of other segments of the colorectum by way of the serosa; for example, invasion of the sigmoid colon by a carcinoma of the cecum. Tumor that is adherent macroscopically to other organs or structures is classified T4. If no tumor is present in the adhesion microscopically, however, the classification should be pT3. The V and L substaging should be used to identify the presence or absence of vascular or lymphatic invasion.

[c]A tumor nodule in the pericolorectal adipose tissue of a primary carcinoma without histologic evidence of residual lymph node in the nodule is classified in the pN category as a regional lymph node metastasis if the nodule has the form and smooth contour of a lymph node. If the nodule has an irregular contour, it should be classified in the T category and also coded as V1 (microscopic venous invasion) or as V2 (if it was grossly evident), because there is a strong likelihood that is represents venous invasion.

in 12.5% of patients in the FOLFOX4 arm versus 0.2% of those in the LV5-FU2 arm. However, the frequency of peripheral sensory neuropathy declined during the follow-up period in patients assigned to FOLFOX4. Additionally, patients in the FOLFOX4 group experienced fewer second cancers compared with those in the LV5-FU2 group. The main side effect of FOLFOX4 was anticipatory sensory neuropathy with grade 3 toxicity affecting 12.4% of patients overall and 18% of patients who received the entire planned 1,020 mg/m^2 dose of oxaliplatin. However, the neurotoxicity proved reversible in the vast majority of patients so that, 12 and 18 months after discontinuation of therapy, only 1.1% and 0.5% of patients, respectively, had residual grade 3 neurotoxicity. Based on the results of the Multicenter International Study of Oxaliplatin/5 Fluorouracil/ Leucovorin in the Adjuvant Treatment of Colon Cancer (MOSAIC) trial, FOLFOX4 was approved by the U.S. Food and Drug Administration (FDA) as the new standard of care in the adjuvant treatment of stage III in 2004 (19).

Another study conducted by the NSABP (NSABP C-07) reported the role of oxaliplatin with bolus administration of 5-FU in the adjuvant setting (20). In this study, 2,407 patients were randomized to either the Roswell Park schedule of 5-FU/LV (500 mg/m^2 of both given weekly for 6 weeks followed by 2 weeks rest for three cycles) versus the same 5-FU/LV regimen and oxaliplatin (FLOX). The oxaliplatin was administered at 85 mg/m^2 every 2 weeks but only on weeks 1, 3, and 5 of the 8-week cycle (cumulative dose 765 mg/m^2). Seventy-three percent of patients received the planned oxaliplatin treatment. The primary end point, 3-year DFS, favored the FLOX arm (76.5% vs 71.6%; HR 0.79, $P = .004$). At 5-year update, the DFS advantage had increased to a 5.2% advantage in the FLOX arm. A trend toward improved survival was seen for patients with stage II or III colon cancer with the addition of oxaliplatin to FULV. Interestingly, when stage II (node negative) patients were teased out, no benefit was seen for them. The benefit of oxaliplatin is independent of the schedule of FULV administration. There were fewer deaths than had been anticipated in this trial. The results of this trial were similar to those reported in the MOSAIC trial, and thus validate those findings. The regimen was tolerable as grade 3 and 4 toxicities were similar in the two arms (grade 3/4: 50%/10% with FLOX vs 41%/9% with 5-FU/LV). Only 8% of patients experienced grade 3 neurotoxicity and, after 12 months, this decreased to 0.5% of patients. Enteritis leading to diarrhea and dehydration was higher in the experimental arm (4.5% vs 2.7%).

■ THERAPEUTICS: ONCOLOGY

IFL and FOLFIRI

Contrary to oxaliplatin addition to 5-FU, irinotecan combinations both with bolus and infusional 5-FU showed no survival advantage in the adjuvant setting as shown in Table 2.

The results from these phase III adjuvant trials demonstrate the superiority of oxaliplatin-containing arms over conventional 5-FU/LV controls. This is in contrast to the less favorable results observed with irinotecan in this group of patients (21–23).

Biologic Agents in Adjuvant Therapy

Recent phase III studies have shown that targeted agents improved survival in patients with advanced CRC. Bevacizumab, a monoclonal antibody targeting vascular endothelial growth factor (VEGF), is the first antiangiogenic drug to show improved efficacy when used in combination with irinotecan and oxaliplatin for first- and second-line treatment of CRC. Cetuximab, another monoclonal antibody targeting epidermal growth factor receptor (EGFR), has shown efficacy in third-line therapy and promising results in first-line phase II studies. There is great interest in whether the biologic agents bevacizumab and cetuximab can improve survival in the adjuvant therapy setting (8).

The NSABP C-08 trial was designed to investigate the safety and effectiveness of adding bevacizumab to modified infusional fluorouracil, leucovorin, and oxaliplatin (FOLFOX) 6 regimen for the adjuvant treatment of patients with stage II

TABLE 2   Randomized studies of irinotecan in adjuvant therapy of colon cancer

Trial	DFS HR	*P* Value	OS HR	*P* Value
CALGB 89803	NR	0.85	NR	0.74
PETACC-3	0.89	0.091	NR	NR
ACCORD-2	1.19	0.22	NR	NR

or III colon cancer. A total of 2,710 patients were randomly assigned to 6 months chemotherapy with FOLFOX6 or 6 months FOLXFOX6 plus bevacizumab plus an additional 6 months bevacizumab after chemotherapy had ended. The primary end point was DFS. Median follow-up was 3 years. At 3 years, 77.4% of patients assigned bevacizumab were alive and free of disease compared with 75.5% of patients assigned standard chemotherapy. There was an absolute difference of 2% in favor of bevacizumab at 3 years, with an HR of 0.89 and a P value that was not statistically significant. Interestingly, at 1 year, there was a 40% reduction in the event rate ($P = .0004$) with bevacizumab. However, after 1 year this effect disappeared. The addition of bevacizumab to standard chemotherapy did not result in an overall statistically significant prolongation in DFS and clearly the prespecified end point of the trial was not met. This study, however, suggests that consideration should be given to clinical trials that use bevacizumab for periods of time well beyond the 1 year that was used in NSABP Protocol C-08 (24). Overall rates of grade 4 or 5 toxicities were nearly identical in the FOLFOX6 and FOLFOX6 plus bevacizumab arms (15.2% and 15.0%, respectively). Six-month mortality rates were 0.96% and 0.90% for the control and experimental groups, respectively. Grade 3+ toxicities that occurred more often in the experimental arm versus control arm included hypertension (12% vs 1.8%, respectively), wound complications (abdominal incisional hernia or infusion port dehiscence/inflammation; 1.7% vs 0.3%, respectively), pain (11.1% vs 6.3%, respectively), and proteinuria (2.7% vs 0.8%, respectively). Grade 2+ neuropathy was increased in the experimental arm versus the control arm (grade 2, 33% vs 29%, respectively; grade 3, 16% vs 14%, respectively; and grade 4, <1% each). In the experimental arm versus control arm, significantly less thrombocytopenia (1.4% vs 3.4%, respectively) and allergic reactions (3.1% vs 4.7%, respectively) were observed. Advanced age was associated with a significantly greater rate of grade 4 and 5 toxicities regardless of treatment.

Currently, AVANT, ECOG 5202, and US NO147 are evaluating the role of these agents (8).

Capecitabine Versus 5-FU

The international, phase III X-ACT trial enrolled 1,987 patients (1,004 patients were randomly assigned to Xeloda; 983 patients were assigned to intravenous 5-FU/LV), who were treated for a period of 24 weeks between 1998 and 2001 at 164 centers worldwide. The primary study objective was to show equivalence in DFS between Xeloda and intravenous 5-FU/LV. Secondary objectives included: relapse-free survival, overall survival (OS), and safety. Xeloda 3-year DFS and relapse-free survival rates demonstrated noninferiority to 5-FU/LV (intent-to-treat analysis, $P < 0.0001$; $P = 0.0407$, respectively). Xeloda was associated with fewer AEs than 5-FU/LV ($P < 0.001$).With a median follow-up of 7 years, updated study results presented at ECCO show 5-year OS rates for Xeloda at 71.4% compared to 68.4% in the 5-FU/LV arm (25). These updated 5-year OS data support that Xeloda can be a safe and effective alternative to the current standard of care for adjuvant CRC. In addition, study also showed that Xeloda is more cost-effective than the Mayo Clinic regimen (the current standard treatment) and is associated with fewer side effects. Additionally, many of the side effects can be easily managed by altering the dose without compromising efficacy.

XELOX

New results for Xeloda in early colon cancer were recently presented at ECCO ESMO. The NO16968 trial (XELOXA) is an open-label, randomized, phase III study of XELOX (oral Xeloda in combination with intravenous oxaliplatin) versus 5-FU/LV as adjuvant therapy for patients with stage III colon cancer who have undergone surgery. It studied the use of XELOX for 6 months. The study included 1,886 patients and was conducted at 226 study sites across 29 countries. The primary end point of the study was to demonstrate the superiority of XELOX versus 5-FU/LV in terms of DFS. Secondary end points included OS, safety profiles, and perceived treatment convenience between the treatment arms. The pivotal NO16968 (XELOXA) study, the largest-ever study of patients with stage III colon cancer, showed that the 3-year DFS for patients receiving XELOX was 70.9%, superior to the 5-FU/LV arm (66.5%) (HR = 0.80 [95% CI: 0.69–0.93], $P = 0.0045$) (26). The DFS result obtained with XELOX is similar to that shown in trials evaluating the use of FOLFOX in patients with stage III colon cancer. These results confirm that patients have an additional option for the treatment of stage III colon cancer. Most treatment-related AEs occurred at similar rates in both treatment arms. However, patients receiving XELOX experienced less all-grade diarrhea, alopecia, and more neurosensory toxicity, vomiting, and hand-foot syndrome than those patients receiving FU/LV. Compared with Mayo, XELOX showed fewer grade 3/4 hematologic AE and more grade 3/4 gastrointestinal AE. Compared with RP, XELOX showed less grade 3/4 gastrointestinal AE and more grade 3/4 hematologic AE. As expected grade 3/4 neurosensory toxicity and grade 3 hand-foot syndrome were higher with XELOX. Treatment-related mortality within 28 days from the last study dose was 0.6% in the XELOX group and 0.6% in the FU/LV group.

Stage I Colon Cancer

Because of its localized nature, stage I colon cancer has a high cure rate. Wide surgical resection and anastomosis is the standard therapy.

Stage II Colon Cancer

The role of adjuvant chemotherapy for patients with stage II colon adenocarcinoma remains controversial (27,28). The high surgical cure rate for patients with "low-risk" stage II CRC ranges from 75% to 80%, and the available clinical trials and metaanalyses provide conflicting recommendations for or against adjuvant chemotherapy for this group of patients (Table 3). For fit "high-risk" stage II patients with characteristics such as intestinal perforation, clinical obstruction, T4 tumors, poorly differentiated tumors, and inadequately pathologically examined (< 13) lymph node and extramural venous or lymphatic invasion, in whom the 5-year survival rate is 60% to 70%, there is little controversy, as these patients are routinely treated with adjuvant chemotherapy (29). In addition to pathologic factors, some molecular factors considered potentially "high risk," including high histologic grade, microsatellite instability, and loss of 18q, have yet to be validated in prospective trials. Currently, more emphasis is placed on those patients with fewer than 12 regional lymph nodes identified in the surgical specimen—these patients have a statistically unclear risk of lymph node involvement (30). These patients might be upgraded to stage III disease if more lymph nodes were sampled, and therefore should receive adjuvant therapy. The decision to use adjuvant chemotherapy to treat low-risk stage II colon cancer patients (no obstruction or perforation) should be an informed decision weighing the magnitude of a net 2% to 5% survival benefit, a 0.5% to 1.0% risk of mortality with chemotherapy in addition to 6 months of chemotherapy-related toxicities, other coexisting patient morbidities, and the anticipated life expectancy of each patient. As adjuvant chemotherapy is therapy addressing local or metastatic microscopic disease, and the effectiveness of systemic and biologically targeted therapy for advanced macroscopic colon cancer continues to improve rapidly, it remains to be determined by clinical trials whether therapies including newer agents such as cetuximab and bevacizumab administered in the adjuvant setting may affect survival for stage II cancer patients. Approximately 30% of stage II patients currently receive adjuvant chemotherapy in the United States. "High-risk" patients may be considered for 5-FU/LV or FOLFOX. For average-risk patients, a discussion of the small benefit of chemotherapy should be conducted, and the patient should be involved in the decision-making process.

Oxaliplatin-based combination chemotherapy may be over treatment in low-risk stage II colon cancer, as neurotoxicity can be prolonged and disabling. Therefore, an honest discussion of risk versus benefit should be carried out to tailor the individual therapy in these patients at this time.

TABLE 3 ASCO recommendations for stage II disease

High-risk subsets exist
Inadequate lymph node sampling
T4 lesions
Perforation/obstruction
Poorly differentiated histology
Honest risk/benefit discussion is in order for all stage II patients

Stage III Colon Cancer

Oxaliplatin-based chemotherapy (FOLFOX) is now the standard of care as adjuvant chemotherapy for stage III colon cancer and for patients with high-risk stage II disease. Based on the clinical studies conducted to date, irinotecan cannot be recommended for use in the adjuvant setting. The oral fluoropyrimidine capecitabine has demonstrated equivalent efficacy to bolus 5-FU/LV as adjuvant treatment, and is a standard of care when fluoropyrimidine therapy is being considered. XELOX now presents an additional option for this stage of patents. The role of biologic agent's bevacizumab and cetuximab in the adjuvant setting is still pending; however, aside from assessing the additional benefit of these monoclonal antibodies over cytotoxic agents, it will be important to address the long-term effects of these agents on cancer survivors, the optimal duration of these agents, and the costs associated with these treatments.

Six months of adjuvant treatment is the current standard duration, and treatment should start within 8 weeks following surgery. Pooled data analyses from numerous clinical trials and registries support the view that chronologic age in itself should not be a selection criterion for adjuvant therapy. Trial data in the very elderly (> 80 years) are more lacking. For all patients, an assessment of other medical problems, functional status, and anticipated life expectancy is necessary. Otherwise-fit elderly patients should be offered one of the standard adjuvant treatment options with a detailed discussion including potential benefits, treatment risks, and patient choice. Less toxic options can be offered to patients who are more frail.

Metastatic Colon Cancer

A combination regimen of 5-FU/LV + oxaliplatin or irinotecan with bevacizumab is the current standard treatment for metastatic colon cancer (4). Recently, addition of anti-EGFR agents to the combination chemotherapy regimens also look promising, especially in patients with liver only metastasis. Factors involved in a treatment decision may include clinical evidence, patient characteristics, previous treatments, patient preferences (e.g., oral vs intravenous [IV]), and financial costs/reimbursements. Patient's characteristics include performance status/comorbid illnesses, age, prior adjuvant therapy, prior pelvic/abdominal irradiation, baseline liver and/or renal function, status of disease, sites of disease, tumor bulk, and tumor-related symptoms.

Cytotoxic Agents

5-Fluorouracil

5-FU had been the only anticancer drug proven to benefit patients with mCRC for 50 years. 5-FU has also been the backbone on which most regimens for treatment of mCRC are built (31). 5-FU, when used alone, has limited activity in advanced disease, rendering a response rate (RR) ranging from 10% to 15%.

5-FU/LCV

A meta-analysis of data incorporating 3,300 patients from 19 clinical trials demonstrated that combining LV (a biomodulating agent) with 5-FU was associated with improved RR up to 21% from 11% ($P < .0001$) and improved survival from 10.5 months to 11.7 months ($P < .004$) (32,33). The 5-FU/LV regimen was recognized as standard first-line treatment of mCRC until more advanced combination therapies containing irinotecan and oxaliplatin were developed. However, optimizing ways in which 5-FU/LV is delivered remains quite debatable. Among several different regimens, the most common bolus schedules are the Mayo regimen, with 5-FU at a dose of 425 mg/m^2 and LV at 20 mg/m^2 every 4 weeks, and a weekly schedule developed by Roswell Park Cancer Institute, with 5-FU at 600 mg/m^2 and LV at 500 mg/m^2 weekly for 6 of 8 weeks. Two randomized trials have demonstrated similar RR, duration of response, progression-free intervals, and median OS between the monthly and weekly schedules of LV-modulated 5-FU (34,35).

Infusional 5-FU

The clinical efficacy of 5-FU/LV has been improved upon by the use of infusional schedules. A metaanalysis that incorporated 1,219 patients from six different randomized trials compared infusional 5-FU with bolus 5-FU revealed that infusional schedules of 5-FU resulted in higher RR than bolus schedules (22% vs 14%; $P < .0002$). Infusional schedules were also associated with less hematologic toxicity compared to that of bolus regimens (4% vs 31%, respectively; $P < .0001$) and less gastrointestinal toxicity (36). Common infusional schedules include the protracted venous infusion (PVI) schedule with 5-FU at 300 mg/m^2 for 28 days; the AIO German regimen of 5-FU at 2,000 to 2,600 mg/m^2 over 24 hours with LV at 500 mg/m^2 administered once weekly for 6 weeks with 1 week of rest; LV5-FU2 (the de Gramont regimen), which is a combination of bolus and infusional 5-FU/LV administered on days 1 and 2 on a biweekly schedule; and a simplified LV5-FU2 schedule with LV 400 mg/m^2 and 5-FU 400 mg/m^2 on day 1, followed by a single 46-hour continuous infusion of 5-FU for a total 5-FU infusion dose of 2,400 mg/m^2 (36–38). Based on recent National Comprehensive Cancer Network guidelines, the PVI 5-FU/LV schedule is a reasonable first-line treatment option for patients who cannot tolerate intensive chemotherapy (39).

Capecitabine

Capecitabine is an oral fluoropyrimidine carbamate prodrug of 5-FU designed to be reliably absorbed intact through the gastrointestinal tract. It then becomes activated by three successive enzymatic steps. The enzyme thymidylate phosphorylase is involved in the final step, and it is also thought to be expressed at a higher level in tumor tissue when compared to corresponding normal tissue. This tumor localization of thymidylate phosphorylase may be the basis for its selective activation of capecitabine in tumors and associated favorable tolerability. In two randomized phase III trials comparing capecitabine with Mayo regimen bolus 5-FU/LV, capecitabine showed similar efficacy. An integrated analysis of the two trials revealed that the overall RR was higher with capecitabine than with bolus 5-FU/LV (25.7% vs 16.7%; $P < .0002$) while time to progression (TTP) and survival were similar. Capecitabine also was associated with fewer side effects (40). Gastrointestinal and hematologic toxicities were significantly lower in incidence in the capecitabine arm compared to that in the bolus 5-FU/LV arm. Hand-foot syndrome was the only side effect that was observed with higher incidence in the capecitabine arm. There have been no randomized clinical trials comparing the efficacy and toxicity of capecitabine with any infusional 5-FU schedules. When compared to historical controls of continuous infusion of 5-FU, capecitabine monotherapy appeared to have similar RR, TTP, and median survival (41). Capecitabine, at a dosage of 1,250 mg/m^2 twice daily for 14 days of every 21-day cycle, was approved in the United States for first-line treatment of mCRC when fluoropyrimidine monotherapy is indicated. However, clinical experience and retrospective analysis indicate that 900 to 1,000 mg/m^2 twice daily may be better tolerated with similar efficacy (41).

Irinotecan

Irinotecan is a topoisomerase I poison (42). Irinotecan monotherapy in 5-FU–refractory mCRC patients showed an improved 1-year OS (36% vs 14%) and improved QoL when compared with best supportive care (BSC). Severe diarrhea is the well-known dose-limiting toxicity of irinotecan (43).

Irinotecan was initially approved for second-line treatment by the FDA; however, three randomized phase III trials provided evidence that a first-line combination regimen including irinotecan and 5-FU/LV rendered improved clinical efficacy, including OS, compared to 5-FU/LV alone (43–45). In Europe,

Douillard et al. compared the clinical efficacy of infusional 5-FU plus irinotecan versus infusional 5-FU/LV alone. In this trial, the irinotecan group was superior in RR (35% vs 22%; $P = .005$), time to treatment failure (6.7 vs 4.4 months; $P = .001$), and OS (17.4 vs 14.2 months; $P = .031$) (44). Köhne et al. compared weekly infusional 5-FU/LV with and without irinotecan and reported that addition of irinotecan improved RRs (54% vs 31.5%; $P < .0001$) and TTP (8.5 vs 6.4 months; $P = .0001$) (45). However, the median survival benefit (10.1 vs 16.9 months; $P = .2279$ log-rank) did not reach the level of statistical significance (45). In the United States, Saltz et al. compared an IFL (bolus 5-FU/LV) weekly schedule versus 5-FU/LV alone, and reported the superiority of the IFL regimen over 5-FU/LV alone in terms of RR (39% vs 21%; $P < .001$), median progression-free survival (PFS) (7.0 vs 4.3 months; $P = .004$), and OS (14.8 vs 12.6 months; $P = .04$) (46).

The weekly IFL regimen resulted in increased incidence of diarrhea, dehydration, and myelosuppression when compared to the infusional schedules of 5-FU/LV (the FOLFIRI or Douillard regimen). Based on this observation, the IFL regimen, which used to be preferred among U.S. oncologists due to their familiarity with it, are now used rarely or used with modification consisting of 2 weeks on and 1 week off. Conversely, the FOLFIRI strategies have been embraced by more U.S. oncologists recently. In fact, based on a recent randomized trial by Fuchs et al., even the modified IFL regimen (m-IFL) should be considered obsolete, and the FOLFIRI regimen should be the regimen of choice when 5-FU is combined with irinotecan in treatment of previously untreated mCRC. In this trial, FOLFIRI showed its superiority over m-IFL with respect to TTP (8.2 vs 6.0 months; $P = .01$) and median OS (23.1 vs 17.6 months; $P = .10$). FOLFIRI was also better tolerated than m-IFL (47).

Capecitabine + Irinotecan (CapeIri)

Investigators are actively evaluating the combination of capecitabine + irinotecan (CapeIri) to take advantage of the convenience and tolerability of the oral capecitabine. Numerous phase II studies have shown the efficacy of CapeIri with a manageable side effect profile (48–50). In one phase II study including (47) patients with metastatic or unresectable CRC, Ahn et al. (48) investigated the combination of capecitabine (1,000 mg/m^2 orally twice daily on days 2–15 of a 3-week cycle) + irinotecan (100 mg/m^2 IV on days 1 and 8). This trial reported an overall RR of 51.4% (19 partial responses [PRs]; 95% CI 35.3–67.5%), median TTP of 7.1 months (95% CI 4.6–9.6 months), and median OS of 24.8 months (95% CI 10.5–39.1 months). This regimen was relatively well tolerated, with grade 3/4 diarrhea (24%) and grade 3/4 neutropenia (11%). There were no treatment-related deaths (48). However, in a recent multicenter, randomized trial comparing FOLFIRI, m-IFL, and CapeIri in a first-line setting of mCRC, CapeIri was inferior in efficacy with higher rate of toxicities compared to the other two regimens (47). Currently, this regimen is not commonly used outside clinical trials due to diarrhea and constant struggle for optimal dose.

Oxaliplatin

Oxaliplatin is a third-generation platinum compound with significant anticancer activity in CRC in combination with 5-FU. Its dose-limiting toxicity is acute and chronic sensory neuropathy. The chronic form is a dose-dependent sensory neuropathy that develops in up to 12% to 15% of patients when the cumulative dose is greater than 850 mg/m^2 (51). The benefit of adding oxaliplatin to 5-FU/LV was reported in a randomized phase III trial by de Gramont et al. (52). The FOLFOX4 regimen (oxaliplatin at a dose of 85 mg/m^2 as a 2-hour infusion on day 1, every 2 weeks, plus LV5-FU2) was compared with LV5-FU2 alone in 420 patients with previously treated mCRC (52). FOLFOX4 resulted in a longer median PFS (9 vs 6.2 months; P = .0003) and a higher RR (50.7% vs 22.3%; P = .0001). The difference in median OS did not reach statistical significance (16.2 vs 14.7 months; P = .12). However, this trial was not sufficiently powered to detect such a difference, and any potential survival difference may have been obscured as both treatment arms were able to receive salvage therapies. Grade 3/4 neutropenia and grade 3/4 diarrhea were more common with FOLFOX4 but were at clearly manageable levels (52).

Capecitabine + Oxaliplatin (CAPOX)

Capecitabine's convenience of being an oral agent with better tolerability than 5-FU/LV led to a series of studies that compared combination of oxaliplatin with either capecitabine or 5-FU/LV. Based on initial studies, including a phase II trial of the combination of capecitabine (1,000 mg/m^2 twice daily from day 1 to 14) and oxaliplatin (130 mg/m^2 IV on day 1)

every 3 weeks that showed an overall RR of 55% and a median OS of 19.5 months led to randomized phase III study (53). Cassidy et al. reported the results of a randomized phase III study of capecitabine plus oxaliplatin compared with fluorouracil/folinic acid plus oxaliplatin as first-line therapy for mCRC (54). The intent-to-treat population comprised 634 patients from the original two-arm portion of the study, plus an additional 1,400 patients after the start of the amended 2 × 2 design, for a total of 2,034 patients. The median PFS was 8.0 months in the pooled XELOX-containing arms versus 8.5 months in the FOLFOX-4-containing arms (hazard ratio [HR], 1.04; 97.5% CI 0.93–1.16). The median OS was 19.8 months with XELOX versus 19.6 months with FOLFOX-4 (HR, 0.99; 97.5% CI 0.88–1.12). FOLFOX-4 was associated with more grade 3/4 neutropenia/granulocytopenia and febrile neutropenia than XELOX, and XELOX with more grade 3 diarrhea and grade 3 hand-foot syndrome than FOLFOX-4. This study confirmed that XELOX is noninferior to FOLFOX-4 as a first-line treatment for mCRC.

Additional Trials Comparing Therapeutic Regimens

FOLFOX4 Versus IFL

Intergroup trial N9741 was a randomized phase III trial that compared FOLFOX, IFL, or oxaliplatin/irinotecan (IROX) (55). This pivotal trial showed that FOLFOX4 was superior to IFL in RR (45% vs 31%; P = .002), TTP (8.7 vs 6.9 months: P = .0001), and median OS (19.5 vs 14.8 months: P = .0001). In addition, when compared to IFL or IROX, FOLFOX4 was associated with a significantly lower incidence of febrile neutropenia and fewer gastrointestinal side effects. Based on this trial, FOLFOX4 was approved in the United States as first-line treatment for patients with mCRC (55).

FOLFIRI Versus FOLFOX

Tournigand et al. conducted a randomized, multicenter, open-label prospective phase III trial in order to answer the question of whether oxaliplatin is a more active agent than FOLFOXes. irinotecan when an identical 5-FU–based schedule is used (Table 4) (56). Patients had equal access to the alternative regimen at progression. This trial used a simplified

TABLE 4 Phase III trial of first-line FOLFIRI versus FOLFOX-6 (GERCOR C97–3)

	Arm A		Arm B		
	FOLFIRI ($n=109$)	FOLFOX6 ($n=81$)	FOLFOX6 ($n=111$)	FOLFIRI ($n=69$)	P Value
ORR (%)	56	15	54	4	0.68
Median PFS (months)	8.5	4.2	8	2.5	–
Median TTP (months)	14.2		10.9		0.64
Median OS (months)	21.5		20.6		0.99

LV5-FU2 regimen with a single 46-hour infusion. In one arm, patients received FOLFIRI (biweekly irinotecan 180 mg/m², LV 200 mg/m², 5-FU 400 mg/m² on day 1 followed by a 46-hour continuous infusion of 5-FU at 2.4 to 3.0 g/m²) followed at progression by FOLFOX6 (biweekly oxaliplatin 100 mg/m² and the same dose and schedule of 5-FU/LV), while patients in the second arm received the reverse sequence of FOLFOX6 as first-line therapy followed by FOLFIRI at the time of progression. The efficacy was similar in terms of RR (54% vs 56% for FOLFOX6 and FOLFIRI, respectively), PFS (8 vs 8.5 months) and median OS (20.6 vs 21.5 months). Both treatment arms were relatively well tolerated. Patients treated with first-line FOLFIRI experienced a higher incidence of grade ¾ nausea and mucositis. The first-line FOLFOX6 group experienced a higher incidence of grade ¾ myelosuppression. Use of oxaliplatin was associated with grade ¾ neurotoxicity (34%). The Tournigand study was important as it demonstrated equivalent clinical efficacy between irinotecan and oxaliplatin in the first-line setting when used with the same de Gramont infusional 5-FU/LV regimen. It also demonstrated that there is not a superior sequence of the two regimens (56). This conclusion was further augmented by another randomized phase III trial that reported no difference in overall RR, TTP, and OS for mCRC patients treated with the FOLFIRI or FOLFOX4 as first-line regimens (57).

CAPIRI Versus CAPOX and FUFOX Versus CAPOX

Based on randomized trial data, CAPOX and a regimen consisting of weekly infusional 5-FU/LV + oxaliplatin (FUFOX) appeared to have similar antitumor activities, but CAPOX was associated with more significant gastrointestinal toxicities and myelosuppression (58). A randomized phase II trial by Grothey et al. compared the combination of capecitabine + irinotecan (CAPIRI) with CAPOX in the first-line setting. Patients from both arms were allowed to cross over at progression (59). There were no difference in OS, and the safety profiles of both regimens were equally manageable (59). These trials further solidified the potential of capecitabine as an alternative to 5-FU/LV in the first-line setting. Intergroup study NO16966 is the first phase III trial to evaluate the efficacy of bevacizumab in combination with FOLFOX4 and XELOX regimens in the first-line treatment of mCRC, as described later in the chapter (60).

Sequential Versus Combination Therapy

Grothey et al. have shown that exposure to all three main anticancer agents during the treatment course of mCRC is a critical predictor of OS (61). A few studies were conducted to assess whether sequential administration of these agents is superior to up-front combination therapy or vice versa. The Fluorouracil, Oxaliplatin, CPT-11 Usage Study (FOCUS) trial was a five-arm randomized phase III trial conducted to compare sequential therapy with up-front use of combination regimens (62). The up-front use of combination regimens such as FOLFOX or FOLFIRI yielded higher RR, PFS, and median OS. Initiation of combination therapy up front would be reasonable in patients with good to excellent performance status, those with aggressive disease, and potential candidates for salvage surgical resection. Conversely, sequential therapy initiated with 5-FU/LV or capecitabine followed by FOLFOX or FOLFIRI as second-line options may be a reasonable approach in relatively asymptomatic patients with less aggressive and unresectable diseases (62).

FOLFOXIRI and XELOXIRI

An approach of initiating combination therapy that contains all three cytotoxic agents (5-FU/LV, oxaliplatin, and irinotecan; FOLFOXIRI) together has been investigated. A phase III trial by Falcone et al. compared FOLFOXIRI with FOLFIRI in a first-line setting followed by an oxaliplatin-containing regimen as a second-line therapy (63). FOLFOXIRI was superior to FOLFIRI, yielding higher overall RR (66% vs 41%; P = .0002), median PFS (9.8 vs 6.9 months; P = .0006), and median OS (22.6 vs 16.7 months; P = .032). More patients in FOLFOXIRI went on to have resection of liver-only metastasis (36% vs 12%; P = .017). FOLFOXIRI was associated with higher incidence of grade 3/4 neuropathy and neutropenia (63). Souglakos et al. (64) conducted a similar trial but with lower FOLFOXIRI doses than Falcone et al.'s (63) trial. This study reported no significant difference in RR, OS, or ability to resect liver-only metastasis (64). FOLFOXIRI may become a reasonable first-line option for a selected group of patients, particularly for potential candidates for definitive liver metastasis resections or for patients in whom biologic agents are contraindicated.

Recently, a dose-finding trial progression-free has demonstrated the feasibility of the combination of irinotecan, oxaliplatin, and capecitabine (XELOXIRI) and established their recommended doses (65). The aim infrequent, of this study was to evaluate the activity of XELOXIRI. A total of 36 patients with unresectable mCRC received irinotecan 165 mg/m^2 and oxaliplatin 85 mg/m^2 on day 1 plus capecitabine 2,000 mg/m^2/day orally in two doses from day 1 to day 7, every 2 weeks. Grade ¾ toxicities were infrequent, except for every neutropenia and diarrhea, which were each observed in 30% of patients. Two CR and twenty-two PRs were obtained, corresponding an to an overall response rate of 67% (95% CI 51.4–82%). After a median follow-up of 17.7 months, the median progression-free high and OS was 10.1 and 17.9 months, respectively. The study showed that the substitution of 5-FU with capecitabine, in combination with irinotecan and oxaliplatin, is feasible and does not impair the activity of the regimen. However, the XELOXIRI combination is associated with a high alternative incidence of diarrhea and, therefore, should be considered as a not preferable alternative to FOLFOXIRI.

Optimal Duration of Chemotherapy

Maughan et al. conducted a randomized study to show that, by treating patients intermittently, toxicities were reduced without difference in OS versus continuous chemotherapy (66). This was evidence that discontinuing chemotherapy after a treatment period and reinitiating the same regimen at disease progression may be an appropriate option in chemotherapy-sensitive disease (66).

The OPTIMOX trial compared FOLFOX7 to FOLFOX4. Patients in the FOLFOX4 arm received the regimen continuously until disease progression, and patients in the FOLFOX7 arm received intermittent exposure to oxaliplatin, allowing a lower cumulative dose of neurotoxic oxaliplatin (67). The FOLFOX7 arm rendered a similar clinical efficacy with improved safety profile when compared to the FOLFOX4 arm. While this trial's outcome may have been obscured by the fact that there was a series of protocol violations in relation to reintroduction of oxaliplatin, it was an important study suggesting that intermittent use of oxaliplatin-based chemotherapy may be a reasonable alternative with improved tolerability to continuous combination chemotherapy (67).

The OPTIMOX2 trial was a large phase II study that compared LV5-FU maintenance therapy until progression to observation until progression after six cycles of FOLFOX7. The maintenance arm was reintroduced to modified FOLFOX7 at the time of progression, and the observation arm was reintroduced to modified FOLFOX7 before the tumor progression reached the baseline measures. The maintenance LV5-FU arm showed longer PFS (8.7 vs 6.9 months; P = .09). However, there was no difference in the duration of disease control (12.9 vs 11.7 months; P = .41). In addition, the chemotherapy-free interval (CFI) was nearly 6 months (68). Another trial was conducted to evaluate whether the same efficacy of continuous chemotherapy can be achieved with intermittent chemotherapy. Labianca et al. compared FOLFIRI scheduled every 2 weeks continuously versus an alternating schedule of FOLFIRI for 2 months and CFI for 2 months (69). This trial reported no significant difference in PFS or median OS between the two treatment arms, supporting the suggestion that intermittent chemotherapy may be a potential alternative to continuous chemotherapy (69) CFI without significant compromise of PFS and OS can potentially have significant impact on QoL of mCRC patients.

The "OPTIMOX" strategy, or optimization of oxaliplatin, aims to limit exposure to oxaliplatin in order to prevent cumulative, and potentially dose-limiting, neurotoxicity while maintaining antitumor benefit. The OPTIMOX1 and subsequent OPTIMOX2 studies confirmed the feasibility of interrupting oxaliplatin after 3 months of therapy while necessarily continuing 5-FU/LV until disease progression, followed by oxaliplatin reintroduction. These studies provide clear support for a stop-and-go approach to oxaliplatin during FOLFOX therapy for metastatic disease. However, an early preplanned total chemotherapy-free holiday, including cessation of 5-FU/LV, was shown to compromise clinical outcome and is not advisable. The impact of a stop-and-go approach for patients on a bevacizumab-containing regimen is currently being explored in the OPTIMOX3-DREAM study.

An alternative approach to reduction of toxicity is to utilize individual agents sequentially, rather than in combination, and reserve combination therapy for second-line treatment following upfront 5-FU/LV. Three recent European studies have reported similar survival in patients initially treated with infusional 5-FU/LV or capecitabine followed by combination therapy (FOLFOX, FOLFIRI, CapeOX) compared to patients that received upfront combination treatment.

Novel Targeted Agents

Bevacizumab

Bevacizumab is a recombinant humanized monoclonal antibody (Fig. 1) targeted against VEGF, which is a proangiogenic growth factor that is overexpressed in CRC as well as in a wide range of solid human cancers. Bevacizumab monotherapy does not appear to have significant activity in mCRC. Conversely, it has considerable activity when used in combination with commonly used chemotherapies, including 5-FU, irinotecan, oxaliplatin, and combination with cetuximab is under investigation (5,69).

IFL + Bevacizumab

Hurwitz et al. reported phase III trial data showing that addition of bevacizumab to IFL led to statistically significant improvement of OS (20.3 vs 15.6 months; $P = .001$), RR (44.8% vs 34.8%; $P = .004$), and PFS (10.6 vs 6.2 months) in patients with mCRC (5). Patients who progressed after IFL plus bevacizumab then went on to receive second-line therapy with an oxaliplatin-based regimen and achieved an OS of 25.1 months, which was the longest median OS rendered by any first- and second-line combination therapy at the time (5).

FOLFOX-4 + Bevacizumab

The Eastern Cooperative Oncology Group 3,200 study, including 820 patients who were previously treated with first-line 5-FU, irinotecan either separately or as a combination regimen without bevacizumab, reported that adding bevacizumab to a second-line FOLFOX4 regimen improved median OS when compared to FOLFOX4 alone (12.5 vs 10.7 months; $P = .002$) (70).

FOLFOX-6 Versus XELOX Versus bFOL + Bevacizumab

Three Regimens of Eloxatin Evaluation (TREE) studies TREE-1 and TREE-2 studies first evaluated patients with mCRC to receive mFOLFOX6 (bolus and infusion FU and LV with oxaliplatin), bFOL (bolus FU and low-dose LV with oxaliplatin), or CapeOx (capecitabine with oxaliplatin), respectively. The study was later modified such that subsequent patients were randomized to the same regimens plus bevacizumab (TREE-2) (71). A total of 150 and 223 patients were randomly assigned in the TREE-1 and TREE-2 cohorts, respectively. Incidence of grade 3/4 treatment-related AEs during the first 12 weeks of treatment were 59%, 36%, and 67% for mFOLFOX6, bFOL, and CapeOx, respectively, (TREE-1) and 59%, 51%, and 56% for the corresponding treatments plus bevacizumab (TREE-2; primary end point). CapeOx toxicity in TREE-1 included grade 3/4 diarrhea (31%) and dehydration (27%); capecitabine dose reduction to 1,700 mg/m^2/day in TREE-2 resulted in improved tolerance. Overall response rates were 41%, 20%, and 27% (TREE-1) and 52%, 39%, and 46% (TREE-2); median OS was 19.2, 17.9, and 17.2 months (TREE-1) and 26.1, 20.4, and 24.6 months (TREE-2). For all treated patients, median OS was 18.2 months (95% CI 14.5–21.6; TREE-1) and 23.7 months (95% CI 21.3–26.8; TREE-2). The study revealed that the addition of bevacizumab to oxaliplatin and fluoropyrimidine regimens is well

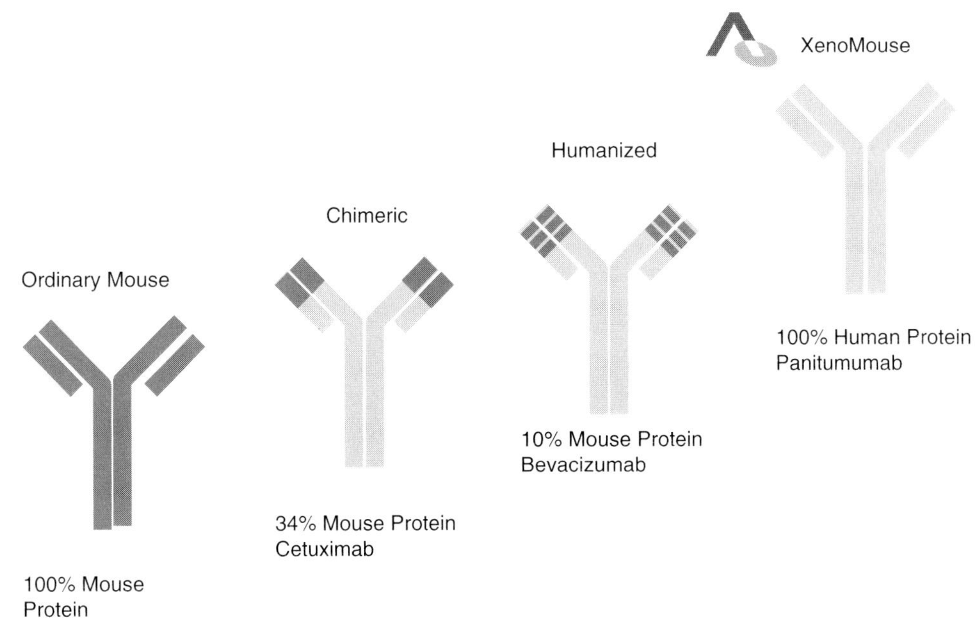

FIGURE 1 Targeted antibodies.

tolerated as first-line treatment of mCRC and does not markedly change overall toxicity. CapeOx tolerability and efficacy is improved with reduced-dose capecitabine. First-line oxaliplatin and fluoropyrimidine-based therapy plus bevacizumab resulted in a median OS of approximately 2 years.

FOLFOX-4 Versus XELOX + Bevacizumab

NO16966 is the first phase III trial to evaluate the efficacy of bevacizumab in combination with FOLFOX4 and XELOX regimens in the first-line treatment of mCRC. In this Intergroup study, 1,401 patients were randomized to receive FOLFOX4 (oxaliplatin and 5-FU/LV as described previously) or XELOX (oxaliplatin 130 mg/m^2 IV + capecitabine 1,000 mg/m^2 twice daily orally on days 1–14, every 3 weeks) plus bevacizumab (5 mg/kg to FOLFOX, 7.5 mg/kg to XELOX) or placebo in a 2 × 2 factorial design (60). The main end point of the recently presented results was PFS. Two primary objectives were: (*a*) XELOX is noninferior to FOLFOX (noninferiority concluded if upper limit of 97.5% CI = 1.23) and (*b*) Bevacizumab + chemotherapy is superior to placebo + chemotherapy (superiority concluded if P = .025). The results presented showed that the median PFS for XELOX-bevacizumab + FOLFOX4-bevacizumab was 9.3 versus 8.0 months for XELOX-placebo + FOLFOX4-placebo (HR 0.83, 97.5% CI,

0.72–0.95, P = .0023). Although the protocol specified the study of drug treatment until progression of disease (PD), only 56% of patients were treated in this manner, and 50% of patients discontinued for reasons unrelated to PD. Median PFS on the specified study treatment was 10.4 months for chemotherapy + bevacizumab versus 8.1 months for chemotherapy + placebo (HR = 0.63, P < .0001). Heterogeneity was detected in subgroups. No unexpected toxicity has been reported. In summary, this large, international phase III trial provided evidence from a first-line CRC phase III trial to show that the addition of bevacizumab to oxaliplatin-based chemotherapy regimens significantly improves PFS. This study further supports the use of bevacizumab in combination with standard first-line chemotherapy (60).

Use of Bevacizumab Beyond Progression

In a large, observational, bevacizumab treatment study (Bevacizumab Regimens: Investigation of Treatment Effects and Safety [BRiTE]) in patients who had mCRC suggested that use of bevacizumab beyond initial progression could improve OS (72). The 1,445 of 1,953 previously untreated patients with mCRC who were enrolled in BRiTE and who experienced PD were classified into three groups: no post-PD treatment (n = 253), post-PD treatment without bevacizumab (no

BBP; $n=531$), and BBP ($n=642$). Relevant baseline and on-study variables, including BBP, were analyzed with a Cox model with respect to their independent effect on survival beyond first PD. Median OS was 25.1 months (95% CI, 23.4–27.5 months), and median PFS was 10.0 months in the overall BRiTE population. Baseline and postbaseline factors were well balanced between the BBP and no-BBP groups. Median OS rates were 12.6, 19.9, and 31.8 months in the no post-PD treatment, no-BBP, and BBP groups, respectively. In multivariate analyses, compared with no BBP, BBP was strongly and independently associated with improved survival (HR=0.48; $P<.001$). Hypertension that required medication was the only bevacizumab-related safety event that occurred more frequently in the BBP group (24.6% vs 19.2%).

Bevacizumab in Third Line

Bevacizumab as a third-line therapy appears to have very limited activity in patients who failed previous treatment with oxaliplatin- or irinotecan-based regimens (73). Optimal duration of bevacizumab, particularly in patients who progressed on first-line combination therapy with bevacizumab, is unclear at this time. The Southwest Oncology Group is conducting a phase II trial in an attempt to answer this question.

Toxicities of Bevacizumab

Bevacizumab is generally well tolerated and has very few overlapping toxicities with chemotherapeutic agents. Hurwitz et al. reported grade 3 hypertension (11%), which was managed with oral medications, and increased risk of gastrointestinal perforation (1.5%) (5). However, there was no significant difference in treatment-related hospitalization, in treatment delay due to toxicity, or in the 60-day rate of death from all causes. Scappaticci (74) by reviewing 1,745 patients who received bevacizumab, noted an approximately twofold increased risk of arterial thromboembolic events. Bevacizumab was also associated with bleeding (2–9.3%), proteinuria (1–2%), and poor wound healing (1–2%) (72). These side effects should be considered when clinicians evaluate patients for the use of bevacizumab. The recommended dose of bevacizumab in treating first-line mCRC is 5 mg/kg IV administered over 90 minutes, while 10 mg/kg IV is the dose for second-line treatment. A dose of 7.5 mg/kg IV every 3 weeks can be used when bevacizumab is used with capecitabine-containing regimens.

Therapeutics: Oncology

Cetuximab

Cetuximab is a recombinant human/mouse chimeric EGFR monoclonal antibody (Fig. 1). EGFR is overexpressed in CRC as well as in a broad range of solid tumors. The efficacy of cetuximab therapy and other anti-EGFR MoAbs is confined to patients with WT K-ras (see chapter on K-ras).

Third-Line Single Agent or + Irinotecan

Cetuximab is approved as a single agent (FDA) or in combination with irinotecan (European Medicines Agency and FDA) for patients with EGFR-expressing tumors who had progressed on a previous irinotecan-based chemotherapy regimen. The approval of cetuximab in this setting followed the positive results of the Bowel Oncology and Cetuximab Antibody (BOND) study that was conducted in 56 centers throughout Europe (74). This study compared the efficacy of cetuximab/irinotecan with cetuximab alone in mCRC refractory to irinotecan-based chemotherapy. A total of 329 patients were randomized in a 2:1 setting to the combination or the cetuximab-alone arm. Upon PD in the cetuximab-alone arm, patients were allowed to be switched to the combination arm. This applied to half of the patients in this group. Patients in the BOND study were heavily pretreated. The efficacy parameters (ORR, disease control rate [DCR], and TTP) showed a statistically significant advantage in favor of the combination arm. Keeping in mind the considerable pretreatment of those patients, a DCR of 32.4% in the cetuximab alone arm and, particularly, 55.5% in the combination arm were convincing results. These encouraging results confirmed data from earlier phase II studies.

The Monoclonal Antibody Erbitux in a European Pre-License (MABEL) study was designed to investigate the combination of cetuximab and irinotecan under BOND-study conditions in a larger community practice setting. A total of 1,147 patients with irinotecan-refractory mCRC from eight European countries were included in this multicenter, uncontrolled trial (76). The ORR was 20%, the DCR was 45%, and the OS at that time was 9.2 months.

Last year, Jonker et al. published the results of a phase III clinical trial comparing cetuximab plus BSC with BSC alone in 572 patients who had mCRC expressing EGFR and who had been previously treated with a fluoropyrimidine, irinotecan, and oxaliplatin or had contraindications to treatment with these drugs (77). The primary end point was to demonstrate an advantage in OS. In comparison with BSC ($n=285$) alone, cetuximab treatment ($n=287$) was associated with a significant improvement in OS ($P=.005$) and in PFS ($P=.001$) (77). The median OS was 6.1 months in the cetuximab group and 4.6 months in the BSC group. PR occurred in 23 patients (8%) in the cetuximab group, but none of the patients in the BSC group had a PR. The disease was stable in an additional 31.4% of patients assigned to cetuximab and in 10.9% of patients assigned to BSC.

Second Line

The Erbitux Plus Irinotecan in Colorectal Cancer (EPIC) trial is a randomized phase III trial investigating the efficacy of second-line irinotecan versus irinotecan plus cetuximab in patients with mCRC after progression or intolerance to a first-line oxaliplatin-based regimen (78). The ORR and PFS were better in the combination arm (16.36% vs 4.15% and 3.98 vs 2.56 months, respectively; $P<.0001$). There were no differences in OS, in part because of the large proportion of patients in the standard arm who received cetuximab upon disease progression.

FOLFIRI + Cetuximab

The phase III CRYSTAL (Cetuximab Combined with Irinotecan in First-Line Therapy for Metastatic Colorectal Cancer) study investigated the effectiveness of cetuximab in combination with the standard FOLFIRI regimen compared with FOLFIRI alone in the first-line treatment of unselected patients with EGFR-expressing mCRC (79). A total of 1,217 patients were included in the study. The addition of cetuximab significantly prolonged PFS (median PFS, 8.9 vs 8 months; $P<.05$), the primary end point of the study, and increased the ORR (47% vs 39%; $P<.005$). The 1-year PFS rate was 34% for the combination arm compared with 23% for the chemotherapy-alone arm (15% risk reduction for progression). A preliminary exploratory analysis showed a 9.8% of hepatic resection rate (R0) in patients with only liver metastasis treated with FOLFIRI plus cetuximab compared with 4.5% in patients treated with chemotherapy alone.

FOLFOX + Cetuximab

Preliminary results of a randomized phase II study by Schuch et al. (OPUS; Oxaliplatin and Cetuximab in first-line treatment of mCRC) have been recently presented, showing an increase in the ORR of patients treated with the combination of cetuximab and FOLFOX4 compared with patients treated with FOLFOX4 alone (80).

Toxicities of Cetuximab

Cetuximab was associated with acneiform rash (up to 88% of all patients) (Fig. 2), severe infusion reaction (3%), interstitial lung disease, and hypomagnesaemia. Cetuximab is administered with a loading dose of 400 mg/m^2 IV over 90 minutes, followed by a maintenance dose of 200 mg/m^2 IV given weekly.

A relationship between the incidence and severity of acne-like rash and response to anti-EGFR therapy has been suggested by numerous investigators. This positive correlation has led to the hypothesis of skin rash being a surrogate marker of the efficacy of EGFR inhibitors. The EVEREST (Evaluation of Various Erbitux Regimens by Means of Skin and Tumor Biopsies) trial tested this hypothesis in patients with irinotecan-refractory EGFR-expressing mCRC (81). In this study, patients were initially treated with cetuximab at the recommended doses in combination with irinotecan. After 3 weeks of treatment, patients who did not develop a grade = 2 skin rash were randomized to receive cetuximab at the same weekly dose (250 mg/m^2) or an escalation of cetuximab until skin toxicity grade > 2 appears up

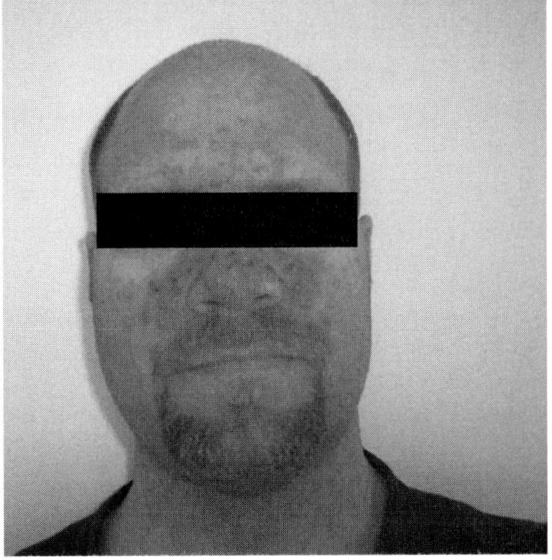

FIGURE 2 Acneiform rash associated with cetuximab and other anti-epidermal growth factor receptors.

to a maximum dose of 500 mg/m². Efficacy data has been recently reported and showed that, in patients who had no or mild skin rash in response to standard cetuximab dose, dose escalation (= 500 mg/m²) improved the response, reaching the ORR experienced by the patients who developed grade = 2 skin rash with the standard cetuximab dose (30% and 34%, respectively). Patients having grade 1 or no skin rash treated with standard cetuximab doses achieved an ORR of 13%.

Panitumumab

Panitumumab is a fully human monoclonal antibody (Fig. 1) to EGFR to enter clinical trials for the treatment of solid tumors. Like cetuximab (Erbitux; BMS), it is directed against the extracellular ligand-binding domain of the receptor and results in blockade of the essential downstream signaling pathways that are known to govern apoptosis, proliferation, and differentiation of both normal and neoplastic cell types in a wide array of tissues. It has a very high affinity for EGFR and has been generally well tolerated and associated with very few infusion reactions. As a fully human agent, panitumumab has not been associated with the formation of any antibodies directed against it that has been evidenced by a very reliable pharmacokinetic profile with possible dosing schedules ranging from 1 to 3 weeks. Similar to other agents targeting the EGFR pathway, a rash has been the primary toxicity and is dose dependent up to 2.5 mg/kg at which dose 100% of all patients have been affected. The antitumor activity of panitumumab has been tested in vitro and in vivo, and inhibition of tumor growth has been observed in numerous cancer models, particularly lung, kidney, and colorectal. It has been efficacious and well tolerated both as monotherapy and in combination with other chemotherapeutic agents. Several phase I trials, two phase II trials, and most recently a phase III trial in pretreated CRC have been carried out to date (82,83).

Third Line

Gibson et al. conducted a randomized phase III trial that compared panitumumab as a single agent to BSC in patients previously treated for mCRC. In this study, panitumumab was shown to be efficacious (46% reduction in the risk of tumor progression and a PR rate of 8%) with a manageable side effect profile (84).

First Line

The Panitumumab Advanced Colorectal Cancer Evaluation (PACCE) study is a phase IIIb randomized, open-label clinical trial evaluating oxaliplatin- and irinotecan-based chemotherapy and bevacizumab with and without panitumumab in the first-line treatment of patients with mCRC (85). The trial is powered to show a 30% reduction in PFS, the primary end point. The PACCE trial enrolled 1,054 patients (824 patients were randomized to receive oxaliplatin-based chemotherapy, and 230 patients were randomized to receive irinotecan-based chemotherapy) at 240 trial sites in the United States between Q1 2005 and Q3 2006. The combination-antibody arm failed to show superiority; in fact, it showed no difference in response rate and worse PFS and OS.

The Panitumumab Randomized Trial in Combination with Chemotherapy for Metastatic Colorectal Cancer to Determine Efficacy (PRIME) study randomized 1,183 patients to receive FOLFOX4 every 2 weeks with or without 6.0 mg/kg of panitumumab (86). KRAS status was identified after enrollment but prior to treatment, and David Reese, MD, executive medical director, Global Development, who heads the Vectibix program at Amgen, said 60% of patients had wild-type KRAS. For these patients, median PFS was 1.6 months longer in the panitumumab group than in the chemotherapy-alone group, at 9.6 versus 8.0 months, respectively ($P = .02$), a significant result. Blinded central review determined that 55% of patients with wild-type KRAS responded to treatment in the combination group compared with 48% of wild-type KRAS patients in the FOLFOX-only group. Median OS was 18.8 months in the group that received only FOLFOX and has not yet been reached in the panitumumab-combination arm. Results with panitumumab were, as expected, inferior in patients with KRAS mutations; the drug's recently revised label advises against using panitumumab in this patient population. AEs were as expected, with more patients in the panitumumab cohort reporting events typically associated with EGFR inhibitors, such as rash, diarrhea, and hypomagnesemia.

Second Line

The multicenter, randomized, phase III trial (study 181) by Amgen involved 1,186 patients who received either 6.0 mg/kg of panitumumab and FOLFIRI every 2 weeks or FOLFIRI alone (87). The primary end points were PFS and OS; secondary end points were objective response rate, TTP, duration of response, and safety by KRAS status. The AEs included skin toxicity, diarrhea, and hypomagnesemia. These results add to the growing body of evidence confirming the utility of KRAS as a predictive biomarker. Originally designed to compare the treatment effect in the overall population, the study was amended to analyze outcomes with respect to the presence or absence of activating mutations in KRAS in the tumor itself. Tumor KRAS status was ascertained in more than 90% of patients enrolled in this trial.

This is the first large, randomized study prospectively analyzed by KRAS status as a predictive biomarker for EGFR treatment in second line mCRC. In patients with WT KRAS tumors, panitumumab significantly improved PFS when added to FOLFIRI (median 5.9 vs. 3.9 months, HR = 0.73, P = 0.004). Response rate was improved in WT KRAS patients with panitumumab (35% vs. 10%). Overall survival was also improved in patients with WT KRAS tumors with the addition of panitumumab to FOLFIRI (median 14.5 vs. 12.5 months, HR = 0.85, P = 0.12).

Combination of Targeted Agents

Following the presentation of evidence of activity for both cetuximab and bevacizumab, the combination of these two agents was explored in a small randomized phase II trial, known as the BOND 2 trial (87). Enrolled patients had failed an irinotecan-based regimen and were naive to both cetuximab and bevacizumab. One cohort was treated with cetuximab, bevacizumab, and irinotecan, and one cohort was treated with the two antibodies alone. Toxicity was as would have been expected from the individual agents alone. Activity appeared favorable compared to historic controls. The promising results from the BOND-2 study (88) are in contradiction with the negative results of the PACCE trial (84). These efficacy data suggest that there is a lack of biologic synergy between panitumumab and bevacizumab in combination with chemotherapy. The contradictory results between the BOND-2 and the PACCE studies support the idea to continue with large trials evaluating this double VEGF and EGFR inhibition strategy.

This finding was further supported by the CAIRO-2 study, a phase III trial which also found similar result for capecitabine, oxaliplatin, bevacizumab plus/minus cetuximab (89). Therefore, neither panitumumab nor cetuximab plus bevacizumab in combination with chemotherapy should be routinely used in clinical practice. A large phase III clinical trial is evaluating the feasibility and efficacy of this approach, the US SWOG 80405 NCI Intergroup study.

The double inhibition of the EGFR by simultaneously blocking the external portion—the ectodomain—of the receptor, and the catalytic TK endodomain is another attractive option. Preclinical evidence suggests that the combination of cetuximab and gefitinib have synergistic activity against EGFR-expressing cell lines. Meaningful clinical activity of the combination of gefitinib and cetuximab was observed in a phase I study presented by Baselga et al. at the 2006 ASCO Annual Meeting (89). In this trial, 43 patients with advanced EGFR-expressing CRC (56%), head and neck cancer (39%), or non–small cell lung cancer (5%), were treated with the combination of gefitinib and cetuximab. The primary objective of the study was to determine the maximum tolerated dose and the recommended dose of the combination. One out of 43 patients (2%) had a complete response (CR, a patient with a head and neck cancer), and 6 patients (14%) had a PR (5 patients with CRC and 1 patient with a head and neck tumor). The median TTP of patients with chemotherapy-refractory CRC included in this study was 3.2 months. Skin rash was the most frequent toxicity of this combination (grade 3 in 23% of the patients). No significant pharmacokinetic interaction between cetuximab and gefitinib was observed. The recommended dose of both agents used in combination was the same as when administered as single agents. The authors concluded that the combination of cetuximab and gefitinib is feasible and that combined anti-EGFR therapy deserves further evaluation.

These combination strategies are now being developed in several trials. The identification of patients more likely to obtain benefit from these treatments in the future might help to improve the efficacy of these therapies. Advances are being made in the identification of biomarkers of sensitivity for targeted agents.

■ METASTESECTOMY

Surgery is the only curative option for patients with liver metastases of CRC, but few patients present with resectable hepatic lesions. Chemotherapy is increasingly used to downstage initially unresectable disease and allow for potentially curative surgery. Standard chemotherapy regimens convert 10% to 20% of cases to resectable disease in unselected populations and 30% to 40% of those with disease confined to the liver (88). One strategy to further increase the number of candidates eligible for surgery is the addition of active targeted agents such as cetuximab and bevacizumab to standard chemotherapy.

Metastesectomy should always be considered in eligible patients because the procedure is potentially curative, with a 5-year survival rate of almost 40% (91). Such patients with metastases to the liver only should be evaluated by a hepatobiliary surgeon with experience in the procedure, with the exception of those patients with extensive multifocal bilobar involvement. The standard approach is to proceed directly to surgery, but there are several potential advantages to neoadjuvant chemotherapy and these should always be discussed as a part of a multidisciplinary approach.

Perioperative FOLFOX given for 3 months before and after surgery showed a benefit in a recent study. PFS at 3 years was improved in a subset of patients considered eligible for resection (36.2% vs 28.1%, $P = .041$) and in those who underwent resection (42.4% vs 33.2%, $P = .025$). Reversible postoperative complications occurred more often after chemotherapy than after surgery (25% vs 16%, $P = .04$) but were overall tolerable (92). This study provides evidence to suggest a therapeutic benefit to perioperative chemotherapy. Whether chemotherapy is best used before or after surgery remains unresolved.

Data from a phase III trial indicate that cetuximab increases the number of patients eligible for secondary hepatic resection, as well as the rate of complete resection when combined with first-line treatment with the FOLFIRI regimen. The safety profiles of preoperative cetuximab or bevacizumab have not been thoroughly assessed, but preliminary evidence indicates that these agents do not increase surgical mortality or exacerbate chemotherapy-related hepatotoxicity, such as steatosis (5-FU), steatohepatitis (irinotecan), and sinusoidal obstruction (oxaliplatin). Secondary resection is a valid treatment goal for certain patients with initially unresectable liver metastases and an important end point for future clinical trials.

Emerging Targets and Therapeutics

The treatment of colon cancer has definitely advanced in the last decade as newer and more active cytotoxic chemotherapy agents as well as targeted monoclonal antibodies have become available. Better understanding of different fundamental molecular changes in carcinogenesis has resulted in the emergence of such therapeutic targets in the treatment of colon cancer. Efforts to identify the critical molecular biomarkers to predict for either clinical response to chemotherapy and/or targeted therapies and/or the drug-specific side effects are warranted. At the same time, many clinical questions remain unanswered.

Can the combination of bevacizumab plus cetuximab provide more benefit than each on its own, when added to chemotherapy? Two negative trials have been reported thus far. CALGB 80405 is a three-arm comparison of chemotherapy, either FOLFOX or FOLFIRI, plus cetuximab, bevacizumab, or both and hopefully will help to answer this question.

Another important question that need further attention is: Is there benefit to continuing bevacizumab beyond first progression? Results from the BRiTE registry suggest there might be, but this is a registry, not a randomized trial, and so the question remains unanswered. The BOND 2.5 study, a single-arm phase II study of cetuximab, bevacizumab, and irinotecan in patients who have progressed through both irinotecan and bevacizumab, will attempt to give some preliminary insight into this question. The SWOG 0600/iBET study follows on this theme. Patients who have progressed following a prior bevacizumab-containing regimen will be randomized to continue bevacizumab or not. Another attempt to further explore the question of continuation of bevacizumab beyond PD, while planning an oxaliplatin interruption, is being addressed in the OPTIMOX3-DREAM study. This randomized phase III trial is studying the interim continuation of bevacizumab plus erlotinib following six cycles of FOLFOX or XELOX plus bevacizumab in patients with stable or responding disease. At the time of PD, patients may resume initial therapy with FOLFOX or XELOX plus bevacizumab.

■ REFERENCES

1. Jemal A, Siegel R, Ward E, Murray T, Xu J, Thun MJ. Cancer statistics, 2007. *CA Cancer J Clin* 2007;57(1):43–66.

2. Wu X, Chen VW, Martin J, et al. Comparative Analysis of Incidence Rates Subcommittee, Data Evaluation and Publication Committee, North American Association of Central Cancer Registries. Subsite-specific colorectal cancer incidence rates and stage distributions among Asians and Pacific Islanders in the United States, 1995 to 1999. *Cancer Epidemiol Biomarkers Prev* 2004;13(7):1215–1222.

3. Meta-Analysis Group in Cancer. Modulation of fl uorouracil by leucovorin in patientswith advanced colorectal cancer: an updated meta-analysis. *J Clin Oncol* 2004;22:3766–3775.

4. Saif MW, Kang SP, Chu E. Treatment of metastatic colorectal cancer: from cytotoxic agents to molecular agents and multitargeted strategies. *Oncology (Williston Park, NY)* 2006;20(14 Suppl 10):11–19.

5. Hurwitz H, Fehrenbacher L, Novotny W, et al. Bevacizumab plus irinotecan, fluorouracil, and leucovorin for metastatic colorectal cancer. *N Engl J Med* 2004;350(23):2335–2342.

6. American Joint Committee on Cancer. Colon and rectum. In American Joint Committee on Cancer: AJCC Cancer Staging Manual, 6th ed. New York: Springer-Verlag, 2002, 113–124.

7. Compton CC, Greene FL. The staging of colorectal cancer: 2004 and beyond. *CA Cancer J Clin* 2004;54(6):295–308.

8. Saif MW. Targeted agents for adjuvant therapy of colon cancer. *Clin Colorectal Cancer* 2006;6(1):46–51.

9. Smith RE, Colangelo L, Wieand HS, Begovic M, Wolmark N. Randomized trial of adjuvant therapy in colon carcinoma: 1-year results of NSABP protocol C-01. *J Natl Cancer Inst* 2004;96(15):1128–1132.

10. Moertel CG, Fleming TR, Macdonald JS, et al. Levamisole and fluorouracil for adjuvant therapy of resected colon carcinoma. *N Engl J Med* 1990;322(6):352–358.

11. Moertel CG, Fleming TR, Macdonald JS, et al. Intergroup study of fluorouracil plus levamisole as adjuvant therapy for stage II/Dukes' B2 colon cancer. *J Clin Oncol* 1995;13(12):2936–2943.

12. O'Connell MJ. A Phase III trial of 5-fluorouracil and leucovorin in the treatment ofadvanced colorectal cancer. A Mayo Clinic/North Central Cancer Treatment Groupstudy. *Cancer* 1989;63(6 Suppl):1026–1030.

13. InternationalMulticentrePooledAnalysisofColonCancer Trials (IMPACT) Investigators. Efficacy of adjuvant fluorouracil and folinic acid in colon cancer. *Lancet* 1995;345:939–944.

14. Haller DG, Catalano PJ, Macdonald JS, et al. Phase III study of fluorouracil, leucovorin, and levamisole in high-risk stage II and III colon cancer: final report of Intergroup 0089. *J Clin Oncol* 2005;23(34):8671–8678.

15. Andre T, Colin P, Louvet C, et al. Semimonthly versus monthly regimen of fluorouracil and leucovorin administered for 24 or 36 weeks as adjuvant therapy in stage II and III colon cancer: results of a randomized trial. *J Clin Oncol* 2003;21(15):2896–2903.

16. Andre T, Quinaux E, Louvet C, et al. Updated results at 6 year of the GERCOR C96.1 Phase III study comparing LV5FU2 to monthly 5FU-leucovorin (mFUfol) as adjuvant treatment for Dukes B2 and C colon cancer patients [Abstract 3522]. *J Clin Oncol* 2005;23(16 Suppl).

17. Chau I, Norman AR, Cunningham D, et al. A randomised comparison between 6 months of bolus fluorouracil/leucovorin and 12 weeks of protracted venous infusion fluorouracil as adjuvant treatment in colorectal cancer. *Ann Oncol* 2005;16(4):549–557.

18. Poplin EA, Benedetti JK, Estes NC, et al. Phase III Southwest Oncology Group 9415/Intergroup 0153 randomized trial of fluorouracil, leucovorin, and levamisole versus fluorouracil continuous infusion and levamisole for adjuvant treatment of stage III and high-risk stage II colon cancer. *J Clin Oncol* 2005;23(9):1819–1825.

19. André T, Boni C, Navarro M, et al. Improved overall survival with oxaliplatin, fluorouracil, and leucovorin as adjuvant treatment in stage II or III colon cancer in the MOSAIC trial. *J Clin Oncol* 2009 Jul 1;27(19):3109–3116.

20. Kuebler JP, Wieand HS, O'Connell MJ, et al. Oxaliplatin combined with weekly bolus fluorouracil and leucovorin as surgical adjuvant chemotherapy for stage II and III colon cancer: results from NSABP C-07. *J Clin Oncol* 2007;25(16):2198–2204.

21. Saltz LB, Niedzwiecki D, Hollis D, et al. Irinotecan plus fluorouracil/leucovorin (IFL) versus fluorouracil/leucovorin alone (FL) in stage III colon cancer (intergroup trial CALGB C89803). *J Clin Oncol* 2004; 22 (July 15 Suppl): 3500.

22. Van Cutsem E, Labianca R, Hossfeld D, et al. Randomized Phase III trial comparinginfused irinotecan/5-fl uorouracil (5-FU) folinic acid (IF) versus 5-FU/FA (F) in stageIII colon cancer patients (pts) (PETACC 3) [Abstract LBA8]. *J Clin Oncol* 2005;23(16Suppl).

23. Ychou M, Raoul JL, Douillard JY, et al. A Phase III randomized trial of LV5FU2 + CPT-11 vs. LV5FU2 alone in adjuvant high risk colon cancer (FNCLCC Accord02/FFCD9802) [Abstract 3502]. *J Clin Oncol* 2005;23(16 Suppl):3502.

24. Wolmark N. #LBA4. Presented at: ASCO 2009 Annual Meeting; May 29–June 2, 2009; Orlando.

25. Twelves C, Scheithauer W, McKendrick J, et al. 5-year overall survival update from the X-ACT trial of capecitabine vs 5-FU/LV as adjuvant treatment for stage III colon cancer [Abstract]. *Eur J Cancer Supplements* 2007;5(6):1.

26. Haller D, Tabernero J, Maroan J, et al. First efficacy findings from a randomized phase III trial of Capecitabine + Oxaliplatin vs. bolus 5-Fu/LV for stage III colon cancer (NO 16968/XELOXA study). *Eur J Cancer* 2009;7(3):4.

27. Gill S, Loprinzi CL, Sargent DJ, et al. Pooled analysis of fluorouracil-based adjuvant therapy for stage II and III colon cancer: who benefits and by how much? *J Clin Oncol* 2004;22(10):1797–1806.

28. Figueredo A, Charette ML, Maroun J, Brouwers MC, Zuraw L. Adjuvant therapy for stage II colon cancer: a systematic review from the Cancer Care Ontario Program in evidence-based care's gastrointestinal cancer disease site group. *J Clin Oncol* 2004;22(16):3395–3407.

29. Benson AB, Schrag D, Somerfield MR, et al. American Society of Clinical Oncology recommendations on adjuvant chemotherapy for stage II colon cancer. *J Clin Oncol* 2004;22(16):3408–3419.

30. Le Voyer TE, Sigurdson ER, Hanlon AL, et al. Colon cancer survival is associated with increasing number of lymph nodes analyzed: a secondary survey of intergroup trial INT-0089. *J Clin Oncol* 2003;21(15):2912–2919.

31. Meyerhardt JA, Mayer RJ. Systemic therapy for colorectal cancer. *N Engl J Med* 2005;352(5):476–487.

32. Poon MA, O'Connell MJ, Moertel CG, et al. Biochemical modulation of fluorouracil: evidence of significant improvement of survival and quality of life in patients with advanced colorectal carcinoma. *J Clin Oncol* 1989;7(10):1407–1418.

33. The Meta-Analysis Group in Cancer. Toxicity of fluorouracil in patients with advanced colorectal cancer: effect of administration schedule and prognostic factors. *J Clin Oncol* 1998;11:3537–3541.

34. Buroker TR, O'Connell MJ, Wieand HS, et al. Randomized comparison of two schedules of fluorouracil and leucovorin in the treatment of advanced colorectal cancer. *J Clin Oncol* 1994;12(1):14.

35. Wang WS, Lin JK, Chiou TJ, et al. Randomized trial comparing weekly bolus 5-fluorouracil plus leucovorin versus monthly 5-day 5-fluorouracil plus leucovorin in metastatic colorectal cancer. *Hepatogastroenterology* 2000;47(36):1599.

36. The Meta-Analysis Group in Cancer. Efficacy of intravenous continuous infusion of fluorouracil compared with bolus administration in advanced colorectal cancer. *J Clin Oncol* 1998;16:301–308.

37. Weh HJ, Wilke HJ, Dierlamm J, et al. Weekly therapy with folinic acid (FA) and high-dose 5-fluorouracil (5-FU) 24-hour infusion in pretreated patients with metastatic colorectal carcinoma. A multicenter study by the Association of Medical Oncology of the German Cancer Society (AIO). *Ann Oncol* 1994;5(3):233–237.

38. de Gramont A, Bosset JF, Milan C, et al. Randomized trial comparing monthly low-dose leucovorin and fluorouracil bolus with bimonthly high-dose leucovorin and fluorouracil bolus plus continuous infusion for advanced colorectal cancer: a French intergroup study. *J Clin Oncol* 1997;15(2):808.

39. Engstrom PF, Arnoletti JP, Benson AB 3rd, et al. National Comprehensive Cancer Network. NCCN Clinical Practice Guidelines in Oncology: Colon cancer. *J Natl Compr Canc Netw.* 2009 Sep;7(8):778–831.

40. Twelves C; Xeloda Colorectal Cancer Group. Capecitabine as first-line treatment in colorectal cancer. Pooled data from two large, phase III trials. *Eur J Cancer.* 2002;suppl(2):15–20.

41. Saif MW. Capecitabine versus continuous-infusion 5-fluorouracil for colorectal cancer: a retrospective efficacy and safety comparison. *Clin Colorectal Cancer* 2005;5(2):89–100.

42. Vanhoefer U, Harstrick A, Achterrath W, Cao S, Seeber S, Rustum YM. Irinotecan in the treatment of colorectal cancer: clinical overview. *J Clin Oncol* 2001;19(5):1501–1518.

43. Cunningham D, Pyrhönen S, James RD, et al. Randomised trial of irinotecan plus supportive care versus supportive care alone after fluorouracil failure for patients with metastatic colorectal cancer. *Lancet* 1998;352(9138):1413.

44. Douillard JY, Cunningham D, Roth AD, et al. Irinotecan combined with fluorouracil compared with fluorouracil alone as first-line treatment for metastatic colorectal cancer: a multicentre randomised trial. *Lancet* 2000;355(9209):1041.

45. Köhne CH, van Cutsem E, Wils J, et al.; European Organisation for Research and Treatment of Cancer Gastrointestinal Group. Phase III study of weekly high-dose infusional fluorouracil plus folinic acid with or without irinotecan in patients with metastatic colorectal cancer: European Organisation for Research and Treatment of Cancer Gastrointestinal Group Study 40986. *J Clin Oncol* 2005;23(22):4856.

46. Saltz LB, Cox JV, Blanke C, et al. Irinotecan plus fluorouracil and leucovorin for metastatic colorectal cancer. Irinotecan Study Group. *N Engl J Med* 2000;343(13):905.

47. Fuchs CS, Marshall J, Barrueco J. Randomized, controlled trial of irinotecan plus infusional, bolus, or oral fluoropyrimidines in first-line treatment of metastatic colorectal cancer: updated results from the BICC-C study. *J Clin Oncol* 2008;26(4):689–690.

48. Ahn KH, Jung YS, Park YH, et al. Phase II trial of irinotecan and capecitabine inpatients with advanced colorectal cancer [Abstract 3714]. *J Clin Oncol* 2005;23(16Suppl):299s.

49. Patt YZ, Leibmann J, Diamondidis D, et al. Capicitabine (X) plus irinotecan (XELIRI)as first-line treatment for metastatic colorectal cancer (MCRC): final safety findings from a Phase II trial [Abstract 3602]. *J Clin Oncol* 2004;22(14 Suppl):271.

50. Bajetta E, Di Bartolomeo M, Mariani L, et al.; Italian Trials in Medical Oncology (I.T.M.O.) Group. Randomized multicenter Phase II trial of two different schedules of irinotecan combined with capecitabine as first-line treatment in metastatic colorectal carcinoma. *Cancer* 2004;100(2):279.

51. Grothey A, Goldberg RM. A review of oxaliplatin and its clinical use in colorectal cancer. *Expert Opin Pharmacother* 2004;5(10):2159–2170.

52. de Gramont A, Figer A, Seymour M, et al. Leucovorin and fluorouracil with or without oxaliplatin as first-line treatment in advanced colorectal cancer. *J Clin Oncol* 2000;18(16):2938.

53. Cassidy J, Tabernero J, Twelves C, et al. XELOX (capecitabine plus oxaliplatin): active first-line therapy for patients with metastatic colorectal cancer. *J Clin Oncol* 2004;22(11):2084.

54. Cassidy J, Clarke S, Díaz-Rubio E, et al. Randomized phase III study of capecitabine plus oxaliplatin compared with fluorouracil/folinic acid plus oxaliplatin as first-line therapy for metastatic colorectal cancer. *J Clin Oncol* 2008;26(12):2006–2012.

55. Goldberg RM, Sargent DJ, Morton RF, et al. A randomized controlled trial of fluorouracil plus leucovorin, irinotecan, and oxaliplatin combinations in patients with previously untreated metastatic colorectal cancer. *J Clin Oncol* 2004;22(1):23.

56. Tournigand C, André T, Achille E, et al. FOLFIRI followed by FOLFOX6 or the reverse sequence in advanced colorectal cancer: a randomized GERCOR study. *J Clin Oncol* 2004;22(2):229.

57. Colucci G, Gebbia V, Paoletti G, et al.; Gruppo Oncologico Dell'Italia Meridionale. Phase III randomized trial of FOLFIRI versus FOLFOX4 in the treatment of advanced colorectal cancer: a multicenter study of the Gruppo Oncologico Dell'Italia Meridionale. *J Clin Oncol* 2005;23(22):4811–4814.

58. Arkenau H, Schmoll H, Kubicka S, et al. Infusional 5-fl uorouracil/folinic acid plusoxaliplatin (FUFOX) versus capecitabine plus oxaliplatin (CAPOX) as fi rst line treatment of metastatic colorectal cancer (MCRC): results of the safety and effi cacy analysis [Abstract 3507]. *J Clin Oncol* 2005;23(16 Suppl):247s.

59. Jordan K, Kellner O, Kegel T, Schmoll HJ, Grothey A. Phase II trial of capecitabine/irinotecan and capecitabine/oxaliplatin in advanced gastrointestinal cancers. *Clin Colorectal Cancer.* 2004; May;4(1):46–50.

60. Saltz LB, Clarke S, Díaz-Rubio E, et al. Bevacizumab in combination with oxaliplatin-based chemotherapy as first-line therapy in metastatic colorectal cancer: a randomized phase III study. *J Clin Oncol* 2008;26(12):2013–2019.

61. Grothey A, Sargent D, Goldberg RM, et al. Survival of patients with advanced colorectal cancer improves with the availability of fluorouracil-leucovorin, irinotecan, and oxaliplatin in the course of treatment. *J Clin Oncol* 2004;22:1209–1214.

62. Maughan T, on Behalf of the NCRI Colorectal Group. Fluorouracil, oxaliplatin, CPT-11 (irinotecan), use and sequencing, in advanced colorectal cancer: the UK MRCFOCUS Trial [Abstract 165]. *J Clin Oncol* 2005;23(16 Suppl).

63. Falcone A, Ricci S, Brunetti I, et al. Gruppo Oncologico Nord Ovest. Phase III trial of infusional fluorouracil, leucovorin, oxaliplatin, and irinotecan (FOLFOXIRI) compared with infusional fluorouracil, leucovorin, and irinotecan (FOLFIRI) as first-line treatment for metastatic colorectal cancer: the Gruppo Oncologico Nord Ovest. *J Clin Oncol* 2007;25(13):1670–1676.

64. Souglakos J, Androulakis N, Syrigos K, et al. FOLFOXIRI (folinic acid, 5-fluorouracil, oxaliplatin and irinotecan) vs FOLFIRI (folinic acid, 5-fluorouracil and irinotecan) as first-line treatment in metastatic colorectal cancer (MCC): a multicentre randomised phase III trial from the Hellenic Oncology Research Group (HORG). *Br J Cancer* 2006;94(6):798–805.

65. J. Maroun, D. Jonker, C. Cripps, R. Goel, D. Lister, G. Chiritescu. Encouraging results from a phase I study of capecitabine (X), irinotecan (I) and oxaliplatin (O) as first-line therapy in patients (pts) with metastatic colorectal cancer (MCRC). *Journal of Clinical Oncology, 2007 ASCO Annual Meeting Proceedings Part I*. Vol 25, No. 18S (June 20 Supplement), 2007:4086.

66. Maughan TS, Kerr J, Ledermann M, et al. Comparison of intermittent and continuouspalliative chemotherapy for advanced colorectal cancer: a multicenter randomizedtrial. *Lancet* 2003;361:457–464.

67. de Gramont A, Cervantes A, Andre T, et al. OPTIMOX study: FOLFOX/LV5FU2compared to FOLFOX 4 in patients with advanced colorectal cancer [Abstract 3525]. *J Clin Oncol* 2004;22(14 Suppl):251.

68. Chibaudel B, Maindrault-Goebel F, Lledo G, et al. Can chemotherapy be discontinued in unresectable metastatic colorectal cancer? The GERCOR OPTIMOX2 Study. *J Clin Oncol* 2009;27(34):5727–5733.

69. Labianca R, Floriani I, Cortesi E, et al. Alternating versus continuous "FOLFIRI" inadvanced colorectal cancer (ACC): a randomized "GISCAD" trial [Abstract 3505]. *J Clin Oncol* 2006;24(18 Suppl):3505.

70. Giantonio BJ, Catalano PJ, Meropol NJ, et al. Eastern Cooperative Oncology Group Study E3200. Bevacizumab in combination with oxaliplatin, fluorouracil, and leucovorin (FOLFOX4) for previously treated metastatic colorectal cancer: results from the Eastern Cooperative Oncology Group Study E3200. *J Clin Oncol* 2007;25(12):1539–1544.

71. Hochester HS, Welles L, Hart L, et al. Safety and effi cacy of bevacizumab whenadded to oxaliplatin/fluoropyrimidine regimens as first line treatment of metastaticcolorectal cancer: TREE 1 & 2 study [Abstract 3515]. *J Clin Oncol* 2005;23(16Suppl).

72. Grothey A, Sugrue MM, Purdie DM, et al. Bevacizumab beyond first progression is associated with prolonged overall survival in metastatic colorectal cancer: results from a large observational cohort study (BRiTE). *J Clin Oncol* 2008;26(33):5326–5334.

73. Chen HX, Mooney M, Boron M, et al. Bevacizumab (BV) plus 5-FU/leucovorin (FU/LV) for advanced colorectal cancer (CRC) that progressed after standard chemotherapies:an NCI Treatment Referral Center trial (TRC-0301) [Abstract 3515]. *J Clin Oncol* 2004;22:249a.

74. Scappatticci FA, Skillings JR, Holden SR, et al. Arterial thromboembolic events in patients with metastatic carcinoma treated with chemotheraphy and bevacizumab. *J Natl Cancer Inst* 2007;99(16):1232–1239.

75. Cunningham D, Humblet Y, Siena S, et al. Cetuximab monotherapy and cetuximab plus irinotecan in irinotecan-refractory metastatic colorectal cancer. *N Engl J Med* 2004;351(4):337–345.

76. Wilke H, Glynne-Jones R, Thaler J, et al. Cetuximab plus irinotecan in heavily pretreated metastatic colorectal cancer progressing on irinotecan: MABEL Study. *J Clin Oncol* 2008;26(33):5335–5343.

77. Jonker DJ, O'Callaghan CJ, Karapetis CS, et al. Cetuximab for the treatment of colorectal cancer. *N Engl J Med* 2007;357(20):2040–2048.

78. Sobrero AF, Maurel J, Fehrenbacher L, et al. EPIC: phase III trial of cetuximab plus irinotecan after fluoropyrimidine and oxaliplatin failure in patients with metastatic colorectal cancer. *J Clin Oncol* 2008;26(14):2311–2319.

79. Van Cutsem E, Nowacki M, Lang I, et al. Randomized phase III study of irinotecan and 5-FU/FA with or without cetuximab in the first-line treatment of patients with metastatic colorectal cancer (mCRC): The CRYSTAL trial. *Journal of Clinical Oncology, 2007 ASCO Annual Meeting Proceedings (Post-Meeting Edition).* Vol 25, No 18S (June 20 Supplement), 2007: 4000.

80. Schuch G, Staroslawska E, Nowacki M, et al. Cetuximab plus 5-FU/FA/oxaliplatin (FOLFOX-4) in the first-line treatment of mCRC: OPUS, a phase II study [Abstract O-0022]. *Ann Oncol* 2007;18(suppl 7):vii18.

81. Tabernero J, Cervantes A, Ciardiello F, et al. *Correlation of efficacy to KRAS status (wt vs. mut) in patients (pts) with metastatic colorectal cancer (mCRC), treated with weekly (q1w) and q2w schedules of cetuximab combined with FOLFIRI.* Presented at: the American Society of Clinical Oncology: 2008 Gastrointestinal Cancers Symposium [Abstract 435]. January 25–27, 2008; Orlando, FL.

82. Saif MW, Mehra R. Incidence and management of bevacizumab-related toxicities in colorectal cancer. *Expert Opin Drug Saf* 2006;5(4):553–566.

83. Saif MW, Cohenuram M. Role of panitumumab in the management of metastatic colorectal cancer. *Clin Colorectal Cancer* 2006;6(2):118–124.

84. Gibson TB, Ranganathan A, Grothey A. Randomized phase III trial results of panitumumab, a fully human anti-epidermal growth factor receptor monoclonal antibody, in metastatic colorectal cancer. *Clin Colorectal Cancer* 2006;6(1):29–31.

85. Hecht JR, Mitchell E, Chidiac T, et al. An update analysis of safety and efficacy of oxaliplatin (Ox)/bevacizumab (bev) N panitumumab (pmab) for fist-line treatment (tx) of metastatic colorectal cancer (mCRC) from a randomized, controlled trial (PACCE). Presented at: the American Society of Clinical Oncology: 2008 Gastrointestinal Cancers Symposium [Abstract 273] January 25–27, 2008; Orlando, FL.

86. Douillard JY, Siena S, Cassidy J, et al. Randomized phase 3 study of panitumumab with FOLFOX compared to FOLFOX alone as first-line treatment (tx) for metastatic colorectal cancer (mCRC): the PRIME trial. Presented at: ECCO 15–34th ESMO Multidisciplinary Congress; September 20–24, 2009; Berlin, Germany.

87. Peeters M, Price T, Hotko Y, et al. Randomized phase 3 study of panitumumab with FOLFIRI vs. FOLFIRI alone as second-line treatment (tx) in patients (pts) with metastatic colorectal cancer (mCRC). Presented at: ECCO 15–34th ESMO Multidisciplinary Congress; September 20–24, 2009; Berlin, Germany.

88. Punt CJ, Tol J, Rodenburg CJ, et al. 2008.Randomized phase III study of capecitabine, oxaliplatin, and bevacizumab with or without cetuximab in advanced colorectal cancer (ACC), the CAIRO2 study of the Dutch Colorectal Cancer Group (DCCG) [Abstract LBA4011]. *J Clin Oncol* 26(May 20 Suppl).

89. Baselga J, Schöffski P, Rojo F, et al. A phase I pharmacokinetic (PK) and molecular pharmacodynamic (PD) study of the combination of two anti-EGFR therapies, the monoclonal antibody (MAb) cetuximab (C) and the tyrosine kinase inhibitor (TKI) gefitinib (G), in patients (pts) with advanced colorectal (CRC), head and neck (HNC) and non-small cell lung cancer (NSCLC) [Abstract 3006]. *J Clin Oncol* 2006;24(18 suppl):122s.

90. Saltz LB, Lenz H, Kindler HL, et al. Randomized phase II trial of cetuximab, bevacizumab, and irinotecan compared with cetuximab and bevacizumab alone in irinotecan-refractory colorectal cancer: The BOND-2 study. *J Clin Oncol.* 2007 Oct 10;25(29):4557–4561.

91. Fong Y, Cohen AM, Fortner JG, et al. Liver resection for colorectal metastases. *J Clin Oncol* 1997;15(3):938–946.

92. Nordlinger B, Sorbye H, Glimelius B, et al. EORTC Gastro-Intestinal Tract Cancer Group; Cancer Research UK; Arbeitsgruppe Lebermetastasen und-tumoren in der Chirurgischen Arbeitsgemeinschaft Onkologie (ALM-CAO); Australasian Gastro-Intestinal Trials Group (AGITG); Fédération Francophone de Cancérologie Digestive (FFCD). Perioperative chemotherapy with FOLFOX4 and surgery versus surgery alone for resectable liver metastases from colorectal cancer (EORTC Intergroup trial 40983): a randomised controlled trial. *Lancet* 2008;371(9617):1007–1016.

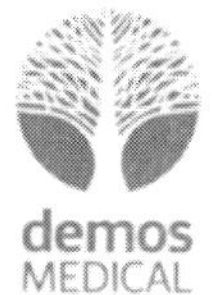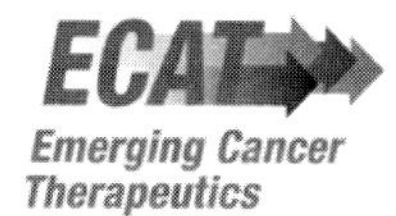

Pancreatic Cancer

M. Wasif Saif and Jonathan Knisely*

Yale Cancer Center, Yale University School of Medicine, New Haven, CT

ABSTRACT

Pancreatic cancer remains the 4th leading cause of death and is responsible for 6% of cancer deaths in the United States. Radical resection remains the only curative therapy, but late diagnoses preclude curative resection in nearly all patients. Radiation therapy and chemotherapy have had only insubstantial effects on pancreatic cancer; overall 5 year survival rates for all stages of disease remain at ~4%. For locally advanced cancers, combined chemotherapy and radiotherapy has not been demonstrated to be undeniably superior to chemotherapy alone, though preoperative combined modality therapy may permit R0 resection of a subset of patients. Radiosurgical treatment of pancreatic cancer may provide improved palliation of local symptoms including pain. Systemic treatment of pancreatic cancer has been hampered by a lack of effective agents. Gemcitabine and 5-fluorouracil (5-FU) improve survival in the adjuvant setting, and gemcitabine appears to have a slightly better toxicity profile. Doublets and triplets including gemcitabine with cytotoxic and targeted agents have not shown remarkably improved outcomes relative to gemcitabine alone. Novel targets and novel agents are needed for making advances in treatment of pancreatic cancer, and the role of radiation therapy will likely remain controversial until more effective systemically administered therapies are developed and tested with or without radiation in the locally advanced and adjuvant settings.

■ INTRODUCTION

The American Cancer Society estimated 18,030 deaths from pancreatic cancer in American men in 2009, fourth after lung, prostate, and colorectal cancer, and 17,210 deaths in women, again fourth after lung, breast, and colorectal cancer. Although pancreatic cancer represents only 2% to 3% of all cancers, it remains the fourth cause of death by cancer since the 1970s in the United States and accounts for over 6% of all cancer deaths (1). A tremendous effort has been focused on this aggressive disease for almost a century;

the only curative option is still the Whipple surgery, named after a surgeon in New York. More than 80% of new cases present at an unresectable stage resulting in 5-year overall survival (OS) for all stages of ~4% (2). Besides the insidious presentation, the high mortality associated with pancreatic cancer is due to debilitating symptoms and *ab initio* chemoresistance. Five-year OS rates for advanced pancreatic cancer are less than 1%. The poor prognosis has been attributed to the inability to diagnose while the tumor is resectable and its propensity toward early vascular and lymphatic dissemination.

One of the greatest challenges in the treatment of pancreatic cancer remains its inherent lack of beneficial response to cytotoxic chemotherapy. In inoperable pancreatic cancer, gemcitabine is the only

*Corresponding author, Medical Oncology and Radiation Oncology, Yale Cancer Center, New Haven, CT
E-mail address: Jonathan.knisely@yale.edu

Emerging Cancer Therapeutics 1 (2010) 137–148.

DOI: 10.5003/2151–4194.1.1.139

cytotoxic agent approved by the U.S. Food and Drug Administration since 1997. Several trials have evaluated whether there is any benefit for gemcitabine-based combinations, including molecular-targeted agents, over gemcitabine alone. Although several of these have shown a higher response rate favoring the combined regimens, a clear benefit in OS has yet to be shown. Despite the benefit of gemcitabine, most patients with advanced disease still do poorly, with a median time-to-tumor progression between 2 and 3 months and median OS of 5 to 6 months. The authors review slow progress and the recent developments with newer chemotherapeutic and molecular-targeted agents in the management of pancreatic cancer.

■ ADJUVANT THERAPY

The high risk of local and systemic disease recurrence, as well as overall poor prognosis, laid down the rationale for adjuvant therapy after resection of pancreatic adenocarcinoma (3,4).

The Gastrointestinal Tumor Study Group (GITSG) trial was the first prospective randomized trial suggesting a survival advantage with postoperative chemoradiotherapy using bolus 5-FU (median survival: 20 vs 11 months; 5-year survival: 18% vs 8%) (5). However, this study was criticized for poor patient accrual, early termination, and small patient numbers, and the radiotherapy dose is most likely suboptimal (currently, a continuous course of fractionated radiotherapy that delivers a dose of ~50 Gy in 5 weeks is regarded as probably optimal).

The European Organization of Research and Treatment of Cancer (EORTC) compared 5-FU with concurrent split-course radiotherapy to 40 Gy with observation only in patients with resected pancreatic and periampullary cancer (6). This trial excluded patients with T3 tumors, and the criteria for distinguishing between pancreatic and periampullary tumors were not explicitly stated, which is important because of the different natural histories and prognoses of these tumors. The posterior (retroperitoneal) resection margin was not rigorously assessed, perhaps contributing to differences in locoregional recurrences. Additionally, a sizeable subset (~20%) of patients assigned to receive postoperative adjuvant chemoradiotherapy did not receive this therapy, perhaps influencing adversely the ability of this small study to detect the impact of the adjuvant therapy on patient outcomes. Additional criticism

arose for the continued use of split-course suboptimal dosed radiotherapy, as well as for its lack of power to detect benefit of 10% to 15% in treated patients. The subgroup analysis looking only at pancreatic cancer patients did show a trend toward benefit with therapy with a median survival of 17.1 versus 12.6 months ($P = 0.099$) (6).

A virulent debate over the role of radiotherapy in the adjuvant therapy of pancreatic cancer was sparked by ESPAC-1 (7). ESPAC-1 was a 2 × 2 factorial designed study comparing adjuvant concurrent chemoradiotherapy (bolus 5-FU/split course radiotherapy to a total of 40 Gy) without additional chemotherapy, chemotherapy alone (5-FU/leucovorin), chemoradiotherapy followed by chemotherapy, and observation. Investigators could randomize patients into two concurrent, separate studies that compared adjuvant chemotherapy to no adjuvant chemotherapy and adjuvant chemoradiotherapy to no therapy. It is uncertain whether bias was introduced by this design. Also, additional anticancer therapy was permitted before patients were entered into these two component studies, and this may also have resulted in unpredictable effects on the study findings. It was found that the chemotherapy-only arm had a statistically significant benefit over observation arm in median survival (20.1 vs 15.5 months; $P = 0.009$). However, the chemoradiotherapy arm showed a worse median survival compared with patients who did not receive chemoradiotherapy (15.9 vs 17.9 months; $P = 0.05$) (7). There were major criticisms made of the trial for possible selection biases as both patients and clinicians were allowed to select which trial to enter, the use of split course, suboptimally dosed radiotherapy, and for allowing the final radiotherapy dose to be left to the judgment of the treating physicians (8).

The CONKO-001 study randomized 368 patients with resected pancreatic cancer to gemcitabine or observation for 6 months (9). This trial showed statistically significant disease-free survival benefit (13.4 vs 6.9 months; $P < 0.001$) of gemcitabine over observation. Gemcitabine rendered a trend toward overall benefit (22.1 vs 20.2 months; $P = 0.06$). This benefit of chemotherapy was consistent with the result from the ESPAC-1 trial, which showed a benefit of 5-FU/leucovorin over no adjuvant therapy in pancreatic cancer patients (median survival of 19.7 vs 14.0 months) who had complete resection (7,9).

RTOG-Intergroup #97–04 was the first American cooperative group study since the GITSG trials and had no observation arm. The study posed the question of whether 5-FU or gemcitabine is the better chemotherapy agent when used before and after chemoradiotherapy using continuous infusion 5-FU (250 mg/m^2/day, and a dose of 50.4 Gy) with respect to: (*a*) OS, (*b*) locoregional disease control, and (*c*) distant disease control and failure patterns. CA 19–9 will be evaluated prospectively to predict outcome (10,11). Patients were randomized to receive chemotherapy with either fluorouracil (continuous infusion of 250 mg/m^2/day; $n = 230$) or gemcitabine (30-minute infusion of 1,000 mg/m^2 once per week; $n = 221$) for 3 weeks prior to chemoradiation therapy and for 12 weeks after chemoradiation therapy. The addition of gemcitabine to adjuvant fluorouracil-based chemoradiation was associated with a survival benefit for patients with resected pancreatic cancer, although this improvement was not statistically significant. Forty-two percent crossed over to gemcitabine (10). Three hundred and eighty-five patients had assessable CA 19–9 levels. The majority had a CA 19–9 level lower than 180 or ≤ 90 ($n = 220$ and 200, respectively), while 34% were Lewis Antigen negative and 33 (9%) and 53 (14%) patients had levels higher than 180 and higher than 90, respectively. When CA 19–9 was analyzed as a dichotomized variable, there was a significant survival difference favoring patients with CA 19–9 lower than 180 (hazard ratio [HR], 3.53; $P < 0001$). This corresponds to a 72% reduction in the risk of death for patients with a CA 19–9 lower than 180. This was also true for patients with CA 19–9 ≤ 90 (HR, 3.4; $P < 0001$). Multivariate analyses confirmed that CA 19–9, when analyzed as both a continuous and a dichotomized variable, is a highly significant predictor of OS in patients with resected pancreatic cancer (11).

Neoptolemos et al. presented the results of the ESPAC-3 study at the annual meeting of ASCO in June 2009 in Orlando, Florida. This is a multicenter, international, open-label, randomized, controlled, phase III trial that aimed at comparing adjuvant 5-fluorouracil/leucovorin (5-FU/LV) versus gemcitabine in patients with resected pancreatic ductal adenocarcinoma (8). Patients with an R0/R1 resection for pancreatic ductal adenocarcinoma were randomized (stratified for resection margin status and country) starting within 8 weeks of surgery to receive either 5-FU/LV (leucovorin, 20 mg/m^2, IV bolus injection followed by 5-FU, 425 mg/m^2, IV bolus injection given 1–5 days every 28 days) or gemcitabine (1,000 mg/m^2 IV infusion at days 1, 8, and 15 every 4 weeks) for 6 months. The primary outcome measure was OS; the secondary measures were toxicity, progression-free survival, and quality of life (12).

ESPAC-3 was revised to version 2 to close the observation arm (12). From July 2000 to January 2007, 1,088 patients from 16 countries were randomized (5-FU/LV, $n = 551$; gemcitabine, $n = 537$). Median age was 63 years, and 55% were men. Thirty-five percent were R1 resections and approximately over 70% were node positive (8). The study confirmed the role of adjuvant chemotherapy. However, OS was similar on both arms, hence showing that gemcitabine is not superior to 5-FU in adjuvant setting. Median OS was 23.0 months (95% CI: 21.1–25.0 months) with 5-FU/FA and it was 23.6 months (95% CI: 21.4–26.4 months) with gemcitabine. There was no significant difference in the effect of treatment across subgroups according to R status ($P = 0.56$). The study also confirmed the role of prognostic factors (whatever adjuvant chemotherapy): grade, stage, nodal status, and resection status (8). The study showed that gemcitabine is not superior to 5-FU in adjuvant setting; however, safety and dose intensity favor gemcitabine. This study is very important because there has been a tendency to reject 5-FU in pancreatic cancer and now it is very much back on the stage (12).

Controversy About the Role of Radiotherapy in Adjuvant Therapy

As stated above, the available randomized and non-randomized clinical trials have failed to resolve the role of adjuvant radiation therapy in the management of resected pancreatic cancer (5,7) Controversies about the appropriateness of continuing to include radiation therapy in the adjuvant management of resected pancreatic cancer provide an opportunity for subjective opinions to be rendered based on selective interpretations of suboptimal data (13).

Briefly put, those who favor the use of postoperative radiation as part of adjuvant therapy wish to use this treatment modality to intensify the locoregional therapy (and improve locoregional control) above and beyond what is possible with systemic therapy alone. Those who would use chemotherapy alone believe that the risk of nonregional failure is substantial enough that there is little advantage to attempts to intensify the locoregional control through the use of radiation to the tumor bed in the adjuvant setting.

In this light, the limitations of the EORTC study (6) detailed above provide fortuitously beneficial support for the use of chemoradiotherapy in the adjuvant setting for cancer of the pancreatic head. Disparagement of the ESPAC-1 trial for poor quality assurance of the radiation therapy and other reasons is common among radiation oncologists, but it is difficult to argue with an interpretation of the study results advocating that delaying full-dose systemic therapy to give locoregional radiation therapy may compromise survival, even though the benefit from systemic drugs is far from great. The 63% local recurrence rate in ESPAC-1 is pointed to as evidence of suboptimal treatment; the local recurrence rate was only 26% in the RTOG 97–04 trial. It is argued that as more effective systemic therapies are developed that are better able to control metastatic disease, the importance of the improved locoregional control that radiation can provide will increase in a proportionate fashion (10).

■ LOCALLY ADVANCED PANCREATIC CANCER

Locally advanced pancreatic cancer is defined as the presence of a surgically unresectable tumor (involving the celiac axis, superior mesenteric artery, or portal veins) or on the basis of bulky peripancreatic lymphadenopathy without evidence of distant metastases (14). Surgery is the only means of cure for pancreatic cancer, fewer than 10% of patients are eligible for resection based on the extent of disease at presentation. According to the Surveillance, Epidemiology and End Results (SEER; http://seer.cancer.gov/statfacts/html/pancreas.html) database, 26% of pancreatic cancer cases are locally advanced at the time of diagnosis, with a 5-year survival rate of 8.7% (15).

Chemoradiotherapy

Chemoradiotherapy with 5-fluorouracil (5-FU) and radiotherapy to a total dose of 50 Gy increases OS and quality of life of patients with locally advanced pancreatic cancer, as supported by the GITSG (16) and the Eastern Cooperative Oncology Group (ECOG) 8282 (17) trials. Most studies have investigated 5-FU-based chemotherapy regimens with radiotherapy. Over the past 10 years, gemcitabine has become the standard of chemotherapy in advanced pancreatic carcinoma and is also a potent radiosensitizer of epithelial cells. Many phase I and II trials have demonstrated the feasibility of combining radiotherapy (to total doses ranging from 24 to 61 Gy) with gemcitabine at weekly doses ranging from 100 to 1,000 mg/m^2; however, results of randomized phase II studies are not sufficient or consistent to recommend such a regimen. Therefore, 5-FU is still the reference chemotherapy in association with radiotherapy for locally advanced pancreatic cancer. The optimal protocol to deliver 5-FU has not been evaluated in comparative trials, and multiple administration schedules have been reported, including weekly bolus (250–600 mg/m^2), bolus on the first 3 days of radiotherapy (350–600 mg/m^2), continuous infusion on the first and fifth weeks of radiotherapy (1,000 mg/m^2), and continuous infusion (200–300 mg/m^2/day).

Even though chemoradiotherapy may be widely used to treat patients with locally advanced pancreatic cancer, its superiority compared to chemotherapy has never been proven. In the Federation Francophone de Cancerologie Digestive-Societe Francaise de Radiotherapie Oncologique (FFCD-SFRO) trial (18), although the chemoradiotherapy regimen used was not optimal (5-FU and cisplatin with 60 Gy external beam radiation therapy), survival was worse in the cohort randomized to receive radiotherapy (median survival 8.6 versus 13 months ($P = 0.03$); 1-year survival was 32% versus 53% (18). This chemoradiotherapy regimen produced unacceptable toxicity rates; the results of this trial were consistent with older studies published in the 1980s.

In the phase III ECOG E4201 study, patients were randomized to receive gemcitabine 1,000 mg/m^2/week for 6 weeks or gemcitabine 600 mg/m^2/week for 6 weeks while radiotherapy to a dose of 50.4 Gy in 5.5 weeks was administered. Consolidative treatment was the same in both arms—gemcitabine 1,000 mg/m^2 weekly for 3 of 4 weeks for 5 cycles. Survival was prolonged in the cohort getting combined modality therapy (median survival 9.2 vs 11.0 months [$P = 0.034$]); 18- and 24-month survivals were tripled in the combined modality arm to 29% and 12%, respectively (19). Although the results of the ECOG E4201 phase III trial (6) were in favor of chemoradiotherapy, however these results should be considered cautiously because of the insufficient number of patients included.

Role of Radiation

Despite the lack of a data-based consensus approach, some difficult-to-refute arguments for the inclusion of radiation in the initial, definitive treatment of *slightly less* locally advanced pancreatic cancer exist. These include the possibility that regression of disease may occur that will make a resection that might have been technically difficult or likely to have had positive margins more readily accomplished with histopathologically negative margins. Also cited is the possibility that while locoregional treatment is delivered, distant metastatic disease may become manifest, changing the risk–benefit ratio for undertaking a major resection. Additionally, the delivery of these treatments preoperatively may decrease operative dissemination of viable tumor stem cells and can ensure that postoperative complications do not delay needed adjuvant therapies (20–22).

Radiation therapy to the pancreas is technically difficult because of the location of the tumor in relation to contiguous normal tissues such as the kidneys, liver, small intestine, and spinal cord. The radiation tolerance of these organs is lower than the dose of radiation that will reliably sterilize macroscopic tumor within the pancreas or regional nodes. Care is required to ensure that the design of the treatment fields will account for not only the tolerance of the normal tissues, but also for possible movement of the tumor and critical normal tissues with respiration (23).

Dose intensification of radiation treatment has been historically pursued with brachytherapy and intraoperative radiation therapy and continues to be pursued through a variety of strategies such as stereotactic radiation therapy, intensity modulated radiation therapy (IMRT), and particle beam therapy. These approaches, by preferentially sparing normal tissue morbidity while increasing the dose delivered to the tumor, may marginally improve locoregional tumor control. At present, these approaches have not been shown in any rigorous evaluation to provide superior survival outcomes.

The historical radiotherapeutic approach for locally advanced disease that treated all regional nodal volumes with the same dose used to treat the primary tumor is now infrequently used relative to an approach in which only the macroscopic tumor burden is targeted (22,24–28). This approach dovetails well with a desire to increase the aggressiveness of concomitant chemosensitization without increasing locoregional normal tissue toxicities. Overly generous field sizes correlated with increased toxicity in RTOG 9704, both during chemoradiotherapy and during maintenance chemotherapy (24), and the volume of the duodenum receiving high-dose radiation was noted to correlate with late duodenal toxicity in single fraction body radiosurgery (28).

Intensity-modulated radiotherapy is a radiation therapy technique that allows for dose intensification with concurrent improved sparing of normal tissues. By dividing the radiation beams into thousands of "pencil beams" of varying intensities, concave dose distributions and very sharp regions of dose fall-off can be created. Gemcitabine is known to be a potent radiation sensitizer, with potential for both enhanced antitumor effects and increased toxicity. Early studies of concurrent gemcitabine and radiotherapy for locally advanced pancreatic cancer showed substantial dose-related gastrointestinal toxicity (29). More recent studies have demonstrated the feasibility of treating only the gross tumor volume with full-dose weekly gemcitabine, omitting the uninvolved lymph node beds and thereby decreasing the amount of normal tissue treated, as summarized in Table 1.

The difference between IMRT and body radiosurgery may perhaps be simply explained by

TABLE 1 Selected results of tumor-only radiation and gemcitabine for pancreatic cancer

Author (Reference)	Radiation Dose	Patient No.	Gemcitabine Dose (mg/m²/week)	Toxicity	Results
Talamonti et al. (25)	36 Gy in 15 fractions	20 preoperative	1,000	5% grade 3 GI toxicity 24% surgical complication rate	5% complete response 15% microscopic residual 65% pathologically node negative
Murphy et al. (26)	36 Gy in 15 fractions	74 inoperable	1,000	22% grade 3+ GI toxicity	5% local failure in nodes 64% 1-year freedom from local progression

the difference in accuracy sought and doses used. Investigators at Stanford gave a 25 Gy dose in a single stereotactic fraction with a millimetric degree of precision, so as to minimize normal tissue exposure to high-dose radiation. Such accuracy cannot be easily achieved for a 5- to 6-week course of radiation therapy, and greater uncertainty in patient positioning and accuracy beam delivery is accepted. The radiosurgical approach used at Stanford has been shown to provide 1-year local control rates of 95%, but is unsuccessful at making locally advanced pancreatic cancer resectable or to improve survival rates compared to conventional chemoradiation therapy (28). They found that by excluding all but the primary tumor from the high-dose volume, acute and delayed local complication rates were acceptably low. The OS rates at 6 and 12 months, calculated from the date of body radiosurgery, were 56% and 21%, respectively. OS for the entire cohort from the date of diagnosis was 11.9 months. It is possible that if survival is improved through improved systemic control, additional significant late complications may be experienced.

Also, this focal radiation approach did not lead to an unacceptably high regional nodal failure rate, though some of the control at these nodal sites were attributed to nonprotocol gemcitabine administration (96% of patients) or regional radiotherapy to 45 to 54 Gy given in addition to the radiosurgical treatment (21% of patients). Several prominent groups have noted that radiotherapy can help palliate the pain associated with locally advanced pancreatic cancer (30,31), and it may be possible that the dose-intensity of radiosurgery provides a more rapid benefit than a 5- to 6-week course of fractionated treatment. Moreover, the radiosurgical approach completes the local therapy promptly so that full-dose systemic therapy can be instituted promptly.

Table 2 summarizes selected phase III randomized clinical trials of chemotherapy and radiation in the treatment of locally advanced pancreatic cancer.

■ ADVANCED OR METASTATIC PANCREATIC CANCER

Before gemcitabine's approval, 5-FU was a routinely used treatment for pancreatic cancer. Rubin et al. performed a phase II study of 5-FU plus leucovorin in 31 patients with pancreatic cancer. No objective response was observed with a median OS of 5.7

months (32). To improve the response, three 5-FU-based regimens were evaluated including doxorubicin and mitomycin. An increased toxicity with no significant increase in response or survival benefit was observed (33).

Earlier studies of gemcitabine showed modest activity with a response rate of 6.3% and 11% and median OS of 6.3 and 5.6 months, respectively (34,35). The median survival reported in gemcitabine trials was akin to that of the 5-FU. However, the Carmichael et al. study did show clinical benefit in terms of improved performance status (17.2%), decreased pain score (28.6%), and decreased nausea (27.3%), and this study might have led to the randomized phase III study (34). Burris et al. performed a multicentered randomized, phase III clinical trial that compared 5-FU to gemcitabine (36). Treatment with gemcitabine resulted in a relative improvement of 36% in median OS compared to 5-FU (5.7 vs 4.2 months) and 1-year survival rates (18% vs 2%). In addition to the survival benefit, gemcitabine was also superior to 5-FU in producing clinical benefit response (24% vs 5%) (Fig. 1). This study led to the approval of gemcitabine as a first-line chemotherapy agent.

Using gemcitabine as the control, several investigational drugs (BAY 12–9566, exatecan, SCH 66336) were compared against gemcitabine and no such agent demonstrated superiority over gemcitabine (Fig. 2) (37–40).

Therefore, the study design for clinical trials for pancreatic cancer was directed toward comparing gemcitabine monotherapy or gemcitabine plus the investigational drug. This trial design allows new drugs to be tested in the first-line setting. Over the last decade, multiple cytotoxic (5-FU, capecitabine, irinotecan, cisplatin, oxaliplatin, etc.) (41–46) and targeted agents (bevacizumab, cetuximab) (47,48) have been combined with gemcitabine in randomized phase III trials and none of these combinations showed superiority over single-agent gemcitabine.

Two large randomized phase III studies in pancreatic cancer have demonstrated the superiority of a gemcitabine-containing combination over single-agent gemcitabine: capecitabine plus gemcitabine versus gemcitabine and erlotinib plus gemcitabine versus gemcitabine (49,50). Preliminary data from a study by Cunningham et al. (49) showed a 7.4-month median survival (95% CI: 6.5–8.5 months) for subjects who received gemcitabine plus capecitabine combination therapy ($n = 267$),

TABLE 2 Selected phase III clinical trials of chemotherapy and radiation for the treatment of locally advanced pancreatic cancer

Trial Author (Reference)	No. of Patients		Chemotherapy	Radiation (Gy)	Median Overall Survival (months)	Median Time to Progression (months)	Grade 3–4 Toxicity
GITSG Moertel et al. (16)	194	Arm A	None	60[a]	5.3	2.9	
		Arm B	5-FU 500 mg/m^2/week bolus days 1–3 + maintenance 5-FU bolus 500 mg/m^2/week until progression	40[a]	7.0	7.0	
		Arm C	5-FU 500 mg/m^2/week bolus days 1–3 + maintenance 5-FU bolus 500 mg/m^2/week until progression	60	7.6	7.6	
					A vs B: $P<0.1$; A vs C: $P<0.1$; B vs C: $P=0.19$	A vs B: $P<0.1$; A vs C: $P<0.1$; B vs C: $P=0.14$	
ECOG 8282 Cohen et al. (17)	108	Arm A	None	59.4	7.1	5.0	24.5%
		Arm B	5-FU 1,000 mg/m^2/day c.i. days 2–5 and days 28–31 + mitomycin-C 10 mg/m^2 day 2	59.4	8.4	5.1	32.7%
					$P=0.16$	$P=0.19$	$P=0.049$
FFCD-SFRO Chauffert et al. (18)	119	Arm A	Gemcitabine 1,000 mg/m^2/week + maintenance gemcitabine until progression	None	13	32% at 1 year	Induction: 27% heme; 18% nonheme Maintenance: 27% heme; 24% nonheme
		Arm B	5-FU 300 mg/m^2/day c.i. 5 days/week + cisplatin 20 mg/m^2/day days 1–5 and days 29–33 + maintenance gemcitabine 1,000 mg/m^2/week until progression	60	8.6	14% at 1 year	Induction: 31% heme; 44% nonheme Maintenance: 71% heme; 30% nonheme
					$P=0.03$		Induction: $P=0.008$ Maintenance: $P=0.001$

continued

TABLE 2   Selected phase III clinical trials of chemotherapy and radiation for the treatment of locally advanced pancreatic cancer (Continued)

Trial Author (Reference)	No. of Patients		Chemotherapy	Radiation (Gy)	Median Overall Survival (months)	Median Time to Progression (months)	Grade 3–4 Toxicity
ECOG 4201 Loehrer et al. (19)	74	Arm A	Gemcitabine 1,000 mg/m^2/week on days 1, 8, 15	None	9.2	6.1	5.7%
		Arm B	Gemcitabine 600 mg/m^2/week + maintenance gemcitabine 1,000 mg/m^2/week on days 1, 8, 15	50.4	11.0	6.3	41.2%
					$P=0.044$	$P=0.34$	$P<0.0001$

[a]Split course.

c.i., continuous infusion.

significantly higher ($P=0.026$) when compared to 6.0 months (95% CI: 5.4–7.1 months) for those who received gemcitabine alone ($n=266$) (HR: 0.80; 95% CI: 0.65–0.98). Moreover, 1-year survival was 19% for subjects on gemcitabine monotherapy and 26% for those receiving the combination. However, the comparison is not equal. The HR compares the entire survival curve and favors the tail-end of the curve, where there were virtually no subjects. Thus, the HR in this trial is based heavily on these preliminary data without many subjects. However, in comparison, Herrmann et al. (43) reported data from a completed phase III trial; results showed that the combination of gemcitabine and capecitabine did not significantly ($P=0.314$) improve OS compared with gemcitabine monotherapy (8.0 vs 7.3 months, respectively). This discrepancy in outcomes from two trials evaluating the gemcitabine and capecitabine combination

indicates that more data are needed before determining the real value of that regimen.

On the other hand, 569 patients were randomly assigned to receive either gemcitabine with or without erlotinib. Patients treated with the combination of gemcitabine and erlotinib had an improved OS with a statistically significant HR of 0.82 (50). The median and 1-year survival rates were better for the combination treatment: 6.24 versus 5.91 months and 23% versus 17%, respectively. This difference, although significant, shows about 12 to 14 days of gain with erlotinib therapy. Is this clinically meaningful? Do we want to add a drug that adds toxicity with only 2 weeks of gain? In most cancers, this difference would be considered as not clinically relevant, but in pancreatic cancer, this difference becomes more meaningful because of the poor outcome of advanced pancreatic cancer, the absence

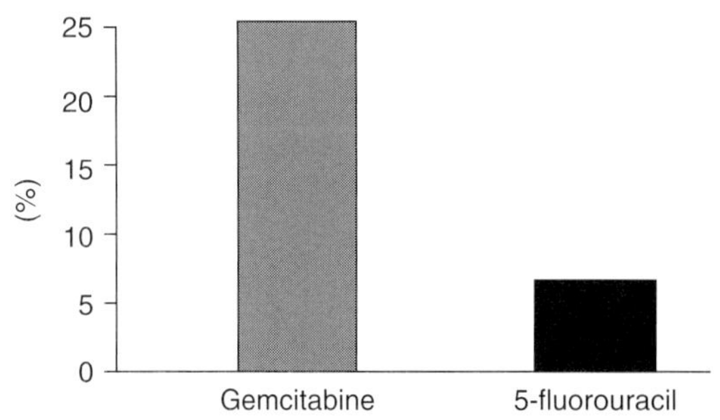

FIGURE 1   Clinical benefit response with gemcitabine. (From Ref. 36.)

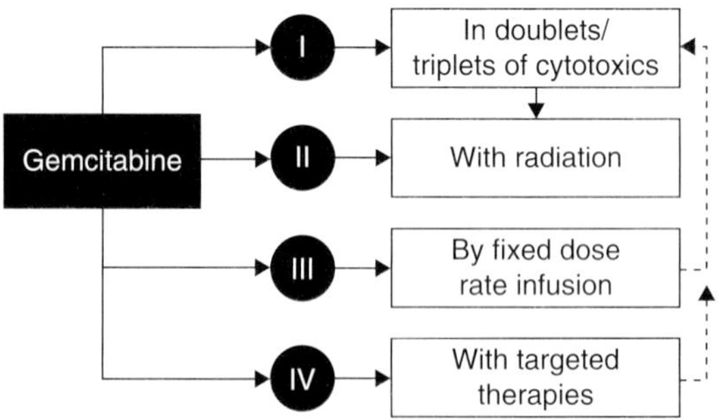

FIGURE 2   Study designs to improve outcome with gemcitabine.

of impact of most other treatment options, the relatively limited impact of the reference treatment of gemcitabine monotherapy, and the acceptable toxicity profile.

Although radiation therapy is not commonly used for advanced pancreatic cancer, it may have a role in the treatment of pain. The investigators at Stanford noted palliation of pain in patients with locally advanced, metastatic, or locally recurrent pancreatic cancer with a single fraction 25 Gy treatment (30) and this procedure's use may to improve quality of life, as well as protein and calorie intake, and thereby possibly also positively influence survival (51).

We definitely need to identify newer agents and newer targets. We need to learn from our mistakes, and patients with locally advanced pancreatic cancer should be studied separately from metastatic pancreatic cancer in future studies. In addition, oncologists need to change their attitudes toward clinical trials. Development of novel agents and approaches are urgently needed in conjunction with improvement in access to clinical trials for patients. In short, there is no current clear standard of care for the treatment of advanced pancreatic cancer.

■ REFERENCES

1. Jemal A, Siegel R, Ward E. Cancer statistics, 2009. *CA Cancer J Clin* 2009;59(4):225–249.
2. Carter SK, Comis RL. The integration of chemotherapy into a combined modality approach for cancer treatment. VI. Pancreatic adenocarcinoma. *Cancer Treat Rev* 1975;2(3):193–214.
3. Mu DQ, Peng SY, Wang GF. Risk factors influencing recurrence following resection of pancreatic head cancer. *World J Gastroenterol* 2004;10(6):906–909.
4. Shibata K, Matsumoto T, Yada K, Sasaki A, Ohta M, Kitano S. Factors predicting recurrence after resection of pancreatic ductal carcinoma. *Pancreas* 2005;31(1):69–73.
5. Kalser MH, Ellenberg SS. Pancreatic cancer. Adjuvant combined radiation and chemotherapy following curative resection. *Arch Surg* 1985;120(8):899–903.
6. Klinkenbijl JH, Jeekel J, Sahmoud T, et al. Adjuvant radiotherapy and 5-fluorouracil after curative resection of cancer of the pancreas and periampullary region: phase III trial of the EORTC gastrointestinal tract cancer cooperative group. *Ann Surg* 1999;230(6):776–82; discussion 782.
7. Neoptolemos JP, Stocken DD, Friess H, et al. A randomized trial of chemoradiotherapy and chemotherapy after resection of pancreatic cancer. *N Engl J Med* 2004;350(12):1200–1210.
8. Koshy MC, Landry JC, Cavanaugh SX, et al. A challenge to the therapeutic nihilism of ESPAC-1. *Int J Radiat Oncol Biol Phys* 2005;61(4):965–966.
9. Oettle H, Post S, Neuhaus P, et al. Adjuvant chemotherapy with gemcitabine vs observation in patients undergoing curative-intent resection of pancreatic cancer: a randomized controlled trial. *JAMA* 2007;297(3):267–277.
10. Regine WF, Winter KA, Abrams RA, et al. Fluorouracil vs gemcitabine chemotherapy before and after fluorouracil-based chemoradiation following resection of pancreatic adenocarcinoma: a randomized controlled trial. *JAMA* 2008;299(9):1019–1026.
11. Berger AC, Garcia M, Hoffman JP, et al. Postresection CA 19–9 predicts overall survival in patients with pancreatic cancer treated with adjuvant chemoradiation: a prospective validation by RTOG 9704. *J Clin Oncol* 2008;26(36):5918–5922.
12. Neoptolemos J, Büchler M, Stocken DD, Ghaneh P, Smith D, C. Bassi C, et al. A multicenter, international, open-label, randomized, controlled phase III trial of adjuvant 5-fluorouracil/folinic acid (5-FU/FA) versus gemcitabine (GEM) in patients with resected pancreatic ductal adenocarcinoma. *J Clin Oncol* 2009; 27(18 Suppl.): Abstract LBA4505.
13. Saif MW. Controversies in the adjuvant treatment of pancreatic adenocarcinoma. *JOP* 2007;8(5):545–552.
14. American Joint Committee on Cancer. Exocrine Pancreas. In: AJCC Cancer Staging Manual. 6th ed. New York, NY: *Springer*, 2002, 157–164.
15. Horner MJ, Ries LAG, Krapcho M, et al. (eds). SEER Cancer Statistics Review, 1975–2006, National Cancer Institute. Bethesda, MD, USA: 2006.
16. Moertel CG, Frytak S, Hahn RG, et al. Therapy of locally unresectable pancreatic carcinoma: a randomized comparison of high dose (6000 rads) radiation alone, moderate dose radiation (4000 rads + 5-fluorouracil), and high dose radiation + 5-fluorouracil: The Gastrointestinal Tumor Study Group. *Cancer* 1981;48(8):1705–1710.
17. Cohen SJ, Dobelbower R, Lipsitz S, et al.; A randomized phase III study of radiotherapy alone or with 5-fluorouracil and mitomycin-C in patients with locally advanced adenocarcinoma of the pancreas: Eastern Cooperative Oncology Group study E8282. *Int J Radiat Oncol Biol Phys* 2005;62(5):1345–1350.
18. Chauffert B, Mornex F, Bonnetain F, et al. Phase III trial comparing intensive induction chemoradiotherapy (60 Gy, infusional 5-FU and intermittent cisplatin) followed by maintenance gemcitabine with gemcitabine alone for locally advanced unresectable pancreatic cancer. Definitive results of the 2000–01 FFCD/SFRO study. *Ann Oncol* 2008;19(9):1592–1599.
19. Loehrer PJ, Powell ME, Cardenes HR, et al. A randomized phase III study of gemcitabine in combination with radiation therapy versus gemcitabine alone in patients with localized, unresectable pancreatic cancer: E4201. *J Clin Oncol* 2008, 26(15 Suppl.): Abstract 4506.
20. Sasson AR, Wetherington RW, Hoffman JP, et al. Neoadjuvant chemoradiotherapy for adenocarcinoma of

the pancreas: analysis of histopathology and outcome. *Int J Gastrointest Cancer* 2003;34(2–3):121–128.

21. Moutardier V, Magnin V, Turrini O, et al. Assessment of pathologic response after preoperative chemoradiotherapy and surgery in pancreatic adenocarcinoma. *Int J Radiat Oncol Biol Phys* 2004;60(2):437–443.

22. Evans DB, Varadhachary GR, Crane CH, et al. Preoperative gemcitabine-based chemoradiation for patients with resectable adenocarcinoma of the pancreatic head. *J Clin Oncol* 2008;26(21):3496–3502.

23. Feng M, Balter JM, Normolle D, et al. Characterization of pancreatic tumor motion using cine MRI: surrogates for tumor position should be used with caution. *Int J Radiat Oncol Biol Phys* 2009;74(3):884–891.

24. Crane CH, Winter K, Regine WF, et al. Phase II study of bevacizumab with concurrent capecitabine and radiation followed by maintenance gemcitabine and bevacizumab for locally advanced pancreatic cancer: Radiation Therapy Oncology Group RTOG 0411. *J Clin Oncol* 2009;27(25):4096–4102.

25. Talamonti MS, Small W, Mulcahy MF, et al. A multi-institutional phase II trial of preoperative full-dose gemcitabine and concurrent radiation for patients with potentially resectable pancreatic carcinoma. *Ann Surg Oncol* 2006;13(2):150–158.

26. Murphy JD, Adusumilli S, Griffith KA, et al. Full-dose gemcitabine and concurrent radiotherapy for unresectable pancreatic cancer. *Int J Radiat Oncol Biol Phys* 2007;68(3):801–808.

27. Ben-Josef E, Griffith K, Francis IR, et al. Phase I radiation dose-escalation trial of intensity-modulated radiotherapy (IMRT) with concurrent fixed dose-rate gemcitabine (FDR-G) for unresectable pancreatic cancer. *J Clin Oncol* 2009, 27(15 Suppl.): Abstract No:4602.

28. Schellenberg D, Goodman KA, Lee F, et al. Gemcitabine chemotherapy and single-fraction stereotactic body radiotherapy for locally advanced pancreatic cancer. *Int J Radiat Oncol Biol Phys* 2008;72(3):678–686.

29. Wolff RA, Evans DB, Gravel DM, et al. Phase I trial of gemcitabine combined with radiation for the treatment of locally advanced pancreatic adenocarcinoma. *Clin Cancer Res* 2001;7(8):2246–2253.

30. Chang DT, Schellenberg D, Shen J, et al. Stereotactic radiotherapy for unresectable adenocarcinoma of the pancreas. *Cancer* 2009;115(3):665–672.

31. Minsky BD, Hilaris B, Fuks Z. The role of radiation therapy in the control of pain from pancreatic carcinoma. *J Pain Symptom Manage* 1988;3(4):199–205.

32. Rubin J, Gallagher JG, Schroeder G, et al. Phase II trials of 5-fluorouracil and leucovorin in patients with metastatic gastric or pancreatic carcinoma. *Cancer* 1996;78(9):1888–1891.

33. Cullinan SA, Moertel CG, Fleming TR, et al. A comparison of three chemotherapeutic regimens in the treatment of advanced pancreatic and gastric carcinoma. Fluorouracil vs fluorouracil and doxorubicin vs fluorouracil, doxorubicin, and mitomycin. *JAMA* 1985;253(14):2061–2067.

34. Carmichael J, Fink U, Russell RC, et al. Phase II study of gemcitabine in patients with advanced pancreatic cancer. *Br J Cancer* 1996;73(1):101–105.

35. Casper ES, Green MR, Kelsen DP, et al. Phase II trial of gemcitabine (2,2'-difluorodeoxycytidine) in patients with adenocarcinoma of the pancreas. *Invest New Drugs* 1994;12(1):29–34.

36. Burris HA, Moore MJ, Andersen J, et al. Improvements in survival and clinical benefit with gemcitabine as first-line therapy for patients with advanced pancreas cancer: a randomized trial. *J Clin Oncol* 1997;15(6):2403–2413.

37. Saif MW. Is there a standard of care for the management of advanced pancreatic cancer? Highlights from the Gastrointestinal Cancers Symposium. Orlando, FL, USA. January 25–27, 2008. *JOP* 2008;9(2):91–98.

38. Moore MJ, Hamm J, Dancey J, et al. Comparison of gemcitabine versus the matrix metalloproteinase inhibitor BAY 12–9566 in patients with advanced or metastatic adenocarcinoma of the pancreas: a phase III trial of the National Cancer Institute of Canada Clinical Trials Group. *J Clin Oncol* 2003;21(17):3296–3302.

39. Cheverton P, Friess H, Andras C, et al. Phase III results of exatecan (DX-8951f) versus gemcitabine (Gem) in chemotherapy-naïve patients with advanced pancreatic cancer (APC). *J Clin Oncol* 2004; ASCO Annual Meeting Proceedings (Post-Meeting Edition) 22(14S, July 15 Suppl):4005.

40. Lersch C, van Cutsem E, Amado R, et al. Randomized phase II study of SCH 66336 and gemcitabine in the treatment of metastatic adenocarcinoma of the pancreas. *Proc Am Soc Clin Oncol* 20: 2001. Abstract No: 608.

41. Berlin JD, Catalano P, Thomas JP, Kugler JW, Haller DG, Benson AB. Phase III study of gemcitabine in combination with fluorouracil versus gemcitabine alone in patients with advanced pancreatic carcinoma: Eastern Cooperative Oncology Group Trial E2297. *J Clin Oncol* 2002;20(15):3270–3275.

42. Reiss H, Helm A, Niedergethmann M, et al. A randomized, prospective, multicenter, phase III trial of gemcitabine, 5-fluorouracil (5-FU), folinic acid vs. gemcitabine in patients with advanced pancreatic cancer. *J Clin Oncol* 2005; ASCO Annual Meeting Proceedings 23(16S, June 1 Suppl):LBA4009.

43. Herrmann R, Bodoky G, Ruhstaller T, et al. Gemcitabine plus capecitabine compared with gemcitabine alone in advanced pancreatic cancer: a randomized, multicenter, phase III trial of the Swiss Group for Clinical Cancer Research and the Central European Cooperative Oncology Group. *J Clin Oncol* 2007;25(16):2212–2217.

44. Rocha Lima CM, Green MR, Rotche R, et al. Irinotecan plus gemcitabine results in no survival advantage compared with gemcitabine monotherapy in patients with locally advanced or metastatic pancreatic cancer despite increased tumor response rate. *J Clin Oncol* 2004;22(18):3776–3783.

45. Louvet C, Labianca R, Hammel P, et al. Gemcitabine in combination with oxaliplatin compared with gemcitabine alone in locally advanced or metastatic

pancreatic cancer: results of a GERCOR and GISCAD phase III trial. *J Clin Oncol* 2005;23(15):3509–3516.

46. Heinemann V, Quietzsch D, Gieseler F, et al. Randomized phase III trial of gemcitabine plus cisplatin compared with gemcitabine alone in advanced pancreatic cancer. *J Clin Oncol* 2006;24(24):3946–3952.

47. Kindler HL, Niedzwiecki D, Hollis D, et al. A double-blind, placebo-controlled, randomized phase III trial of gemcitabine (G) plus bevacizumab (B) versus gemcitabine plus placebo (P) in patients (pts) with advanced pancreatic cancer (PC): a preliminary analysis of Cancer and Leukemia Group B (CALGB) 80303. ASCO Gastrointestinal Cancers Symposium 2007. Abstract No: 108.

48. Philip PA, Benedetti J, Fenoglio-Preiser C, et al. Phase III study of gemcitabine [G] plus cetuximab [C] versus gemcitabine in patients [pts] with locally advanced or metastatic pancreatic adenocarcinoma [PC]: SWOG S0205 study. *J Clin Oncol* 2007; ASCO Annual Meeting Proceedings Part I 25(18S, June 20 Suppl):LBA4509.

49. Cunningham D, Chau I, Stocken C, et al. Phase III randomized comparison of gemcitabine (GEM) versus gemcitabine plus capecitabine (GEM-CAP) in patients with advanced pancreatic cancer. *Eur J Cancer* 2005; Suppl 3:12. Abstract PS11.

50. Moore MJ. Goldstein D, Hamm J, et al. Erlotinib plus gemcitabine compared to gemcitabine alone in patients with advanced pancreatic cancer. A phase III trial of the National Cancer Institute of Canada Clinical Trials Group (NCIC-CTG). *J Clin Oncol* 2005; 23(16S part I). Abstract No: 1.

51. Lillemoe KD, Cameron JL, Kaufman HS, Yeo CJ, Pitt HA, Sauter PK. Chemical splanchnicectomy in patients with unresectable pancreatic cancer. A prospective randomized trial. *Ann Surg* 1993;217(5):447–455.

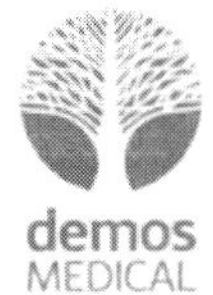

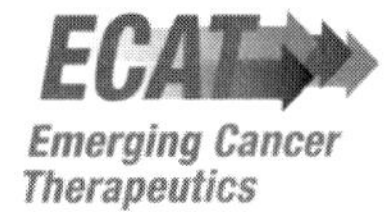

Gastrointestinal Stromal Tumors

Bilal Ahmed and Tanios Bekaii-Saab*
The Ohio State University, Columbus, OH

■ ABSTRACT

Gastrointestinal stromal tumors (GIST) are mesenchymal tumors of the gastrointestinal (GI) tract. They are found most commonly in the stomach and small intestine but can present anywhere in the GI tract from the esophagus to the anus including adjacent mesentery and omentum. The story of GIST has been that of great scientific achievement. From the initial recognition of this entity to the identification of molecular pathogenesis, development of targeted therapies such as imatinib and sunitinib and improvement in surgical techniques, the past two decades have seen remarkable progress in this disease. Targeted therapies have transformed the prognosis with about half of the patients with advanced GIST surviving beyond 5 years. Ongoing research studies exploring new pathways and enriching for specific mutations are underway to help continue improving the outcome of patients with this uncommon cancer.

■ INTRODUCTION

Gastrointestinal stromal tumors (GISTs) are mesenchymal tumors of the gastrointestinal (GI) tract. They are found most commonly in the stomach and small intestine but can present anywhere in the GI tract from the esophagus to the anus including adjacent mesentery and omentum (1).

■ HISTORICAL EVOLUTION OF DIAGNOSIS

Historically, on the basis of light microscopy, these tumors were considered to be of smooth muscle origin and often considered as leiomyoma, leiomyosarcoma, or leiomyoblastoma (2). Appleman did ultrastructural and immunohistochemical studies confirming that component cells from these tumors were basically undifferentiated, and that there was only occasional emergence of smooth muscle features. Other tumors also had features of Schwann cells (3). Mazur and Clark analyzed 28 gastric wall tumors that initially diagnosed as leiomyoma or leiomyosarcoma by light microscopy, establishing the fact that these tumors were not derivatives of smooth muscle (4). The majority of those tumors stained negative for S100, a marker for neuroectodermal differentiation, while others showed evidence of nerve sheath origin; none of those tumors had ultrastructural findings suggestive of smooth muscle origin (4). As such, they were the first to coin the term gastrointestinal stromal tumors or GIST recognizing a distinct clinical entity.

In the 1990s, immunohistochemical analysis of GIST revealed that about 70% were positive for CD34, differentiating them from leiomyomas or schwannomas, and emphasizing their distinct identity (5). A significant breakthrough about the origin of GIST was achieved through the discovery of their

*Corresponding author, The Ohio State University, Arthur James Cancer Hospital, Columbus, OH
E-mail address: Tanios.Bekaii-Saab@osumc.edu

Emerging Cancer Therapeutics 1 (2010) 149–162.

DOI: 10.5003/2151–4194.1.1.151

near universal expression of the CD117 antigen (6). CD117 is part of the KIT transmembrane receptor tyrosine kinase (RTK) which is a product of the c-kit proto-oncogene (6). In addition, most GISTs were found to have c-Kit gain of function mutations. A more recent study looked at sequencing the c-kit complementary DNA that encodes for a proto-oncogenic RTK KIT in GIST (7).The study demonstrated the presence of mutations in the region between the transmembrane and tyrosine kinase domains (7). The mutant KIT proteins were constitutively active without the KIT ligand or the stem cell factor (SCF), thus enabling oncogenic signaling in GIST cells (7).

The immunohistochemical characteristics of GISTs were compared with those of the interstitial cells of Cajal (ICCs) that regulate autonomous contraction in the GI tract. ICCs are located in and around the circular muscle layer of the stomach and small and large intestines. Several features were found to be common with GIST, including double positivity for KIT and CD34, expression of embryonic smooth muscle heavy chain and the presence of the intermediate filament nestin (8,9). This implies that GIST originate from CD34 positive stem cells in the gut wall and eventually differentiate toward ICC (10). Benign GIST does not typically express CD34, hinting that it may be a more mature form of ICC, whereas malignant GIST tends to express CD34 and therefore is more likely to be dedifferentiated ICC (10).

■ EPIDEMIOLOGY

The annual incidence of GIST is 10 to 20 per million. The first big population based study to understand the epidemiology of GIST is the Surveillance, Epidemiology, and End Results registry (SEER) of the National Cancer Institute that helped identify all cases of malignant GIST diagnosed between the years 1992 and 2000. The age-adjusted incidence was 0.68 per 100,000 and the mean age at diagnosis was 63. The incidence rate was higher in men and African Americans. The majority of tumors originate from the stomach and the small intestine (51% and 36%, respectively) with the rest originating from the colon (7%) and rectum (5%) (11). The incidence rate has likely been overestimated in this study given that KIT immunopositivity was not taken into account when making the diagnosis, and other mesenchymal tumors were possibly included. A retrospective

analysis including all patients diagnosed with GIST was performed in a province of western Sweden over a period of 17 years (12). In this study, immunoreactivity to CD117 was used as an absolute inclusion criterion for entry. The incidence of GIST was determined to be 14.5 per million and its incidence 129 per million (12). Another study analyzed 100 stomachs resected from patients with gastric cancer and examined them for microscopic GIST (13). In 35 of those stomachs, 50 microscopic GIST were found with positivity for KIT and/or CD34 (13). Considering that the presumed annual incidence is much lower, only few microscopic GISTs may grow into a size that would lead to a malignant potential. More recently, a study from Israel evaluating 93 patients with c-KIT expressing GISTs (14) found that 40.9% were malignant, 39.8% benign, and 19.4% of uncertain malignant potential. In this study, 60% of those tumors were located in the stomach, 31% in the small intestine, and the rest in the colon, duodenum, and rectum. The mean overall survival (OS) time for malignant gastric GISTs was determined to be 102.2 months (14). The belief is that given the indolent behavior of a number of GISTs which likely never present with symptoms, the true incidence of GIST may be significantly higher than reported in literature.

■ HISTOPATHOLOGY

GISTs are typically well circumscribed, generally unencapsulated and can be submucosal, intramural, or subserosal. Sixty to seventy percent of all tumors are comprised of a uniform population of spindle cells (Fig. 1), while the rest are dominated by epithelioid cells (Fig. 2), or a combination of both in variable proportions. Some of the spindle cell–shaped tumors have a prominent nerve sheath tumor-like nuclear palisade pattern, while others show prominent perinuclear vacuolization (15). GISTs with an epithelioid appearance correspond to the previous designation of leiomyoblastoma and may have either a solid or a myxoid pattern, with an occasional paraganglioma or carcinoid-like compartmental pattern (1). The nuclear features range from a monotonous oval/spindle-like appearance to a pleomorphic appearance and contain nucleoli of variable prominence with multinucleation seen occasionally (16). Multinucleation and nuclear atypia are more common in the epithelioid histology and are typically accompanied by other malignant

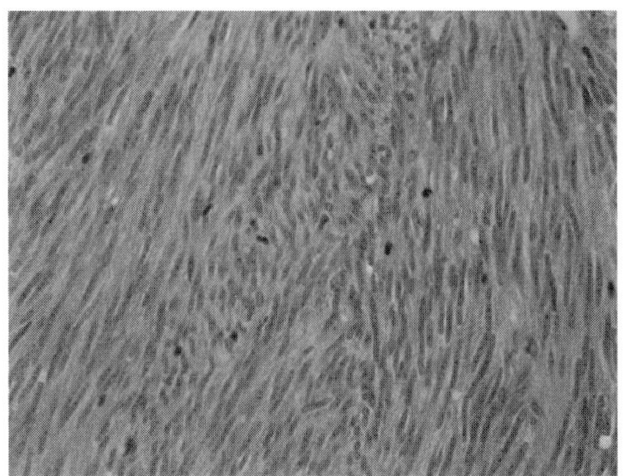

FIGURE 1 Hematoxylin and eosin (H&E) stain at 40x showing a uniform population of spindle cells in a GIST patient.

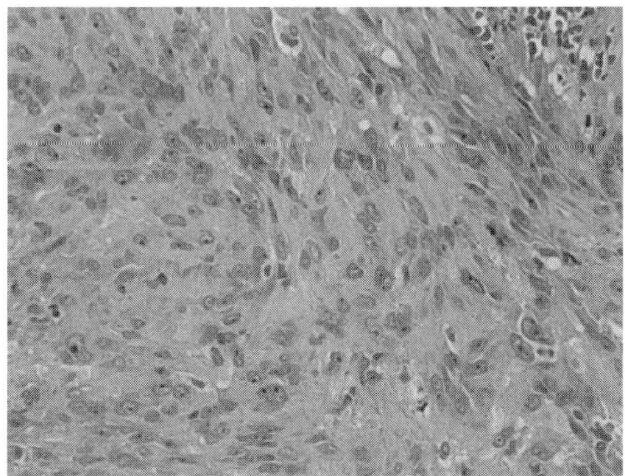

FIGURE 2 H&E stain at 40x showing epitheloid histology of GIST.

features. Mitotic activity can be varied depending on the aggressiveness of the tumor (15). Many GISTS may have a marked lymphocytic infiltrate while others (5%) may have prominent myxoid stroma (15).

■ MOLECULAR AND GENETIC MARKERS

The most biologically relevant, specific, and practical diagnostic criterion for GIST is KIT expression (CD117) as established by immunohistochemistry (17). KIT is an RTK composed of an intracellular tyrosine kinase, a juxtamembrane region, and an extracellular domain with a ligand binding site (Fig. 3). The extracellular region has three immunoglobulin domains classified as a subclass, three tyrosine kinases bearing close homology to other RTKs of subclass 3 such as receptors of platelet-derived growth factor (PDGF), macrophage colony stimulating factor, and FLT3 ligand (18). SCF is a known ligand for the KIT receptor (19). Binding of SCF to KIT induces receptor dimerization followed by activation of the tyrosine kinase enabling it to phosphorylate other proteins in the signal transduction pathway that carry the proliferation signal into the cell (19).

In GIST, KIT mutations lead to ligand-independent activation of the KIT receptor resulting in constitutive signaling for cell proliferation and survival (20). These mutations are reported to occur at a frequency range of 20% to 92% (20). More recent studies have shown a higher incidence of mutations given the likely improved detection techniques including the use of denaturing high-pressure liquid chromatography or systematic sequencing of the entire cDNA KIT coding sequence (21). Exon 9 codes for the extracellular domain, exon 11 for the juxtamembrane domain, and exon 13 for the first part of the split tyrosine kinase domain of the RTK (Fig. 8.2). A recent study of 48 patients with GISTs initially diagnosed based on histologic analysis including high KIT positivity by immunohisto-chemistry found that 44 (92%) patients had c-KIT mutations based on genomic DNA sequencing and cDNA sequencing (22). Out of those, 71% had exon 11 mutations, 13% had exon 9 mutations, and another 4% had mutations in exon 13 or 17 (22). Activating mutations in the juxtamembrane domain region result in constitutive activation of the tyrosine kinase independently of ligand binding (7).

A number of reports assessed the impact of exon 9, 11, and 13 mutations on the clinical behavior and prognosis of GIST. A study of 43 benign or malignant GISTs showed that mutations in exon 11 occurred predominantly in the malignant (62%) versus benign (16%) phenotypes (23). Martin et al. showed a significant decrease in the relapse-free survival in patients with GIST treated with imatinib in the presence of exon 11 mutations, and more specifically those with deletions involving exon 557–558 of c-KIT (24). In another study, it was shown that patients with GIST treated with imatinib had a significantly reduced progression-free survival (PFS) in the presence of deletions/insertions in exon 11 when

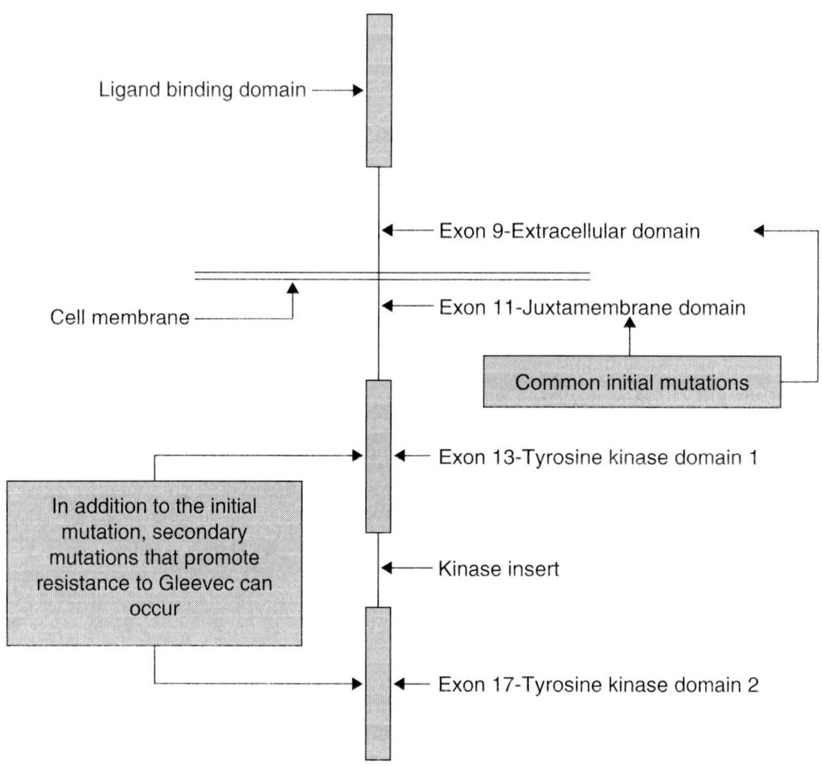

FIGURE 3 Diagram of a receptor tyrosine kinase composed of an intracellular tyrosine kinase, a juxtamembrane region and an extracellular domain with a ligand binding site. Shown are the common primary and secondary mutations.

compared to those with missense mutations in that same exon (22). In another small study, genomic sequencing of tumors of eight patients with GIST showed six of them with exon 9 mutations and two with homozygous exon 13 missense mutations (25). Further studies from Western Europe and Asia confirmed the presence of exon 9 mutations in a small percentage of the GIST patients (26). Exon 9 mutations seem to define a distinct subset of GIST, with most cases showing a duplication of six nucleotides encoding Ala-Tyr and nongastric location with a poorer outcome (27). All these studies suggest that in addition to somatic mutations in the juxtamembrane region (exon 11), mutations in the extracellular domain (exon 9) and kinase portion (exon 13) of the RTK are likely to be important to the pathogenesis of GIST. Gain of function mutations in other exons, such as exon 17, have been reported, although they are exceedingly rare (28,29).

A majority of GISTs lacking KIT mutations have instead activating mutations in related tyrosine kinases such as platelet-derived growth factor receptor alpha (PDGFRα). The signal transduction pathway for PDGFRα-mutant tumors is indistinguishable from KIT-mutant tumors, suggesting that it may substitute for KIT in the molecular pathogenesis of KIT wild-type tumors. It was also observed that KIT and PDGFRα mutations are alternating and mutually exclusive in GIST (30).

■ CLINICAL PRESENTATION

Based on the earlier described histological, epidemiological, and molecular features, GISTs were defined as tumors involving the intestinal tract or adjacent to it, with either spindle shaped or epithelioid histology, and unequivocal immmunoreactivity for CD117.

The most common presenting symptoms include GI bleeding, abdominal pain, and bloating (31). In a recent study from China, 55% of the patients presented with abdominal pain or distension, 31% presented with a palpable abdominal mass, and 17% with reported melena or hematemesis (32). A study from Sweden found that 69% of patients were diagnosed based on clinical symptoms, 21% were incidentally found while the rest of the 10% were found on autopsy (12). There are also case reports of a rare phenomenon of nonislet cell tumor–induced hypoglycemia associated with large metastatic GIST, with rapid resolution of hypoglycemia with tumor resection (33,34). Another retrospective review observed that GIST were likely to be located by order of frequency in the stomach (54%), small intestine (36%), colon (6%), and retroperitoneum or mesentery (4%) (35).

■ DIAGNOSTIC WORKUP

Diagnostic Imaging

In patients with GIST, imaging with CT or MRI is used for diagnosis, staging, monitoring response to therapy, and surveillance (36). Primary GISTs typically appear as large, hypervascular enhancing masses on contrast CT scans and are often heterogeneous because of necrotic, hemorrhagic, and/or cystic components (37). GISTs usually displace adjacent organs and vessels but infrequently invade adjacent structures. Occasionally, and especially in large GISTs, it is difficult to determine the origin of the tumor. Small GISTs are typically homogenous, endoluminal, and polypoid in appearance (38). Lymph nodes are rarely involved with GIST (39). GIST usually spreads to the liver and peritoneal cavity with the CT appearance of metastatic disease showing similarities to that of the primary tumor. Fluorodeoxyglucose (FDG) positron emission tomography (PET) scan has a high sensitivity but a low specificity and therefore has a limited role in the diagnosis of GIST, although it plays an important role in following response to treatment.

Following suspicion of a diagnosis of GIST on imaging, endoscopy is often useful in direct visualization of gastric or colorectal masses if present. Endoscopic ultrasonography is another useful modality for the evaluation of GIST in the upper GI tract as it not only helps delineate with staging, but also with diagnosis through getting a biopsy if needed (40). The need for a preoperative biopsy is a very controversial topic. The main concern is that given the hypervascular nature of GIST tumors, the risk of rupture and eventual seeding or bleeding can be significant (41). Therefore, there are only limited indications for a biopsy such as planned neoadjuvant therapy or suspicion of a non-GIST diagnosis (e.g., lymphoma).

Imaging for Response Assessment

Response evaluation criteria in solid tumor (RECIST) using tumor size has significant limitations when monitoring patients with GIST on treatment with imatinib (42,43). However, FDG-PET was found to be highly sensitive in detecting early response as well as predicting long-term response to imatinib in patients with metastatic GIST (43). A more widespread use of PET scanning is limited by the lack of availability and cost constraints. As such, modified CT criteria have been suggested by Choi et al. to help identify treatment response with a higher accuracy. A recent study included measurements on 173 tumors in 36 patients showing that while 70% of tumors had evidence of improvement on PET scan and decrease in tumor density, only 75% of the tumors showed stable disease as best response per RECIST criteria. Evaluation of CT scan results was then performed based on changes in overall tumor status (OTS), which is a combination of tumor size, density, and vascularization. When compared to results from PET scans, there was a high level of correlation found between the OTS on CT and standardized uptake value (SUV) (44). Another study showed as well the limitations in applying RECIST criteria in patients with GIST treated with imatinib. This study showed that by assessing tumor response as a decrease in tumor size of more than 10% or a decrease in tumor density of more than 15%, sensitivity is 97%, and specificity 100% when compared to PET scan results (42). On the other hand, a more recent study suggested that the absence of progression per RECIST provides an accurate predictive marker for PFS and OS. Additionally, the investigators from this study observed that patients with no change on CT scan did as well as the ones that had a measured response (45).

In conclusion, RECIST criteria do have certain limitations in assessing tumor response. However, more work needs to be done to identify more accurate and reliable response criteria such as the ones suggested by Choi and colleagues.

■ PROGNOSTIC MARKERS

Histological Characteristics

GIST has a wide spectrum of clinical behavior varying from indolent to highly aggressive and malignant. Identifying prognostic predictors for GIST has been an area of active research. A recent study from China attempted to identify histological features associated with poor overall- and disease-free survival. The study suggested that mitotic counts greater than 10 to 50 per high power field (HPF), muscularis propria infiltration, coagulative necrosis, perivascular growth, and severe nuclear atypia were all poor prognostic features (46). In 2002, a consensus approach to define prognostic markers for GIST was established (47). This consensus approach attempted to differentiate between the spectrum of disease between benign and malignant GIST. Two important morphologic characteristics considered to be of relevance included tumor size and mitotic rate. Tumors less than 2 cm with a mitotic rate of less than 5 per HPF were unlikely to be malignant whereas tumors with either a high mitotic rate or a size greater than 10 cm were more likely to be malignant (47). In a recent multivariate analysis, tumor size failed to be an independent predictor when adjustments were made for mitotic rate and histological subtype (22). However, this study suggested that high mitotic rate and a mixed spindle/epitheloid subtype have adverse prognostic features (22).

Mutational Analysis

Historically, tumors with KIT mutations were believed to behave more aggressively than their counterparts without a mutation. In one study, the 5-year recurrence-free survival was shown to be greater for patients without the KIT mutation when compared to those with the mutation. The study also showed that recurrence-free survival was longer in patients with an exon 11 mutation when compared to other identifiable mutations (22). Interestingly, the study also showed that tumors with deletions/insertions in exon 11 have a significantly reduced PFS when compared to those with missense mutation in that same exon (22).

Anatomic Location

The anatomic site of GIST is also believed to be an independent prognostic factor. A recent study determined a statistically significant difference in the 10-year OS varying between 50% and 70% based on the location of the tumor. OS was best for those patients with tumors confined to the esophagus and stomach, and worst for those whose tumors originated in the small bowel and omentum. The differences in survival among groups were significant ($P = 0.00109$) with 10-year survivals varying between 50% and 70% (48). Similarly, another study showed that the more common gastric GIST has generally a better prognosis than the less common small intestinal GIST when controlling for size and mitotic rate (49).

■ TREATMENT OF GIST

Historically, surgical resection was the mainstay of treatment with no proven role for cytotoxic therapy whether in the adjuvant setting or the more advanced disease. The response rate to cytotoxic treatment has historically been lower than 10% (50). Of course, one of the main challenges in assessing the true response rate is that historically GISTs were not differentiated from other sarcomas of the GI tract. One study with patients with advanced malignant GISTs and advanced leiomyosarcomas treated with dacarbazine, mitomycin, doxorubicin, and cisplatin (DMAP) plus GM-CSF showed an objective response rate in only 1 of 21 patients with GIST and 11 of 18 (61%) patients with leiomyosarcomas (51).

The role of systemic targeted therapy for GIST emerged from drug development in chronic myelogenous leukemia. ST1571 (imatinib) is a small, phenylaminopyrimidine derivative molecule that selectively inhibits the enzymatic activity of several tyrosine kinases including PDGF receptor and the product of the c-kit gene. The first patient to receive the drug in GIST was a 54-year-old Finnish patient with metastatic disease who had a dramatic radiological and pathological response (52). This led to opening the way for further development of imatinib in GIST.

The current treatment of GIST is considered as one of the greatest success stories that helped revolutionize the concept of targeted therapy in solid tumor oncology.

Treatment of Early GIST

Surgery

In this section, we will briefly review basic surgical principles involved in the management of these patients. There is no consensus on the management of tumors less than 2 cm, and it is not known whether surgery is a better option than watchful waiting. All tumors >2 cm should be resected. The goal of a surgery with a curative intent is the complete resection of the tumor including the preservation of an intact pseudocapsule. In one study, the 5-year survival rate after a complete resection is 42% compared to 9% after an incomplete resection (53). Another study observed that for patients with resectable disease, the 5-year survival rate was similarly 54% and the tumor size was considered as the most important determinant for outcome (54). Local recurrence is more common when a peritumoral resection is performed, even in the presence of negative resection margins (55). Therefore, the recommendation is to avoid peritumoral resection and prefer instead segmental resection. For example, in GIST involving the stomach, a partial or total gastrectomy is preferred over wedge gastric resection. Similarly, in GIST involving the rectum, an anterior rectal resection is preferable to transanal rectal excision (55).

In the preimatinib era, patients with tumor rupture despite removal of all gross disease had a similar prognosis than those with incomplete resections (56). Therefore, laparotomy is preferred over laparoscopic surgery, especially when careful handling is not possible with the latter. At laparotomy, careful exploration should be performed with special attention paid to the liver and peritoneal surfaces to exclude any metastatic disease (55). Lymph node sampling or dissection is not necessary, as GIST rarely involves them (55).

Adjuvant Treatment

Surgery is the mainstay of treatment for localized GIST. Unfortunately, and despite complete resections, this disease has a high recurrence rate. A recent study showed that 33% of patients with GIST ($n = 93$) who were able to undergo complete resections had eventual disease recurrence, with a 5-year survival rate of 54% (54). The high rate of recurrence and the encouraging results seen with imatinib in advanced GIST paved the way for its use in the adjuvant setting. The results of the ACOSOG randomized phase 3 double-blind study of patients with GIST receiving placebo versus imatinib (400 mg once daily given for a year) following surgical resection were recently presented (57). With a median follow-up of 19.7 months, 20% of patients on placebo and 8% on imatinib had tumor recurrence, respectively. Imatinib significantly improved

recurrence-free survival at 1 year over placebo (98% vs 83%, respectively). The risk of recurrence was more pronounced in tumors larger than 10 cm (57). The OS was similar in the two arms, although this was attributed to the fact that patients were allowed crossover from the placebo to imatinib upon progression (57). This eventually led to the Food and Drug Administration (FDA) approval of imatinib in the adjuvant setting for GIST in December 2008. The main criticism for this study was that the improvement in the recurrence-free survival was minimal for tumors less than 10 cm; hence, whether there should be uniform use of imatinib for all tumors greater than 3 cm remains unanswered (58). Another study evaluated the use of adjuvant imatinib in high risk patients only (59). High risk was based on tumor size (mean tumor size: 9.4 cm, range 2–35 cm) and high mitotic rate (Ki67 2%–10%). Only 1 out of 23 patients (4%) in the adjuvant treatment group developed recurrent disease compared to 32 out of 48 (67%) in the historical control group (59).

In conclusion, although the use of imatinib in adjuvant setting is approved for use in GIST larger than 3 cm, most of the benefit is seen in tumors measuring more than 10 cm. For tumors measuring between 3 and 10 cm, prognostic features such as mitotic rate, histology, site of the tumor, and specific mutations should be taken into consideration in the decision-making process. The recommended duration of therapy is 1 year. A consideration for a higher dose of imatinib (800 mg) in the adjuvant setting for patients with an exon 9 mutation could be justified based on recently published data in the advanced setting (60).

Neoadjuvant Treatment

The use of imatinib in the neoadjuvant setting is also being explored in GIST, especially in patients with locally advanced or surgically unresectable tumors. A small study assessed the efficacy of imatinib in 15 patients with locally advanced GIST showing that all patients exhibited some level of tumor shrinkage with a median size reduction of 34% (61). One patient had a complete radiological response, 3 patients initially deemed unresectable underwent complete resection, and 7 patients who initially were thought to require extensive surgery went on to have more conservative resection. PFS at 3 years was 77% (61). A current phase 2 study is evaluating the safety and efficacy of neoadjuvant imatinib in patients with either primary GIST measuring more than 5 cm (group A) or metastatic/recurrent disease measuring more than 2 cm (group B). In group A, the use of neoadjuvant therapy enabled a high percentage (77%) of complete resection and more function sparing resections. The estimated 2-year PFS in both groups combined is 80.5%, 82.7% in group A, and 77.3% in group B (62). The reduction in the size of GIST allowed for less invasive resections, which is especially useful in sites such as the esophagus and the rectum. For example, downsizing of rectal GIST allowed for more low anterior resections leading to preservation of sphincter activity (63). For now, one can only recommend the use of imatinib in the preoperative setting in borderline resectable disease. Large randomized trials are required to validate further the role of this approach in clearly resectable GIST.

■ ADVANCED GIST

Medical Treatment

First-Line Therapy
Findings that imatinib is a selective inhibitor of c-kit tyrosine kinase activity (64) led to the interest in developing imatinib in GIST. Imatinib was first used on compassionate grounds in a patient with advanced GIST with evidence of remarkable results (52). This was followed by a European Organization for Research and Treatment of Cancer (EORTC) phase 1 study of 40 patients with advanced GIST receiving doses ranging from 400 to 1,000 mg (65). Eighteen patients on this study had a partial response, while 11 had stable disease and the rest had disease progression. Dose-limiting toxicities included nausea, edema, and rash. The maximum tolerated dose was determined to be 400 mg given orally twice a day. A multicenter clinical trial to assess the efficacy and safety of imatinib in patients with unresectable or metastatic GIST followed. A total of 147 patients were randomly assigned to receive either 400 or 600 mg of imatinib orally every day. Overall response rate for the combined group was 53.7% with another 27.9% of the patients experiencing stable disease. There were no significant differences in toxicity or response rate between the two doses tested. The drug was well tolerated with the most common toxicities including edema, diarrhea, and fatigue (66). Patients were followed up long term with the results of the 4-year extension study showing a median OS of 57 months and a 5-year OS

rate close to 50% (67). Historically, patients with advanced GIST who were not treated by imatinib had a reported median survival of 19 months (54). Another trial assessed imatinib doses of 400 versus 800 mg/day without showing any statistically significant difference in objective response rates, PFS, or OS between the two doses (60). Thus, it seemed reasonable to establish the use of an initial dose of 400 mg daily as a standard of care in the initial treatment of advanced GIST.

Recently, development of alternative agents or strategies (such as combining novel agents with imatinib) in first-line treatment has gained a lot of interest. Masitinib mesylate, a novel tyrosine kinase inhibitor, has shown greater potency and selectivity in vitro against c-KIT when compared to imatinib. A recent phase 2 study of 30 patients with advanced untreated GIST who received masitinib therapy showed a response rate of 20% at 2 months according to the RECIST and 84.6% according to the PET criteria (68). The median PFS was 27.2 months. The results compare historically favorably to imatinib prompting a phase 3 study (NCT00812240) comparing imatinib to masitinib.

Second Line and Beyond
Resistance eventually develops in metastatic GIST patients treated with imatinib. Only a small fraction of patients will exhibit resistance in the first 2 months (primary resistance), with most patients showing a response of at least 6 months (69). A study of 818 patients looking at the patterns of resistance to imatinib suggested that primary resistance was recorded in only 12% of assessable patients (67). Another study suggested a similar incidence of primary resistance (11%) in patients with GIST treated with imitanib (70).

Multiple mechanisms have been proposed as potentially responsible for the development of resistance to imatinib treatment in GIST:

1. Amplification of the gene leading to overexpression of KIT receptor or PDGFRα (71)
2. Activation of alternative RTKs (71)
3. Development of activating mutations in the KIT receptor and PDFGRα rendering them resistant to imatinib (55). New KIT mutations probably change the conformation of the receptor which modifies the adenosine triphosphate (ATP)-binding pocket and inhibit imatinib binding to the receptor.

Increasing the Dose of Imatinib

In an early dose finding study, 9 patients on a 400-mg dose were allowed to crossover to 600 mg daily resulting in one partial response and an additional two patients with stable disease (66). This was substantiated by a large European study applying a dose increase of imatinib to 800 mg daily in patients previously receiving 400 mg daily, resulting in 3 patients (2%) with a partial response and another 36 (27%) with stable disease. The median PFS was 81 days with 18.1% of patients alive and progression-free 1 year after crossover (72). The increase in dose proved to be relatively tolerable (72), with increasing fatigue and anemia only while the incidence of other toxicities stayed about the same. Another study confirmed that 33% of patients who received the higher dose after resistance to the lower dose had either a partial response or stable disease. Patients who crossed over had an additional median PFS of 5 months (60).

Therefore, the first approach to a patient who progressed on a standard dose of imatinib (400 mg orally every day) is to increase the dose unless there is evidence of intolerance to the drug.

Sunitinib

Sunitinib is a small molecule that exhibits antitumor and antiangiogenic properties by inhibiting multiple tyrosine kinases including KIT, PDGFRα and β, vascular endothelial growth factor (VEGFR1, VEGFR2, and VEGFR3), and a few others (73). Secondary mutations conferring resistance to imatinib are usually located in the ATP-binding pocket of the RTKs (74). Sunitinib was shown to have inhibitory activity in GIST cell lines with V654A and T670I mutations (mutations in the ATP pocket) providing the basis for using sunitinib in imatinib refractory GIST (74).

In one study, 312 patients with imatinib refractory disease were randomized to receive either sunitinib or placebo (75). Results of this study suggest a significant advantage with sunitinib over placebo with a median time to tumor progression of 27.3 versus 6.4 weeks, respectively (76). OS was also improved with sunitinib versus placebo (HR = 0.49; 95% CI 0.29–0.83; $P = 0.007$) (75). This study led to an accelerated approval by the FDA on January 26, 2006, of sunitinib for the treatment of patients with refractory or intolerant to imatinib in GIST (75).

Other Biologics

Other novel therapeutic strategies are being investigated for patients who are either intolerant or progress on first-line imatinib and second-line sunitinib. One of those agents is nirlotinib, a novel tyrosine kinase inhibitor targeting both KIT and PDGFR showing significant in vitro activity in both imatinib-sensitive or -resistant cell lines (77). A recent European study assessed the efficacy and safety of nirlotinib given orally at 400 mg twice daily in 52 patients with GIST who had progressed on both imatinib and sunitinib (78). The study suggested activity with nirlotinib in those refractory patients with a 10% response rate and 37% stable disease rate (78). Median PFS of nirlotinib treatment was 12 weeks and median OS was 34 weeks (78). There are a number of other agents being studied in the treatment of GIST refractory to imatinib and sunitinib including sorafenib and dasatinib, both of which have shown to inhibit various tyrosine kinases including KIT (79,80).

In conclusion, in case of primary or secondary resistance, either dose escalation or switching to sunitinib is indicated based on the patient's tolerance.

Genetic Predictors of Efficacy in the Treatment of GIST

Various KIT and PDGFRα mutations can be predictive of response to imatinib therapy in advanced GIST. GISTs lacking a detectable kinase mutation were found to have no response to imatinib (81). Tumors with exon 11 mutations were found to have a higher tumor response (83.5%) than those with exon 9 mutation (47.8%). The same advantage was true when looking at event-free survival and OS (81). Patients that harbored exon 11 mutations were also found to have a higher objective response to imatinib (86%) than patients who had either an exon 9 mutation (48%) or no detectable mutation in KIT or PDGFRα (0%) (67). On the other hand, the results of the EORTC phase 3 trial suggest that patients with exon 9 mutations may have a superior PFS when initially treated with a higher dose of imatinib (800 vs 400 mg daily) (60).

A great majority of patients treated on imatinib have a response; however, most of them eventually acquire resistance to treatment (82). We suggest complete molecular profiling whenever possible and starting the patient on an initial dose of 400 mg daily except in those with exon 9 mutation where we suggest 800 mg daily.

A number of studies attempted to correlate specific KIT mutations with the efficacy of sunitinib. A study evaluating the effect of KIT mutations on sunitinib efficacy showed that response rates for sunitinib were observed to be higher in patients with KIT exon 9 mutations when compared to patients with exon 11 mutations (83). Secondary KIT mutations in patients with imatinib resistance are clustered in exon 13 and 14 (ATP-binding pocket of the receptor) or in exon 17 which encodes the kinase activation loop (83). This study confirmed the in vitro findings showing the efficacy of sunitinib in patients with ATP-binding site mutation and relative ineffectiveness in the presence of exon 17 or 18 (i.e., activation loop) mutations (83). Another recent study investigated the mechanism of resistance to sunitinib and found a cis mutation in the activation loop to be a potential culprit (84). However, sunitinib has potent antiangiogenic effects in addition to inhibiting KIT or PDGFR inhibition and thus may confer additional antitumor activity even in the presence of these mutations

Surgery for Advanced or Metastatic GIST

Surgical resection in advanced GIST after treatment with first-line treatment with imatinib or second-line treatment with sunitinib has been looked at recently. In a study 40 patients with metastatic GIST were treated with either imatinib or sunitinib and then underwent surgical resection (85). Twenty patients who had disease responsive to medical therapy had a 2-year PFS of 61% and 2-year OS of 100%. In contrast, the 13 patients with focal resistance (1 tumor growing) had a median PFS of 12 months and the 2-year OS was 36%. There were seven patients with multifocal resistance (more than 1 tumor growing) and they progressed postoperatively at a median of 3 months and had a 1-year OS of 36% (85). Another study involved 69 patients with advanced GIST who underwent surgical resection after initial treatment with imatinib and switching over to sunitinib upon progression (86). The patients were divided into those who had stable disease, limited progression, or generalized progression on medical treatment. The 1-year PFS was 80%, 33%, and 0% for patients with stable disease, limited progression, and generalized progression ($P = .0001$), respectively. One-year OS was 95%, 86%, and 0%, respectively, for patients with stable disease, limited progression, and generalized progression ($P = .0001$) (86). Surgical resection may prove to confer a survival advantage from either the removal of the tumor mass before the development of secondary resistance or from excision of highly resistant tumors (87). Of course, this needs to be further validated on larger randomized studies.

We suggest surgical referral in advanced GIST patients who have had either a response or stable disease after a few months of tyrosine kinase inhibitor (TKI) therapy and have a chance at complete resection.

■ CONCLUSION

The story of GIST has been one of the most successful in translational therapeutics eventually leading to significant improvements in the outcome of patients with GIST in the last two decades. The remarkable progress in GIST spanned across all areas from the development of diagnostic and prognostic markers to remarkable advances in therapy. A lot of work still needs to be done including improving the ability to differentiate between indolent and aggressive disease, continuously refining therapy, and developing a more individualized approach to the systemic treatment of GIST.

■ REFERENCES

1. Miettinen M, Lasota J. Gastrointestinal stromal tumors—definition, clinical, histological, immunohistochemical, and molecular genetic features and differential diagnosis. *Virchows Arch* 2001;438(1):1–12.
2. Stout AP. Tumors of the Stomach. *Bull N Y Acad Med* 1947;23(2):101–108.
3. Appelman HD. Smooth muscle tumors of the gastrointestinal tract. What we know now that Stout didn't know. *Am J Surg Pathol* 1986;10(Suppl 1):83–99.
4. Mazur MT, Clark HB. Gastric stromal tumors. Reappraisal of histogenesis. *Am J Surg Pathol* 1983;7(6):507–519.
5. Miettinen M, Virolainen M, Maarit Sarlomo R. Gastrointestinal stromal tumors—value of CD34 antigen in their identification and separation from true leiomyomas and schwannomas. *Am J Surg Pathol* 1995;19(2):207–216.
6. Rubin BP, Fletcher JA, Fletcher CD. Molecular Insights into the Histogenesis and Pathogenesis of Gastrointestinal Stromal Tumors. *Int J Surg Pathol* 2000;8(1):5–10.
7. Hirota S, Isozaki K, Moriyama Y, et al. Gain-of-function mutations of c-kit in human gastrointestinal stromal tumors. *Science* 1998;279(5350):577–580.
8. Tsujimura T, Makiishi-Shimobayashi C, Lundkvist J, et al. Expression of the intermediate filament nestin in gastrointestinal stromal tumors and interstitial cells of Cajal. *Am J Pathol* 2001;158(3):817–823.

9. Sakurai S, Fukasawa T, Chong JM, Tanaka A, Fukayama M. Embryonic form of smooth muscle myosin heavy chain (SMemb/MHC-B) in gastrointestinal stromal tumor and interstitial cells of Cajal. *Am J Pathol* 1999;154(1):23–28.

10. Wang L, Vargas H, French SW. Cellular origin of gastrointestinal stromal tumors: a study of 27 cases. *Arch Pathol Lab Med* 2000;124(10):1471–1475.

11. Tran T, Davila JA, El-Serag HB. The epidemiology of malignant gastrointestinal stromal tumors: an analysis of 1,458 cases from 1992 to 2000. *Am J Gastroenterol.* Jan 2005;100(1):162–168.

12. Nilsson B, Bümming P, Meis-Kindblom JM, et al. Gastrointestinal stromal tumors: the incidence, prevalence, clinical course, and prognostication in the preimatinib mesylate era—a population-based study in western Sweden. *Cancer* 2005;103(4):821–829.

13. Kawanowa K, Sakuma Y, Sakurai S, et al. High incidence of microscopic gastrointestinal stromal tumors in the stomach. *Hum Pathol* 2006;37(12): 1527–1535.

14. Rabin I, Chikman B, Lavy R, et al. Gastrointestinal stromal tumors: a 19 year experience. *Isr Med Assoc J* 2009;11(2):98–102.

15. Corless CL, Fletcher JA, Heinrich MC. Biology of gastrointestinal stromal tumors. *J Clin Oncol* 2004;22(18):3813–3825.

16. Graadt van Roggen JF, van Velthuysen ML, Hogendoorn PC. The histopathological differential diagnosis of gastrointestinal stromal tumours. *J Clin Pathol* 2001; 54(2):96–102.

17. Fletcher CD, Berman JJ, Corless C, et al. Diagnosis of gastrointestinal stromal tumors: A consensus approach. *Hum Pathol* 2002;33(5):459–465.

18. Rousset D, Agnès F, Lachaume P, André C, Galibert F. Molecular evolution of the genes encoding receptor tyrosine kinase with immunoglobulinlike domains. *J Mol Evol* 1995;41(4):421–429.

19. Kitamura Y, Hirota S, Nishida T. Molecular pathology of c-kit proto-oncogene and development of gastrointestinal stromal tumors. *Ann Chir Gynaecol* 1998;87(4):282–286.

20. Emile JF, Théou N, Tabone S, et al., Clinicopathologic, phenotypic, and genotypic characteristics of gastrointestinal mesenchymal tumors. *Clin Gastroenterol Hepatol* 2004;2(7):597–605.

21. Corless CL, McGreevey L, Haley A, Town A, Heinrich MC. KIT mutations are common in incidental gastrointestinal stromal tumors one centimeter or less in size. *Am J Pathol* 2002;160(5):1567–1572.

22. Singer S, Rubin BP, Lux ML, et al. Prognostic value of KIT mutation type, mitotic activity, and histologic subtype in gastrointestinal stromal tumors. *J Clin Oncol* 2002;20(18):3898–3905.

23. Lasota J, Jasinski M, Sarlomo-Rikala M, Miettinen M. Mutations in exon 11 of c-Kit occur preferentially in malignant versus benign gastrointestinal stromal tumors and do not occur in leiomyomas or leiomyosarcomas. *Am J Pathol* 1999;154(1):53–60.

24. Martín J, Poveda A, Llombart-Bosch A, et al. Deletions affecting codons 557–558 of the c-KIT gene indicate a poor prognosis in patients with completely resected gastrointestinal stromal tumors: a study by the Spanish Group for Sarcoma Research (GEIS). *J Clin Oncol* 2005;23(25):6190–6198.

25. Lux ML, Rubin BP, Biase TL, et al. KIT extracellular and kinase domain mutations in gastrointestinal stromal tumors. *Am J Pathol* 2000;156(3):791–795.

26. Sakurai S, Oguni S, Hironaka M, Fukayama M, Morinaga S, Saito K. Mutations in c-kit gene exons 9 and 13 in gastrointestinal stromal tumors among Japanese. *Jpn J Cancer Res* 2001;92(5):494–498.

27. Antonescu CR, Sommer G, Sarran L, et al. Association of KIT exon 9 mutations with nongastric primary site and aggressive behavior: KIT mutation analysis and clinical correlates of 120 gastrointestinal stromal tumors. *Clin Cancer Res* 2003;9(9):3329–3337.

28. Hirota S, Nishida T, Isozaki K, et al. Familial gastrointestinal stromal tumors associated with dysphagia and novel type germline mutation of KIT gene. *Gastroenterology* 2002;122(5):1493–1499.

29. Kinoshita K, Isozaki K, Hirota S, et al. c-kit gene mutation at exon 17 or 13 is very rare in sporadic gastrointestinal stromal tumors. *J Gastroenterol Hepatol* 2003;18(2):147–151.

30. Heinrich MC, Corless CL, Duensing A, et al. PDGFRA activating mutations in gastrointestinal stromal tumors. *Science* 2003;299(5607):708–710.

31. Chou FF, Eng HL, Sheen-Chen SM. Smooth muscle tumors of the gastrointestinal tract: analysis of prognostic factors. *Surgery* 1996;119(2):171–177.

32. Qin HD, Zhang DW, Yang WL. [Clinical analysis of gastrointestinal stromal tumor: a report of 29 patients]. *Zhonghua Wei Chang Wai Ke Za Zhi* 2006;9(2):139–141.

33. Guiteau J, Fanucchi M, Folpe A, Staley CA, Kooby DA. Hypoglycemia in the setting of advanced gastrointestinal stromal tumor. *Am Surg* 2006;72(12):1225–1230.

34. Escobar GA, Robinson WA, Nydam TL, et al. Severe paraneoplastic hypoglycemia in a patient with a gastrointestinal stromal tumor with an exon 9 mutation: a case report. *BMC Cancer* 2007;7:13.

35. Lin SC, Huang MJ, Zeng CY, Wang TI, Liu ZL, Shiay RK. Clinical manifestations and prognostic factors in patients with gastrointestinal stromal tumors. *World J Gastroenterol* 2003;9(12):2809–2812.

36. Hersh MR, Choi J, Garrett C, Clark R. Imaging gastrointestinal stromal tumors. *Cancer Control* 2005;12(2):111–115.

37. Horton KM, Juluru K, Montogomery E, Fishman EK. Computed tomography imaging of gastrointestinal stromal tumors with pathology correlation. *J Comput Assist Tomogr* 2004;28(6):811–817.

38. Hong X, Choi H, Loyer EM, Benjamin RS, Trent JC, Charnsangavej C. Gastrointestinal stromal tumor: role of CT in diagnosis and in response evaluation and surveillance after treatment with imatinib. *Radiographics* 2006;26(2):481–495.

39. Kingham TP, DeMatteo RP. Multidisciplinary treatment of gastrointestinal stromal tumors. *Surg Clin North Am* 2009;89(1):217–33, x.

40. Tio TL, Tytgat GN, den Hartog Jager FC. Endoscopic ultrasonography for the evaluation of smooth muscle tumors in the upper gastrointestinal tract: an experience with 42 cases. *Gastrointest Endosc* 1990;36(4): 342–350.

41. Gelmini R, Bertolini F, Rossi G, Luppi G, Saviano M, Conte PF. Laparoscopic approach of gastric gastrointestinal stromal tumors (GISTs): is it still a courageous choice? Report of two cases. *Surg Laparosc Endosc Percutan Tech* 2007;17(2):133–137.

42. Choi H, Charnsangavej C, Faria SC, et al. Correlation of computed tomography and positron emission tomography in patients with metastatic gastrointestinal stromal tumor treated at a single institution with imatinib mesylate: proposal of new computed tomography response criteria. *J Clin Oncol* 2007;25(13):1753–1759.

43. Basu S, Mohandas KM, Peshwe H, Asopa R, Vyawahare M. FDG-PET and PET/CT in the clinical management of gastrointestinal stromal tumor. *Nucl Med Commun* 2008;29(12):1026–1039.

44. Choi H, Charnsangavej C, de Castro Faria S, et al. CT evaluation of the response of gastrointestinal stromal tumors after imatinib mesylate treatment: a quantitative analysis correlated with FDG PET findings. *AJR Am J Roentgenol* 2004;183(6):1619–1628.

45. Le Cesne A, Van Glabbeke M, Verweij J, et al. Absence of progression as assessed by response evaluation criteria in solid tumors predicts survival in advanced GI stromal tumors treated with imatinib mesylate: the intergroup EORTC-ISG-AGITG phase III trial. *J Clin Oncol* 2009;27(24):3969–3974.

46. Hou YY, Lu SH, Zhou Y, et al. Predictive values of clinical and pathological parameters for malignancy of gastrointestinal stromal tumors. *Histol Histopathol* 2009;24(6):737–747.

47. Fletcher CD, Berman JJ, Corless C, et al. Diagnosis of gastrointestinal stromal tumors: a consensus approach. *Int J Surg Pathol* 2002;10(2):81–89.

48. Emory TS, Sobin LH, Lukes L, Lee DH, O'Leary TJ. Prognosis of gastrointestinal smooth-muscle (stromal) tumors: dependence on anatomic site. *Am J Surg Pathol* 1999; 23(1):82–87.

49. Miettinen M, El-Rifai W, H L Sobin L, Lasota J. Evaluation of malignancy and prognosis of gastrointestinal stromal tumors: a review. *Hum Pathol* 2002;33(5):478–483.

50. Dematteo RP, Heinrich MC, El-Rifai WM, Demetri G. Clinical management of gastrointestinal stromal tumors: before and after STI-571. *Hum Pathol* 2002;33(5):466–477.

51. Edmonson JH, Marks RS, Buckner JC, Mahoney MR. Contrast of response to dacarbazine, mitomycin, doxorubicin, and cisplatin (DMAP) plus GM-CSF between patients with advanced malignant gastrointestinal stromal tumors and patients with other advanced leiomyosarcomas. *Cancer Invest* 2002;20(5–6):605–612.

52. Joensuu H, Roberts PJ, Sarlomo-Rikala M, et al. Effect of the tyrosine kinase inhibitor STI571 in a patient with a metastatic gastrointestinal stromal tumor. *N Engl J Med* 2001;344(14):1052–1056.

53. Pierie JP, Choudry U, Muzikansky A, Yeap BY, Souba WW, Ott MJ. The effect of surgery and grade on outcome of gastrointestinal stromal tumors. *Arch Surg* 2001;136(4): 383–389.

54. DeMatteo RP, Lewis JJ, Leung D, Mudan SS, Woodruff JM, Brennan MF. Two hundred gastrointestinal stromal tumors: recurrence patterns and prognostic factors for survival. *Ann Surg* 2000;231(1):51–58.

55. Aparicio T, Boige V, Sabourin JC, et al. Prognostic factors after surgery of primary resectable gastrointestinal stromal tumours. *Eur J Surg Oncol* 2004;30(10):1098–1103.

56. Ng EH, Pollock RE, Munsell MF, Atkinson EN, Romsdahl MM. Prognostic factors influencing survival in gastrointestinal leiomyosarcomas. Implications for surgical management and staging. *Ann Surg* 1992;215(1): 68–77.

57. Dematteo RP, Ballman KV, Antonescu CR, et al. Adjuvant imatinib mesylate after resection of localised, primary gastrointestinal stromal tumour: a randomised, double-blind, placebo-controlled trial. *Lancet* 2009;373(9669):1097–1104.

58. Hohenberger P. Adjuvant imatinib in GIST: a self-fulfilling prophecy, or more? *Lancet* 2009;373(9669):1058–1060.

59. Nilsson B, Sjölund K, Kindblom LG, et al. Adjuvant imatinib treatment improves recurrence-free survival in patients with high-risk gastrointestinal stromal tumours (GIST). *Br J Cancer* 2007;96(11):1656–1658.

60. Blanke CD, Rankin C, Demetri GD, et al. Phase III randomized, intergroup trial assessing imatinib mesylate at two dose levels in patients with unresectable or metastatic gastrointestinal stromal tumors expressing the kit receptor tyrosine kinase: S0033. *J Clin Oncol* 2008;26(4):626–632.

61. Fiore M, Palassini E, Fumagalli E, et al. Preoperative imatinib mesylate for unresectable or locally advanced primary gastrointestinal stromal tumors (GIST). *Eur J Surg Oncol* 2009;35(7):739–745.

62. Eisenberg BL, Harris J, Blanke CD, et al. Phase II trial of neoadjuvant/adjuvant imatinib mesylate (IM) for advanced primary and metastatic/recurrent operable gastrointestinal stromal tumor (GIST): early results of RTOG 0132/ACRIN 6665. *J Surg Oncol* 2009;99(1):42–47.

63. Ebihara Y, Okushiba S, Kawarada Y, Kitashiro S, Katoh H, Kondo S. Neoadjuvant imatinib in a gastrointestinal stromal tumor of the rectum: report of a case. *Surg Today* 2008;38(2):174–177.

64. Heinrich MC, Griffith DJ, Druker BJ, Wait CL, Ott KA, Zigler AJ. Inhibition of c-kit receptor tyrosine kinase activity by STI 571, a selective tyrosine kinase inhibitor. *Blood* 2000;96(3):925–932.

65. van Oosterom AT, Judson IR, Verweij J, et al. Update of phase I study of imatinib (STI571) in advanced soft tissue sarcomas and gastrointestinal stromal tumors: a

report of the EORTC Soft Tissue and Bone Sarcoma Group. *Eur J Cancer* 2002;38(Suppl 5):S83–S87.

66. Demetri GD, von Mehren M, Blanke CD, et al. Efficacy and safety of imatinib mesylate in advanced gastrointestinal stromal tumors. *N Engl J Med* 2002;347(7):472–480.

67. Blanke CD, Demetri GD, von Mehren M, et al. Long-term results from a randomized phase II trial of standard- versus higher-dose imatinib mesylate for patients with unresectable or metastatic gastrointestinal stromal tumors expressing KIT. *J Clin Oncol* 2008; 26(4):620–625.

68. Le Cesne JB, Bui NB, Bouché O, et al. Masatinib mesylate in imatinib-naive locally advanced or metastatic gastrointestinal stromal tumor (GIST): Results of the French Sarcoma Group phase II trial. ASCO meeting. 2009 [Abstract 10507] *J Clin Oncol* 2009;27:15s.

69. Van Glabbeke M, Verweij J, Casali PG, et al. Initial and late resistance to imatinib in advanced gastrointestinal stromal tumors are predicted by different prognostic factors: a European Organisation for Research and Treatment of Cancer-Italian Sarcoma Group-Australasian Gastrointestinal Trials Group study. *J Clin Oncol* 2005;23(24):5795–5804.

70. Verweij J, Casali PG, Zalcberg J, et al. Progression-free survival in gastrointestinal stromal tumours with high-dose imatinib. randomised trial. *Lancet* 2004;364(9440): 1127–1134.

71. Liegl B, Kepten I, Le C, et al. Heterogeneity of kinase inhibitor resistance mechanisms in GIST. *J Pathol* 2008;216(1):64–74.

72 Zalcberg JR, Verweij J, Casali PG, et al., Outcome of patients with advanced gastro-intestinal stromal tumours crossing over to a daily imatinib dose of 800 mg after progression on 400 mg. *Eur J Cancer* 2005;41(12):1751–1757.

73. Cassier PA, Dufresne A, Arifi S, et al. Novel approaches to gastrointestinal stromal tumors resistant to imatinib and sunitinib. *Curr Gastroenterol Rep* 2008;10(6):555–561.

74. Prenen H, Cools J, Mentens N, et al. Efficacy of the kinase inhibitor SU11248 against gastrointestinal stromal tumor mutants refractory to imatinib mesylate. *Clin Cancer Res* 2006;12(8):2622–2627.

75. Goodman VL, Rock EP, Dagher R, et al. Approval summary: sunitinib for the treatment of imatinib refractory or intolerant gastrointestinal stromal tumors and advanced renal cell carcinoma. *Clin Cancer Res* 2007;13(5):1367–1373.

76. Demetri GD, van Oosterom AT, Garrett CR, et al. Efficacy and safety of sunitinib in patients with advanced gastrointestinal stromal tumour after failure of imatinib: a randomised controlled trial. *Lancet* 2006;368(9544):1329–1338.

77. Sevinc A. Activity of nilotinib (AMN-107) alone in advanced gastrointestinal stromal tumors progressing on imatinib and sunitinib. Case report. *Chemotherapy* 2009;55(2):132–136.

78. Montemurro M, Schoffski P, Reichardt P, et al. Nilotinib in the treatment of advanced gastrointestinal stromal tumours resistant to both imatinib and sunitinib. *Eur J Cancer.* Sep 2009;45(13):2293–2297.

79. Guo T, Agaram NP, Wong GC, et al. Sorafenib inhibits the imatinib-resistant KITT670I gatekeeper mutation in gastrointestinal stromal tumor. *Clin Cancer Res* 2007;13(16):4874–4881.

80. Dewaele B, Wasag B, Cools J, et al. Activity of dasatinib, a dual SRC/ABL kinase inhibitor, and IPI-504, a heat shock protein 90 inhibitor, against gastrointestinal stromal tumor-associated PDGFRAD842V mutation. *Clin Cancer Res* 2008;14(18):5749–5758.

81. Heinrich MC, Corless CL, Demetri GD, et al. Kinase mutations and imatinib response in patients with metastatic gastrointestinal stromal tumor. *J Clin Oncol* 2003;21(23): 4342–4349.

82. Sanborn RE, Blanke CD. Gastrointestinal stromal tumors and the evolution of targeted therapy. *Clin Adv Hematol Oncol* 2005;3(8):647–657.

83. Heinrich MC, Maki RG, Corless CL, et al. Primary and secondary kinase genotypes correlate with the biological and clinical activity of sunitinib in imatinib-resistant gastrointestinal stromal tumor. *J Clin Oncol* 2008;26(33):5352–5359.

84. Nishida T, Takahashi T, Nishitani A, et al., Sunitinib-resistant gastrointestinal stromal tumors harbor cis-mutations in the activation loop of the KIT gene. *Int J Clin Oncol* 2009;14(2):143–149.

85. DeMatteo RP, Maki RG, Singer S, Gonen M, Brennan MF, Antonescu CR. Results of tyrosine kinase inhibitor therapy followed by surgical resection for metastatic gastrointestinal stromal tumor. *Ann Surg* 2007;245(3):347–352.

86. Raut CP, Posner M, Desai J, et al. Surgical management of advanced gastrointestinal stromal tumors after treatment with targeted systemic therapy using kinase inhibitors. *J Clin Oncol* 2006;24(15):2325–2331.

87. Pantaleo MA, Di Battista M, Catena F, et al. Surgical debulking of gastrointestinal stromal tumors: is it a reasonable option after second-line treatment with sunitinib? *J Cancer Res Clin Oncol* 2008;134(5):625–630.

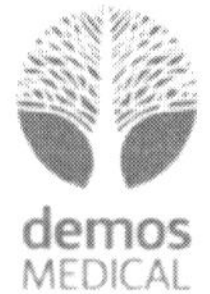

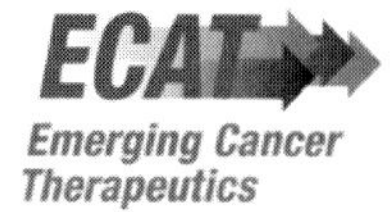

Current Management of Anal Cancer

David Grew[a], M. Wasif Saif[b], and Bryan Chang[b]*

[a]Tulane University School of Medicine, New Orleans, LA

[b]Yale Cancer Center, YaleUniversity School of Medicine, New Haven, CT

■ ABSTRACT

Anal cancer is a rare malignancy, with about 4,000 cases per year in the United States. Individuals with a history of receptive anal intercourse and human papillomavirus (HPV) infection are at increased risk of developing anal cancer. The standard of care for management of localized anal cancer is definitive combined-modality therapy with concurrent chemotherapy and radiation. While toxic, this treatment results in 60–70% long-term disease-free survival. Randomized trials have demonstrated that chemoradiation is superior to radiation alone, and that inclusion of mitomycin C (MMC) improves colostomy-free survival. Intensity-modulated radiation therapy (IMRT) is a promising new radiation technique that may be able to reduce the acute and late morbidity of chemoradiation. Abdomino-perineal resection (APR) is reserved for salvage after local recurrence, while metastatic disease is managed with systemic therapy alone.

■ EPIDEMIOLOGY

Cancer of the anal canal is a rare malignancy. It is estimated that in the United States in 2009 there will be 5,290 new cases and 710 deaths due to anal carcinoma (1). Anal cancer is more common in women; however, the difference in incidence between sexes has been decreasing. Importantly, the overall incidence of anal cancer is increasing among both sexes. In 2002 there were approximately 3,900 new cases of anal cancer, and in 2006, there were an estimated 4,650 (2,3). According to the Surveillance, Epidemiology, and End Results database, 5-year survival for patients who present with distant disease

and those with localized disease is 18% and 78%, respectively (4).

■ ETIOLOGY/RISK FACTORS

Environmental factors play a significant role in the carcinogenesis of anal cancer. A history of receptive anal intercourse, a higher number of sexual partners, and a history of sexually transmitted infections, specifically human papillomavirus (HPV), increase the risk of anal cancer. HPV serotype 16 can be found in 84% of anal cancer specimens (5). The same HPV serotypes associated with cervical cancer (HPV-16, HPV-18) are believed to lead to anal intraepithelial neoplasia, a precursor to anal cancer. Additional risk factors include a known history of cervical, vulvar or vaginal cancer, immunosuppression after solid organ transplantation, HIV infection, and a history of cigarette smoking.

---

*Corresponding author, Department of Therapeutic Radiology, Yale University School of Medicine, New Haven, CT

E-mail address: bryan.chang@yale.edu

Emerging Cancer Therapeutics 1 (2010) 163–170.

DOI: 10.5003/2151-4194.1.1.165

■ PATHOLOGY: ANATOMY, HISTOLOGY, LYMPHATIC, AND VENOUS DRAINAGE

The anal canal is the distal end of the gastrointestinal tract. Approximately 4 to 5 cm in length, it extends proximally from the anorectal ring to the anal verge. The entire anal canal can usually be appreciated on digital rectal exam. Superiorly, the anorectal ring is marked by the structures that intersect there: the puborectalis sling, distal longitudinal bowel, and deep external sphincter muscles. Inferiorly, the anal verge is identified as the point at which nonkeratinized squamous epithelium meets the hair-bearing keratinized perianal skin.

Histologically, the anal canal is divided by the dentate line, an area of epithelial transition. Proximal to the dentate line, the anal lumen is lined by glandular mucosa. Distally, the mucosal surface is mostly modified squamous epithelium, lacking glandular structures and hair follicles. Within the transition zone, the epithelium bears features of urothelial, rectal, and squamous epithelium. The most common cell type involved in anal cancer is squamous, representing approximately 75% to 80% of anal carcinomas (6). Most squamous cell carcinomas of the anus arise from keratinizing squamous cells. Nonkeratinizing squamous carcinomas consist of basaloid, cloacogenic, and transitional histologic variants. Adenocarcinomas typically arise from the proximal anal canal and anal glands. Other less common histologies include lymphoma, melanoma, and Kaposi sarcoma. This chapter will focus on the management of squamous cell carcinoma of the anal canal.

The dentate line also marks a division in lymphatic drainage. Proximal to and around the dentate line, lymphatics drain to nodes in the internal iliac system and inferior mesenteric system. Distal to the dentate line, including the lining of the anal canal, the anal verge, and the perianal skin, tissues predominantly drain to the superficial inguinal nodes, with some drainage to the femoral and external iliac nodes (7). These distinctions represent generalizations; cross drainage and variations in anatomy are not uncommon and may lead to different patterns of lymphatic spread.

Venous drainage of the anal canal feeds into both the portal and the systemic circulation. The anal mucosa and skin of the anal verged are enshrouded by network of venous plexuses. Superior portions of the anal canal drain into the portal system via the inferior mesenteric vein, while inferior portions drain into systemic circulation via the internal pudendal veins.

■ ROUTES OF SPREAD

Anal carcinoma may spread by direct invasion, through lymphatic drainage, or, less commonly, hematogenously. Spread by direct invasion may involve any organs in close proximity to the anal canal, including rectal mucosa, perianal tissues, anorectal fat, external anal sphincter, perineum, bladder, urethra, prostate, cervix, vagina, or uterus. The overall risk of lymphatic spread at the time of diagnosis is approximately 25% (6). One series reports tumor invasion of superior hemorrhoidal nodes in 25% of patients, external iliac, obturator or hypogastric nodes in 20%, and inguinal nodes in 16% of patients (8). Hematogenous dissemination, the least common route of anal carcinoma metastasis, occurs in less than 10% of patients. Distant metastatic lesions are most commonly found in the liver and lungs (7).

■ CLINICAL PRESENTATION

Symptoms associated with anal cancer can be nonspecific and may mimic benign conditions, sometimes leading to a delay in diagnosis. The most common presenting symptoms are bleeding and anal discomfort, occurring in about half of patients (9). Other presenting symptoms include the sensation of an anal mass, discharge, anal pruritus, diarrhea, and constipation. An anal mass is sometimes found incidentally on rectal exam, or in the workup for a suspicious inguinal lymph node. One quarter of patients with squamous cell carcinoma of the anus are asymptomatic at the time of diagnosis (10).

■ DIAGNOSIS AND WORKUP

The diagnostic workup for anal cancer should include a thorough history and physical examination. Special attention should paid to a history of weight loss, tenesmus, anal receptive intercourse, and HIV risk factors. A complete physical exam should include palpation and evaluation of the superficial inguinal lymph nodes, examination of the perineum, and digital rectal exam. Anoscopy may be indicated for complete evaluation of the tumor location, size, and distance from the anal verge. In women, a complete pelvic exam and Pap smear are necessary to rule out vaginal extension of the primary tumor or a concurrent cervical tumor.

Diagnosis is confirmed by biopsy of the anal mass. Pathologic evaluation of suspicious lymph nodes may be done by fine needle aspirate.

Various radiologic tests are necessary for complete staging of anal cancer, including transanal ultrasound for evaluation of local extension and perirectal adenopathy, computed tomography or magnetic resonance imaging of the abdomen and pelvis, positron emission tomography–computed tomography scan, and chest radiograph.

Laboratory tests should include complete blood counts, complete metabolic panel, including liver function tests, and a HIV test and CD4 count.

■ STAGING/PROGNOSTIC FACTORS

The American Joint Committee on Cancer (AJCC) tumor–node–metastasis staging system is commonly used in clinical practice (Table 1) (11).

The most important prognostic factor in localized anal cancer is the size of the primary tumor (12). Lymphatic spread is another negative prognostic factor for survival (13). Distant metastatic spread portends the worst prognosis; the median survival of stage IV disease is 12 months (14–16).

■ TREATMENT

Historical Approach, Current Standard Treatment

In the past, abdominoperineal resection (APR) was the standard therapy for anal carcinoma. However, APR necessitates a permanent colostomy, imposes perioperative morbidity and mortality, and is associated with a 5-year survival ranging from 40% to 80% (6). These disappointing outcomes led to the exploration of alternative treatment options. In the first step toward modern management of anal cancer, Nigro et al. initiated a study in which patients received preoperative chemoradiation (17). They found that three patients had no evidence of residual disease upon surgical resection. The authors concluded that combined radiation therapy and 5-flourouracil (5-FU) and mitomycin chemotherapy could serve as a definitive, organ-

sparing alternative to surgery for anal carcinoma. This finding has been replicated by numerous randomized trials since it was originally reported in 1974.

There are four major studies that lay the framework for the current standard therapy for anal cancer. One study by the United Kingdom Coordinating Committee on Cancer Research (UKCCR) aimed to clarify the role of chemotherapy in the definitive treatment of anal cancer (18). In this trial, patients were randomized to receive either RT alone or RT with 5-FU/mitomycin. Good responders received an RT boost, while poor responders underwent salvage surgery. Results showed that patients in the combined modality group had better local control and disease-free survival, but there was no difference in 3-year survival. A similarly designed study by the European Organization for the Research and Treatment of Cancer (EORTC) also showed the benefit of combined RT with 5-FU/mitomycin in terms of local control and disease-free survival, but there was no significant advantage in overall survival at 3 years (19). Results of these trials are summarized in Table 2.

Given the fact that mitomycin leads to significant hematologic toxicity, the Radiation Therapy Oncology Group (RTOG) and Eastern Cooperative Oncology Group (ECOG) initiated a trial to evaluate the benefit of mitomycin in multimodal therapy (20). Patients were randomized to either RT with 5-FU/mitomycin C (MMC) or RT and 5-FU alone. Results showed that patients in the mitomycin arm, while experiencing more hematologic toxicities, had significantly better disease-free survival and colostomy rates. There were no differences in overall survival. The authors concluded that despite the increased risk of hematologic toxicity, mitomycin should be included in chemoradiation regimens for anal cancer because of the benefit in disease-free survival.

Chemoradiation with cisplatin has proven effective against squamous cell cancers at other sites (21,22). The RTOG 98–11 study was designed to evaluate whether cisplatin-based chemoradiation would result in a superior disease-free survival when compared to standard therapy with radiation, 5-FU, and mitomycin (23). Patients were randomized to receive either chemoradiation with 5-FU/mitomycin or induction therapy with 5-FU/cisplatin followed by chemoradiation with 5-FU/cisplatin. There was no significant difference in 5-year disease-free survival, local control, or overall survival between the two groups. Patients in the cisplatin arm not only had less toxicity but also a significantly higher colostomy rate of 19% versus 10% in the control arm.

TABLE 1 AJCC classification of anal canal tumors

Primary Tumor (T)

TX	Primary tumor cannot be assessed
T0	No evidence of primary tumor
Tis	Carcinoma in situ
T1	Tumor $\leq$2 cm in greatest dimension
T2	Tumor >2 cm but $\leq$5 cm in greatest dimension
T3	Tumor >5 cm in greatest dimension
T4	Tumor of any size invades adjacent organ(s); vagina, urethra, bladder (involvement of sphincter muscle, rectal wall perirectal skin, or subcutaneous tissues is not T4)

Lymph Node (N)

NX	Regional lymph nodes cannot be assessed
N0	No regional lymph node metastases
N1	Metastasis in perirectal lymph node(s)
N2	Metastasis in unilateral internal iliac and/or inguinal lymph node(s)
N3	Metastasis in perirectal and inguinal lymph nodes and/or bilateral internal iliac and/or inguinal lymph nodes

Distant Metastasis (M)

MX	Distant metastases cannot be assessed
M0	No distant metastases
M1	Distant metastases

Grade (G)

GX	Grade cannot be assessed
G1	Well differentiated
G2	Moderately differentiated
G3	Poorly differentiated
G4	Undifferentiated

Stage Groupings

Stage 0	Tis	N0	M0
Stage I	T1	N0	M0
Stage II	T2	N0	M0
	T3	N0	M0
Stage IIIA	T1–3	N1	M0
	T4	N0	M0
Stage IIIB	T4	N1	M0
	Any T	N2–3	M0
Stage IV	Any T	Any N	M1

This study established a lack of benefit for induction chemotherapy and again confirmed radiation, 5-FU, and mitomycin as the standard of care (Table 3.)

These four studies establish radiation therapy combined with 5-FU and MMC as the treatment of choice for patients with localized anal carcinoma. Long-term disease-free survival is generally 50% to 60% and 5-year survival is approximately 70%. APR is reserved for instances of local treatment failure.

Toxicity of Chemoradiation

The acute toxicities of chemoradiation can be severe and include desquamation, anemia, thrombocytopenia, diarrhea, infection, electrolyte abnormalities, pain, and fatigue. Some studies have shown that long (greater than 2-week) treatment breaks may lead to inferior local control (24). Therefore, extended breaks should be avoided whenever possible. Long-term chemoradiation toxicities may include fibrosis, anal stenosis, lymphedema, fistulae, bleeding, sexual dysfunction, sterility, femoral neck fractures, and injury to the small bowel. A recent single institution series suggests that, with careful monitoring, HIV-positive patients can be successfully treated with standard therapy (25).

Intensity-Modulated Radiation Therapy

Historically, radiation therapy was planned in 2D based on bony landmarks and plain films. With the widespread availability of CT scans over the last two decades, 3D planning became common in clinical practice, offering an advantage in target volume coverage and avoidance of normal structures. More recently, the use of intensity-modulated radiation therapy (IMRT) has offered further advantage in avoiding normal structures. In IMRT, dose restriction values are assigned to normal tissues and prescription doses are assigned to target volumes. Software programs using "inverse planning" algorithms based on these values aid the radiation oncologist in designing the final treatment plan. Computerized optimization of the intensity profile of each beam allows for sharp gradients of dose and the ability to conform isodose curves to concave target volumes (Fig. 9.1). Ultimately, IMRT can be used to reduce the dose to normal tissues while still delivering the prescription dose to the target volume.

As the acute toxicity from chemoradiation for anal cancer can be substantial, there has been considerable interest in using IMRT to spare normal structures such as the bowel, bladder, skin, and bone marrow. Dosimetric studies have demonstrated improved normal tissue-sparing with IMRT compared to conventional 3D planning (26). In a multiinstitutional phase II study, Salama et al. report that patients treated with IMRT had similar disease-related outcomes compared to those treated with conventional radiation (27). Additionally, there was a reduction in severe dermatologic toxicity among those treated with IMRT compared to recent RTOG trials. The authors concluded that IMRT is a reasonable treatment

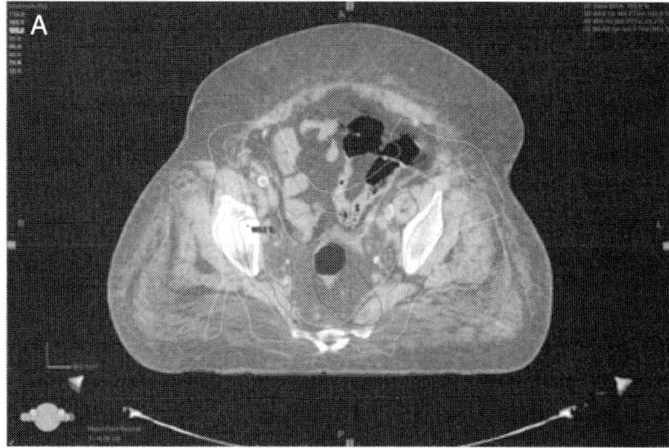

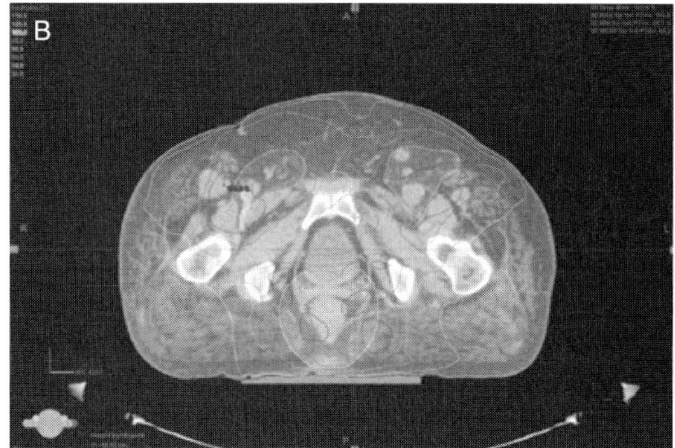

FIGURE 1 Anal Cancer IMRT Plan. A 74-year-old woman presented with a bleeding anal mass. She was found to have a T3N0 squamous cell carcinoma of the anal canal. Treatment consisted of chemoradiation with 5-FU, mitomycin, and IMRT. The 95% isodose line conforms to the pelvic and inguinal nodal volumes (A) and the perirectal target volume (B) while sparing the bowel, bladder, skin, and pelvic bones. The patient had a clinical complete response and remains disease-free 1 year after.

alternative to conventional radiation therapy for the sake of toxicity reduction.

Dose Escalation

Despite extensive research and multiple randomized clinical trials, there has not been a significant improvement in overall survival and local control with combined chemoradiation since the Nigro trials in the 1970s where patients were treated to 30 Gy. Radiation dose escalation has been shown to improve local control in other solid tumors (28,29). Rich et al. reported that patients treated to >60 Gy achieved a local control rate of 83%, patients treated between 50 and 54 Gy had 73% local control, and among patients receiving <45 Gy, only 50% achieved local

TABLE 2 Randomized controlled trials: radiation therapy alone versus chemoradiation

Author Group	Arm	N	Complete Response (%)[a]	Crude Metastasis Rate (%)	3-Year Local Control (%)[b]	3-Year Survival (%)
UKCCCR	RT alone	285	30	17	39[c]	58
	RT+5FU/MMC	292	39	10	61	65
EORTC	RT alone	52	54	21	55[c]	64
	RT+5FU/MMC	51	80	18	69	69

EORTC, European Organization for the Research and Treatment of Cancer; 5-FU, 5-flourouracil; MMC, mitomycin C; N, total number of patients enrolled; RT, radiation therapy; UKCCCR, United Kingdom Coordinating Committee on Cancer Research.

[a]Local control was assessed 6 weeks after RT (60–65 Gy) in the UKCCCR trial and 6 weeks after initial therapy (45 Gy) but before boost in the EORTC trial.
[b]Patients who received salvage surgery after RT or for RT-related morbidity in the UKCCCR study were considered local failures, and patients who received surgery for the sake of local control after RT were considered locally controlled in the EORTC trial.
[c]Statistically significant difference, $P < 0.05$.

control (30). The dosimetric advantages of IMRT have the potential to make dose escalation more tolerable. However, dose escalation in the setting of chemoradiation clearly has the potential to cause increased acute and long-term toxicity. Studies have yet to show a clear benefit to dose escalation above 50 to 60 Gy with 5-FU and mitomycin. The daily fraction size should be 2 Gy or less to avoid severe toxicity.

Follow-Up

During the first 3 years after treatment, patients should be seen every 3 months. For the following 2 years, patients should be seen every 6 months, and annually thereafter. On each visit, a careful history and physical examination should be performed, including digital rectal exam and palpation of the inguinal lymph nodes. Follow-up labs should include

TABLE 3 Randomized controlled trials: radiation therapy with 5-FU and MMC versus other chemoradiation regimens

Trial Name	Arm	N	Toxicity	Colostomy Rate (%)	Disease-Free Survival (%)	Overall Survival (%)
RTOG/ ECOG	RT/5-FU	145	8% grade 4–5	22	51	67
	RT/5-FU/MMC	146	26% grade 4–5	9	73	76
RTOG 98–11	Induction 5-FU/ CDDP, then RT/5-FU/CDDP	320	75% nonheme, 47% heme grade 3–4	19	56	69
	RT/5-FU/MMC	324	76% nonheme, 67% heme grade 3–4	10	48	69

CDDP, cisplatin; ECOG, Eastern Cooperative Oncology Group; 5-FU, 5-flourouracil; heme, hematologic; MMC, mitomycin C; RT, radiation therapy; RTOG, Radiation Therapy Oncology Group.

a complete blood count and liver function tests. Patients should also undergo a chest radiograph annually and a CT of the pelvis every 6 to 12 months for the first 3 years. The median time of tumor regression is 12 weeks after completion of combined therapy, but may take even longer when patients are treated with radiation therapy alone. Residual tumor should not be biopsied unless it is noted to persist without regressing on serial examinations.

■ SUMMARY

Anal cancer is rare, but the incidence has increased over the past several decades. The development of anal squamous cell cancer is linked to HPV infection. The standard of care for localized disease is radiation therapy with concurrent 5-FU and mitomycin. APR is reserved for salvage of local failures. Recent advances in IMRT techniques may help decrease the toxicity of treatment.

■ REFERENCES

1. American Cancer Society. <www.Cancer.org> Accessed September 27, 2009.
2. Jemal A, Siegel R, Ward E, Murray T, Xu J, Thun MJ. Cancer statistics, 2007. *CA Cancer J Clin* 2007;57(1):43–66.
3. Jemal A, Thomas A, Murray T, Thun M. Cancer statistics, 2002. *CA Cancer J Clin* 2002;52(1):23–47.
4. Johnson LG, Madeleine MM, Newcomer LM, Schwartz SM, Daling JR. Anal cancer incidence and survival: the surveillance, epidemiology, and end results experience, 1973–2000. *Cancer* 2004;101(2):281–288.
5. Frisch M, Glimelius B, van den Brule AJ et al. Sexually transmitted infection as a cause of anal cancer. *N Engl J Med* 1997;337(19):1350–1358.
6. Myerson RJ, Karnell LH, Menck HR. The National Cancer Data Base report on carcinoma of the anus. *Cancer* 1997;80(4):805–815.
7. Cummings BJ, Briesley JD. Anal cancer. In: Halperin EC, Perez CA, Brady LW, eds. *Principles and Practice of Radiation Oncology.* Philadelphia: Lippincott Williams & Wilkins;2008:1383–1396.
8. Stearns MW, Urmacher C, Sternberg SS, Woodruff J, Attiyeh F. Cancer of the anal canal. *Curr Probl Cancer* 1980;4(12):1–44.
9. Wolfe HR, Bussey HJ. Squamous-cell carcinoma of the anus. *Br J Surg* 1968;55(4):295–301.
10. Beahrs OH, Wilson SM. Carcinoma of the anus. *Ann Surg* 1976;184(4):422–428.
11. Sobin LH, Wittekind C. *TNM Classification of Malignant Tumours,* 6th ed. New York: *Wiley-Liss,* 2002.
12. Cummings BJ. Anal cancer. In: Gospodarowicz MK, O'Sullivan B, Sobin LH, eds. *Prognostic Factors in Cancer,* 3rd ed. Hoboken, NJ: John Wiley & Sons, 2006;139–142.
13. Cummings BJ, Keane TJ, O'Sullivan B, et al. Epidermoid anal cancer: treatment by radiation and 5-fluorouracil with and without mitomycin C. *Int J Radiat Oncol Biol Phys* 1991;21:1115–1125.
14. Greenall MJ, Quan SH, DeCosse JJ. Epidermoid cancer of the anus. *Br J Surg* 1985;72:S97–103.
15. Tanum G. Treatment of relapsing anal carcinoma. *Acta Oncol* 1993;32(1):33–35.
16. Tanum G, Tveit K, Karlsen KO, Hauer-Jensen M. Chemotherapy and radiation therapy for anal carcinoma. Survival and late morbidity. *Cancer* 1991;67(10):2462–2466.
17. Nigro ND, Vaitkevicius VK, Considine B. Combined therapy for cancer of the anal canal: a preliminary report. *Dis Colon Rectum* 1974;17(3):354–356.
18. UKCCCR Anal Canal Cancer Trial Working Party. Epidermoid anal cancer: results from the UKCCCR randomized trial of radiotherapy alone versus radiotherapy, 5-fluorouracil and mitomycin C. *Lancet* 1996;348:1049–1054.
19. Bartelink H, Roelofsen F, Eschwege F, *et al.* Concomitant radiotherapy and chemotherapy is superior to radiotherapy alone in the treatment of locally advanced anal cancer: results of a phase III randomized trial of the European Organization for Research and Treatment of Cancer Radiotherapy and Gastrointestinal Cooperative Groups. *J Clin Oncol* 1997;15(5):2040–2049.
20. Flam M, John M, Pajak TF, *et al.* Role of mitomycin in combination with fluorouracil and radiotherapy, and of salvage chemoradiation in the definitive nonsurgical treatment of epidermoid carcinoma of the anal canal: results of a phase III randomized intergroup study. *J Clin Oncol* 1996;14(9):2527–2539.
21. Cooper JS, Guo MD, Herskovic A, *et al.* Chemoradiotherapy of locally advanced esophageal cancer: long-term follow-up of a prospective randomized trial (RTOG 85–01). Radiation Therapy Oncology Group. *JAMA* 1999;281(17):1623–1627.
22. Forastiere AA, Goepfert H, Maor M, *et al.* Concurrent chemotherapy and radiotherapy for organ preservation in advanced laryngeal cancer. *N Engl J Med* 2003;349(22):2091–2098.
23. Ajani JA, Winter KA, Gunderson LL, *et al.* Fluorouracil, mitomycin, and radiotherapy vs fluorouracil, cisplatin, and radiotherapy for carcinoma of the anal canal: a randomized controlled trial. *JAMA* 2008;299(16):1914–1921.
24. John M, Pajak T, Flam M, *et al.* Dose escalation in chemoradiation for anal cancer: preliminary results of RTOG 92–08. *Cancer J Sci Am* 1996;2(4):205–211.
25. Chiao EY, Giordano TP, Richardson P, El-Serag HB. Human immunodeficiency virus-associated squamous cell cancer of the anus: epidemiology and outcomes in the highly active antiretroviral therapy era. *J Clin Oncol* 2008;26(3):474–479.

26. Mell LK, Schomas DA, Salama JK, *et al.* Association between bone marrow dosimetric parameters and acute hematologic toxicity in anal cancer patients treated with concurrent chemotherapy and intensity-modulated radiotherapy. *Int J Radiat Oncol Biol Phys* 2008;70(5):1431–1437.

27. Salama JK, Mell LK, Schomas DA, *et al.* Concurrent chemotherapy and intensity-modulated radiation therapy for anal canal cancer patients: a multicenter experience. *J Clin Oncol* 2007;25(29):4581–4586.

28. Bartelink H, Horiot JC, Poortmans PM, *et al.* Impact of a higher radiation dose on local control and survival in breast-conserving therapy of early breast cancer: 10-year results of the randomized boost versus no boost EORTC 22881–10882 trial. *J Clin Oncol* 2007;25(22):3259–3265.

29. Pollack A, Zagars GK, Starkschall G, *et al.* Prostate cancer radiation dose response: results of the M. D. Anderson phase III randomized trial. *Int J Radiat Oncol Biol Phys* 2002;53(5):1097–1105.

30. Rich TA, Ajani JA, Morrison WH, Ota D, Levin B. Chemoradiation therapy for anal cancer: radiation plus continuous infusion of 5-fluorouracil with or without cisplatin. *Radiother Oncol* 1993;27(3):209–215.

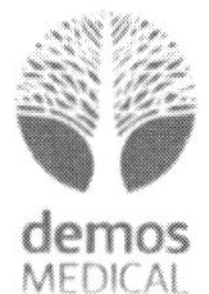

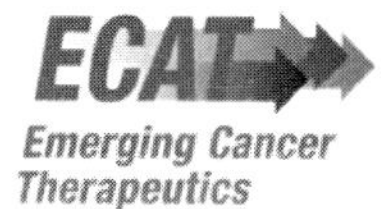

Small Bowel Adenocarcinoma

Jia Li* and M. Wasif Saif

Yale Cancer Center, Yale University School of Medicine, New Haven, CT

■ ABSTRACT

The small bowel cancer (SBC) is rare disease with generally poor prognosis. SBC accounts for less than 2% of all gastrointestinal (GI) malignancies. Small bowel adenocarcinoma (SBA) is the most common histology, accounting for 40% of all SBC. SBA shares some pathological and etiological features with colorectal cancer. Sequential development of genetic abnormalities is believed to be the mechanism of SBA. Major risk factors are similar to those seen in colorectal cancer, such as inflammatory bowel disease, familial adenomatosis polyposis (FAP), hereditary nonpolyposis colorectal cancer (HNPCC) et al. SBC usually presents with nonspecific vague abdominal symptoms. How to diagnose SBC had been a challenge traditionally given the hard-to-reach location. However, newer techniques such as video capsule endoscopy (VCE), double balloon endoscopy (DBE) have overcome some limitations and offered better visualization of the entire small bowel. The staging of SBC is according to the colorectal American Joint Commitee on Cancer TNM system. Surgery remains the mainstream of treatment for local, early stage SBC. There are no standard adjuvant or neo-adjuvant therapies for SBC. Palliative chemotherapy especially 5-fluorouracil (5-FU) based regimens seems to be beneficial for locally advanced or metastatic disease from early phase trials or retrospective experience. Large randomized trials to test therapies in either adjuvant or metastatic settings are highly encouraged. Patients with early stage disease have better prognosis. In general, patients with non-metastatic diseases had median overall survival (OS) of 29 months, while patients with metastatic disease had median OS of 11 months.

This chapter will review the epidemiology, histology, etiology, diagnostic modality as well as the current trends of treatment of SBC, primarily focusing on small bowel adenocarcinoma (SBA).

■ EPIDEMIOLOGY

SBC is rare despite its anatomic location between the stomach and the colon which are at much higher risk of developing neoplasms. SBC accounts for less than 2% of all gastrointestinal (GI) malignancies; in contrast, the incidences of esophageal/gastric and colorectal cancers are approximately 20% and 80%, respectively (1). According to the American Cancer Society, in 2009 there will be 6,230 estimated new cases in the United States, and 146,970 new cases of colorectal cancer and 37,600 gastroesophageal cancers (1).

■ HISTOLOGY

There are approximately 40 different histological subtypes of SBC. SBA is the most common one, accounting for approximately 40% of all SBCs. Other common subtypes include carcinoid tumors

---

*Corresponding author, Yale Cancer Center, Department of Oncology, New Haven, CT
E-mail address: jia.li@yale.edu

Emerging Cancer Therapeutics 1 (2010) 171–176.

DOI: 10.5003/2151–4194.1.1.173

(30%), sarcomas and gastrointestinal stromal tumors (15%), and lymphomas (<5%) (2,3). The duodenum is the most frequently affected location, followed by the jejunum and the ileum (2,3). Adenocarcinomas arising from the ampulla of Vater and the periampullary region are often included as SBA, while adenocarcinomas arising from the ileocecal valve, appendix, and Meckel diverticulum are generally excluded according to the tumor–node–metastasis (TNM) classification.

SBAs demonstrate similar pathologic features to colorectal cancers. Most SBAs are solitary, sessile lesions often appearing in association with adenomas. Immunohistochemical staining is often positive for carcinoembryonic antigen (CEA), carbohydrate antigen 19–9 (CA19–9), p53, and almost always positive for acid mucin. Positivity of c-erbB2, ki-67, tenascin, and neuroendocrine markers was also described in cases (4).

■ ETIOLOGY

Similar to colorectal cancer, SBA is believed to develop as a result of multiple, sequential genetic abnormalities starting from hyperplasia, dysplasia to malignant transformation and eventually tumor invasion and metastasis. The min (multiple intestinal neoplasia) mouse model was one of the first models used to study the pathogenesis of GI cancers (5). The min mutant mice tend to have small intestinal tumors morphologically similar to familial adenomatosis polyposis (FAP) in human.

According to an analysis of the Surveillance, Epidemiology, and End Results (SEER) database, patients with a personal history of either small bowel or large bowel adenocarcinoma are at increased risk of developing a second cancer at either intestinal site. The inherited genetic cancer syndromes of hereditary nonpolyposis colorectal cancer (HNPCC) and FAP result in an increased risk for both large and small intestine adenocarcinoma (6).

In general, risk factors associated with SBA are similar to those seen in colorectal cancer:

- Inflammatory bowel disease—Crohn disease (40–100-fold increase in relative risk) (7)
- FAP (50–300-fold increase in relative risk)
- HNPCC (greater than 100-fold increase in relative risk)
- Celiac disease, cystic fibrosis, and peptic ulcer (8)

- Environmental exposures such as benzopyrene, 7,12-dimethylbenzanthracene (DMBA), smoking, and ethanol
- Other gene mutations related with SBA include K-ras at codon 12, p53 genes (9,10).

■ CLINICAL PRESENTATION

The clinical presentation of SBA is usually nonspecific and vague. Depending on the location of the primary tumor and the involvement of the disease, SBC may present with anemia, bleeding, abdominal pain, nausea and vomiting, obstruction, and/or perforation.

The nonspecific presentations of SBA lead to more advanced stage upon diagnosis compared to colorectal cancer. For example, among 217 patients from the MD Anderson Cancer Center 4% had stage I disease, 20% had stage II disease, 39% had stage III disease, and 35% had stage IV disease (11). The majority of patients with SBA present with disease in the duodenum (52%); the jejunum (25%) and the ileum (13%) are less common sites of presentation (11). Common sites of metastases include locoregional lymph nodes, liver, peritoneum, and lungs.

■ STAGING AND PROGNOSIS

SBAs are staged according to the American Joint Committee on Cancer (AJCC) TNM system used for colorectal cancer (Table 10.1). Staging is based on the extent to which the tumor is present in the bowel wall, the regional nodal status, and the presence or absence of distant metastasis.

The prognosis of SBC is generally considered poor due to the advanced stage upon presentation and diagnosis, partly because of lack of effective diagnostic imaging techniques and partly because of lack of treatment options for metastatic disease. Resectability is a key prognostic factor. Data from the M.D. Anderson Cancer Center demonstrated that the 5-year overall survival (OS) of all patients was 26% with a median survival (MS) time of 20 months. Early stage diseases have better 5-year OS rate (OSR). Patients with stage I–III had median OS (mOS) of 29 months and 5-year OSR of 35%. In contrast, patients with stage IV disease had mOS of 11 months with 5-year OSR of 5% (11).

Other prognostic factors include age, performance status, histology (well differentiated vs moderately differentiated vs undifferentiated), tumor location, and presence of distant metastatses. The prognostic significance of lymph node status for survival is controversial.

■ DIAGNOSTIC TESTS

Small bowel is divided into three regions—duodenum, jejunum, and ileum—and represents 75% of the length of the GI tract and covers over 90% of the mucosal surface. Due to the anatomic features and length of the small bowel, diagnosis of SBA with standard radiological imaging modalities (computed tomography [CT] or magnetic resonance imaging [MRI]) is challenging. Screening like colorectal cancer strategy is also not practical given the low incidence of SBC.

Traditionally, if there is a suspicious small bowel neoplasm, the small bowel follow-through (SBFT) is generally the first test to be ordered. Barium is swallowed and X-ray images of the small bowel are taken subsequently. The patients have to change positions during the imaging time in order to facilitate views at different angles for best quality. However, the overlapping of the loops of small bowel can still lead to false-negative results.

Contrast and water-enhanced multidetector CT scan is more sensitive than SBFT in detecting small bowel lesions. CT can detect abnormalities in 97% of cases with accuracy of approximately 80% (12). More importantly, CT allows the examination of any extraluminal or distant metastases. Like the limitations of SBFT, CT cannot overcome the overlapping loops of small bowel either. Subtle changes of the small bowel mucosa and small tumors can also be missed.

Endoscopic techniques can be used to directly visualize small bowel and detect early or subtle changes of the mucosa. In addition, the endoscopic approach allows diagnostic tissue biopsy as well as therapeutic resection of small tumors. However, standard upper endoscopy is unable to visualize beyond the duodenum and the proximal jejunum, and a standard colonoscopy can only reach the terminal ileum. A big portion of the small bowel is missed with the standard approach (13).

Newer endoscopic techniques such as push enteroscope, intraoperative endoscopy, video capsule endoscopy (VCE), and double balloon endoscopy (DBE) have conquered some of the above-described limitations and offered better visualization of the entire small bowel.

TABLE 1 Staging of SBA is based on the tumor-node-metastasis (TNM) staging system

Tx	No description of the tumor's extent is possible because of incomplete information.
T0	No pathological evidence of tumor
Tis	The cancer is in the earliest stage. It involves only the mucosa.
T1	The cancer has grown through the muscularis mucosa and extends into the submucosa.
T2	The cancer has grown through the submucosa and extends into the muscularis propria.
T3	The cancer has grown completely through the muscularis propria into the subserosa but not to any surrounding organs or tissues.
T4	The cancer has spread completely through the wall of the small intestine into nearby tissues or organs.
Nx	Nodes not evaluated
N0	No regional nodes involvement
N1	1–3 lymph node metastases
N2	4 or more lymph node metastases
Mx	Metastases not evaluated
M0	No metastases
M1	Distant metastases
Stage 0	Tis N0 M0
Stage I	T1 or 2N0 M0
Stage II	T3 or 4N0 M0
Stage III	Any TN1 or 2M0
Stage IV	Any T Any NM1

- Push endoscopy extends the view to the mid-jejunum.
- Intraoperative endoscopy essentially allows complete visualization of the entire small bowel (13). The disadvantage is that it can only be done in an operating room by an experienced surgeon; patients also need general anesthesia and must undergo laparotomy.
- VCE is a relatively noninvasive approach which permits a pill-sized camera to take continuous images of the small bowel. This technique has been proven to be more sensitive than radiologic imaging in several studies (14). However, unlike endoscopic approach, tissue biopsy or resection cannot be provided at the same time.

- DBE utilizes two balloons to reduce looping and allows easy view of the entire small bowel (15).

The algorithm for working up small bowel neoplasms is to start with noninvasive techniques such as CT scan or VCE. If the yield is negative, then move to the next step with invasive ones such as push enteroscopy or DBE. The last two can also allow tissue biopsy and surgical resection of small tumors.

Although tumor markers such as CEA, CA19–9, or CA125 levels are often elevated in the setting of malignancies, none of them offers diagnostic value over the above-described modalities.

■ TREATMENT

Surgery

For patients with stage I, II, or III SBA, surgery is the mainstay of therapy. Depending on the sites of the primary tumor, the surgical approach can be significantly varied. For instance, pancreaticoduodenectomy (Whipple procedure) is required for adenocarcinomas arising from the first and second portions of duodenum; wide resection of the involved segment of small bowel along with the adjacent mesentery and lymph nodes is usually for adenocarcinomas arising from the third and fourth portions of the duodenum and jejunum; ileal resection and right hemicolectomy are performed for adenocarcinomas of the ileum. Small mucosal tumors can also be effectively and safely resected endoscopically (16).

Several studies demonstrated that a surgical approach provides a curative resection in 40% to 65% of patients with 5-year survival rates of 40% to 60%. In contrast, the 5-year survival rate of nonresected tumors is only 15% to 30% (17,18).

Chemotherapy and Radiation

Adjuvant or Neoadjuvant Setting

Due to the rarity of SBA, there are no large randomized trials to study the benefits of chemotherapy or radiation therapy in the adjuvant setting. The clear benefit of adjuvant chemotherapy used for colorectal, gastric, and pancreatic cancer seemed to be a strong rationale to offer postoperative chemotherapy to patients with SBA. However, several small studies appear to be against this assumption.

However, in patient with advanced unresectable duodenal carcinoma, palliative radiation therapy may be of some benefit in controlling chronic blood loss.

- A retrospective study of 217 patients of the M.D. Anderson Cancer Center conducted by Dabaja et al. showed no benefits of chemotherapy after curative resection when compared with untreated patients ($P = 0.49$) (11). Of the 217 patients, 146 underwent definitive primary surgical resection and 27% received adjuvant chemotherapy. Unfortunately the detailed information regarding the regimens were not released in the article. Interestingly, in a subset analysis of this study, palliative chemotherapy did improve OS for patients who did not undergo surgery or had stage IV disease compared with untreated patients (mOS 12 vs 2 months, $p = 0.02$).
- Another retrospective study conducted by Fishman et al. demonstrated a similar outcome in a small patient population. Among the 113 cases from 1986 to 2004, 60 patients underwent surgical resection, 25% of them received adjuvant therapy, including one patient who received adjuvant chemoradiotherapy (19). For patients who received adjuvant therapy, the median time to progression (TTP) was 9 months, while for patients who did not receive adjuvant therapy, it was 20 months.
- Experience from the Mayo Clinic on 491 patients failed to demonstrate survival benefit from neither adjuvant chemoradiation nor chemotherapy after complete resection. Of 491 patients, 40 patients received chemoradiation and 33 patients received 5-fluorouracil (5-FU)–based chemotherapy (20).
- Experience from the Georgetown Lombardi Cancer Center showed that 12 patients had adjuvant chemotherapy with FOLFOX (bolus 5-FU, leucovorin plus oxaliplatin, followed by a continuous infusion of 5-FU over 46 hours, repeated every 14 days). Four patients also received 5-FU concurrent with radiation after completion of chemotherapy. The disease-free survival (DFS) for patients who did not require adjuvant therapy (most of whom had early stage disease) was 28 months; in contrast, the 12 who received adjuvant chemotherapy had DFS of 18 months, although those who also received radiation afterward had DFS of 34 months (21).
- Coia et al. reported a potential role of neoadjuvant chemoradiotherapy. Four patients with resectable

duodenal adenocarcinoma received 5-FU, mitomycin C concurrent with radiation as part of a clinical study for pancreatic cancer at the Fox Chase Cancer Center (22). The regimen consisted of two cycles of 5-FU at a dose of 1 g/m^2/day for 4 days on days 2 to 5 and days 29 to 32 and mitomycin C at a dosage of 10 mg/m^2 on day 2 with concurrent radiation administered at a dose of 1.8 Gy/day to a total dose of 50.4 Gy. Surgical resection was performed 4 to 6 weeks after completion of chemoradiation. All four patients underwent surgical resection and achieved complete pathological response. At a median follow-up of 4.5 years, all patients were alive without recurrence, with actual survival duration of 12, 23, 35, and 90 months, respectively.

Although there are no prospective randomized large trials for SBA, the above retrospective studies all suggest no role of postoperative chemotherapy after a complete resection. Although radiation in the adjuvant setting is generally not considered a treatment modality given the mobile nature of the small bowel and difficulty to define the target field, adjuvant or neoadjuvant chemoradiation may be beneficial. The Georgetown experience and Coia study suggest a potential role for radiation.

Locally Advanced or Metastatic Setting

The OS for patients with locally advanced or metastatic SBA is usually less than 12 months. Surgery in this setting is only limited to palliation or urgent need for cancer-related bowel obstruction, perforation, or bleeding.

Similar to the situation in adjuvant setting, no large randomized trials evaluated the effectiveness of systemic chemotherapy in advanced disease. However, unlike the adjuvant setting, systemic chemotherapy appeared to be beneficial for locally advanced or metastatic diseases in several studies. The choice of chemotherapeutic agents and the actual efficacy of such treatment in metastatic disease are often extrapolated from colorectal data. 5-FU–based therapies, either alone or in combination, such as FOLFOX or FOLFIRI (bolus 5-FU plus irinotecan, followed by a continuous infusion of 5-FU over 46 hours, repeated every 14 days), are the most commonly used regimens. Other regimens include tegafur, thiotepa, mitomycin C, cisplatin, anthracyclines, or alkylating agents.

- Ouriel and Adams reported six patients treated with 5-FU–based therapy with an mOS of 10.7 months, while untreated patients ($n = 59$) had an mOS of 4 months (23). Similar benefit was later seen in other studies, although all studies tend to be underpowered due to small sample sizes (19,24).
- ECF regimen (epirubucin, cisplatin, and 5-FU) was tested in a small group of patients with advanced SBC at the Royal Marsfen Hospital ($n = 8$) (25). The regimen consisted of epirubicin at 50 mg/m^2, cisplatin at 60 mg/m^2 every 3 weeks with continuous venous infusion of 5-FU at 200 mg/m^2. The overall response rate was 37.5% (3/8). The median progression free survival (mPFS) was 7.8 months (range 0–15) with a mOS of 13 months (range 1–28).
- Overman et al. conducted a prospective phase II trial to treat 30 patients (12 of whom had adenocarcinoma of the ampulla of vater) with capecitabine and oxaliplatin (CAPOX) (26). CAPOX was administered every 3 weeks with oxaliplatin at 130 mg/m^2 on day 1 and capecitabine 750 mg/m^2 twice a day on days 1–14. A total of 31 patients were enrolled in this trial. The response rate (RR) and OS were 50% and 20.4 months, respectively. These results are encouraging when compared with any historical data. Randomized studies should further evaluate the effectiveness of CAPOX in a larger patient population.

In summary, due to lack of prospective randomized trials, it is difficult to recommend any therapies over the others. The decision to treat should be individualized, and the risks and benefits should be carefully explained to the patient. Among all tested regimens, treatment with 5-FU and a platinum agent resulted in a higher response rate (46% vs 16% with other regimens; $p = 0.01$) and longer mPFS (8.7 vs 3.9 months; $p \leq 0.01$). However, OS benefit was not statistically significant (14.8 vs 12 months; $p = 0.1$) (27). CAPOX is a highly active one with an mOS of 15 months in patients with metastatic disease.

■ CONCLUSION

SBA is a rare disease with often delayed diagnosis and generally poor prognosis. Its presentation is usually vague and nonspecific. With the advancement of diagnostic tools, such as CVE and DBE, earlier detection is possible. However, effective adjuvant chemotherapy after a complete resection remains undefined.

The role of radiation in adjuvant and neoadjuvant setting is worth further investigation. Palliative systemic chemotherapy for advanced or metastatic disease provides survival benefit. Nevertheless, large randomized trials in both adjuvant and metastatic settings are urgently needed. This may require the collaboration and cooperation of multiple institutions given the disease incidence is only 0.1% to 0.3% of all malignancies.

■ REFERENCES

1. Jemal A, Siegel R, Ward E, Hao Y, Xu J, Thun MJ. Cancer statistics, 2009. *CA Cancer J Clin* 2009;59(4):225–249.
2. Bilimoria KY, Bentrem DJ, Wayne JD, Ko CY, Bennett CL, Talamonti MS. Small bowel cancer in the United States: changes in epidemiology, treatment, and survival over the last 20 years. *Ann Surg* 2009;249(1):63–71.
3. Howe JR, Karnell L, Menck HR, Scott-Conner C. The American College of Surgeons Commission on Cancer and the American Cancer Society. Adenocarcinoma of the small bowel: review of the National Cancer Data Base, 1985–1995. *Cancer* 1999;86(12):2693–2706.
4. Vaidya P, Yosida T, Sakakura T, Yatani R, Noguchi T, Kawarada Y. Combined analysis of expression of c-erbB-2, Ki-67 antigen, and tenascin provides a better prognostic indicator of carcinoma of the papilla of Vater. *Pancreas* 1996;12(2):196–201.
5. Moser AR, Pitot HC, Dove WF. A dominant mutation that predisposes to multiple intestinal neoplasia in the mouse. *Science* 1990;247(4940):322–324.
6. Neugut AI, Santos J. The association between cancers of the small and large bowel. *Cancer Epidemiol Biomarkers Prev* 1993;2(6):551–553.
7. Persson PG, Karlén P, Bernell O, et al. Crohn's disease and cancer: a population-based cohort study. *Gastroenterology* 1994;107(6):1675–1679.
8. Neugut AI, Marvin MR, Rella VA. The epidemiology of cancer of the small bowel. *Cancer Epidemiol Biomarkers Prev* 1998;7(3):243–251.
9. Younes N, Fulton N, Tanaka R, Wayne J, Straus FH, Kaplan EL. The presence of K-12 ras mutations in duodenal adenocarcinomas and the absence of ras mutations in other small bowel adenocarcinomas and carcinoid tumors. *Cancer* 1997;79(9):1804–1808.
10. Park SH, Kim YI, Park YH, et al. Clinicopathologic correlation of p53 protein overexpression in adenoma and carcinoma of the ampulla of Vater. *World J Surg* 2000;24(1):54–59.
11. Dabaja BS, Suki D, Pro B, et al. Adenocarcinoma of the small bowel: presentation, prognostic factors, and outcome of 217 patients. *Cancer* 2004, 101:518–526.
12. Horton KM, Fishman EK. Multidetector-row computed tomography and 3-dimensional computed tomography imaging of small bowel neoplasms: current concept in diagnosis. *J Comput Assist Tomogr* 2004;28(1):106–116.
13. Van Dam J, Brugge WR. Endoscopy of the upper gastrointestinal tract. *N Engl J Med* 1999;341(23):1738–1748.
14. Maglinte DD, Sandrasegaran K, Chiorean M, Dewitt J, McHenry L, Lappas JC. Radiologic investigations complement and add diagnostic information to capsule endoscopy of small-bowel diseases. *AJR Am J Roentgenol* 2007;189(2):306–312.
15. Pasha SF, Leighton JA, Das A, et al. Double-balloon enteroscopy and capsule endoscopy have comparable diagnostic yield in small-bowel disease: a meta-analysis. *Clin Gastroenterol Hepatol* 2008;6(6):671–676.
16. Friedrich-Rust M, Ell C. Early-stage small-bowel adenocarcinoma: a review of local endoscopic therapy. *Endoscopy* 2005;37(8):755–759.
17. Bauer RL, Palmer ML, Bauer AM, Nava HR, Douglass HO. Adenocarcinoma of the small intestine: 21-year review of diagnosis, treatment, and prognosis. *Ann Surg Oncol* 1994;1(3):183–188.
18. Rose DM, Hochwald SN, Klimstra DS, Brennan MF. Primary duodenal adenocarcinoma: a ten-year experience with 79 patients. *J Am Coll Surg* 1996;183(2):89–96.
19. Fishman PN, Pond GR, Moore MJ, et al. Natural history and chemotherapy effectiveness for advanced adenocarcinoma of the small bowel: a retrospective review of 113 cases. *Am J Clin Oncol* 2006;29(3):225–231.
20. Halfdanarson TR, Quevedo F, McWilliams RR. Small bowel adenocarcinoma: A review of 491 cases. *J Clin Oncol*, 2006;24:4127
21. Zouhairi ME, Venner A, Charabaty A, Pishvaian MJ. Small bowel adenocarcinoma. *Curr Treat Options Oncol* 2008;9(4–6):388–399.
22. Coia L, Hoffman J, Scher R, et al. Preoperative chemoradiation for adenocarcinoma of the pancreas and duodenum. *Int J Radiat Oncol Biol Phys* 1994;30(1):161–167.
23. Ouriel K, Adams JT. Adenocarcinoma of the small intestine. *Am J Surg* 1984;147(1):66–71.
24. Czaykowski P, Dui H. Chemotherapy for small bowel adenocarcinoma (SBA): experience over a 10- year period at the BC Cancer Agency [abstract 109]. 2004 Gastrointestinal Cancers Symposium; 2004.
25. Crawley C, Ross P, Norman A, Hill A, Cunningham D. The Royal Marsden experience of a small bowel adenocarcinoma treated with protracted venous infusion 5-fluorouracil. *Br J Cancer* 1998;78(4):508–510.
26. Overman MJ, Varadhachary GR, Kopetz S, et al. Phase II study of capecitabine and oxaliplatin for advanced adenocarcinoma of the small bowel and ampulla of Vater. *J Clin Oncol* 2009;27(16):2598–2603.
27. Overman MJ, Kopetz S, Wen S, et al. Chemotherapy with 5-fluorouracil and a platinum compound improves outcomes in metastatic small bowel adenocarcinoma. *Cancer* 2008;113(8):2038–2045.

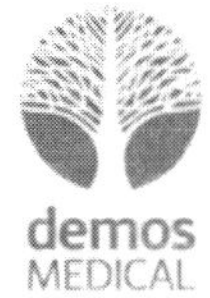

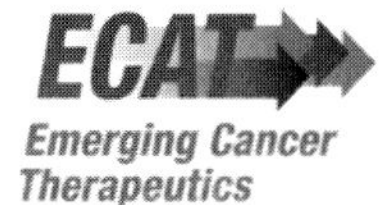

Novel and Targeted Agents for Gastrointestinal Tumors

Mohammed Almubarak[a*] and Michael Newton[b]

[a]Mary Babb Randolph Cancer Center, West Virginia University Hospital, Morgantown, WV

[b]School of Pharmacy, West Virginia University, Morgantown, WV

◾ ABSTRACT

Gastrointestinal (GI) malignancies are common, and despite recent advancements in treatment, they still cause considerable morbidity and mortality worldwide. The development of new cytotoxic agents and targeted agents in the past decade has dramatically increased the number of treatment options available for these patients. These agents can have substantial benefit, often resulting in reduction of recurrences, increases in survival and improvements in quality of life. In addition, treatments may also be individualized to the specific patient based on the biology of the tumor and mechanism of the agent. We present in detail recent advances in the chemotherapeutic treatment of GI malignancies, and provide insight into many agents currently being investigated for these diseases.

◾ INTRODUCTION

Fluoropyrimidines (eg, 5-fluorouracil or 5-FU) have been the backbone of the treatment of many gastrointestinal (GI) cancers for decades. The cytotoxic effect of fluorouracil is a result of several mechanisms. An active fluorouracil metabolite (FdUMP) interferes with DNA synthesis by inhibiting thymidylate synthase, an enzyme required for biosynthesis of the pyrimidine base deoxythymidine triphosphate. Metabolites of fluorouracil also incorporate into nucleic acids (FUTP into RNA and FdUTP into DNA) (1, 2). Several major clinical trials explored the optimal method of 5-FU administration. Regimens utilizing bolus doses of 5-FU were standard for many years. However, infusional 5-FU increases the time that tumor cells are exposed to 5-FU and allows for increased dose. Regimens combining a bolus dose of 5-FU followed by protracted intravenous (IV) infusion have emerged as a favorite method of administration in many institutions due to greater efficacy and tolerable side effect profile (3, 4, 5, 6). Leucovorin (or folinic acid) improves tumor killing of 5-FU by binding to thymidylate synthase to form a stable complex, and thus prolongs its inhibition (7).

The last decade has brought forth major advances in the treatment of GI cancers. The addition of newer cytotoxic agents such as irinotecan and oxaliplatin to fluoropyrimidine-based regimens has improved outcomes in the treatment of colorectal cancer (8). Despite these advances the prognosis remains poor in metastatic GI malignancies. Furthermore, many of the available cytotoxic drugs are not selective for

---

*Corresponding author, West Virginia University Hospital, Morgantown, WV

E-mail address: malmubarak@hsc.wvu.edu

Emerging Cancer Therapeutics 1 (2010) 179–188.

DOI: 10.5003/2151-4194.1.1.179

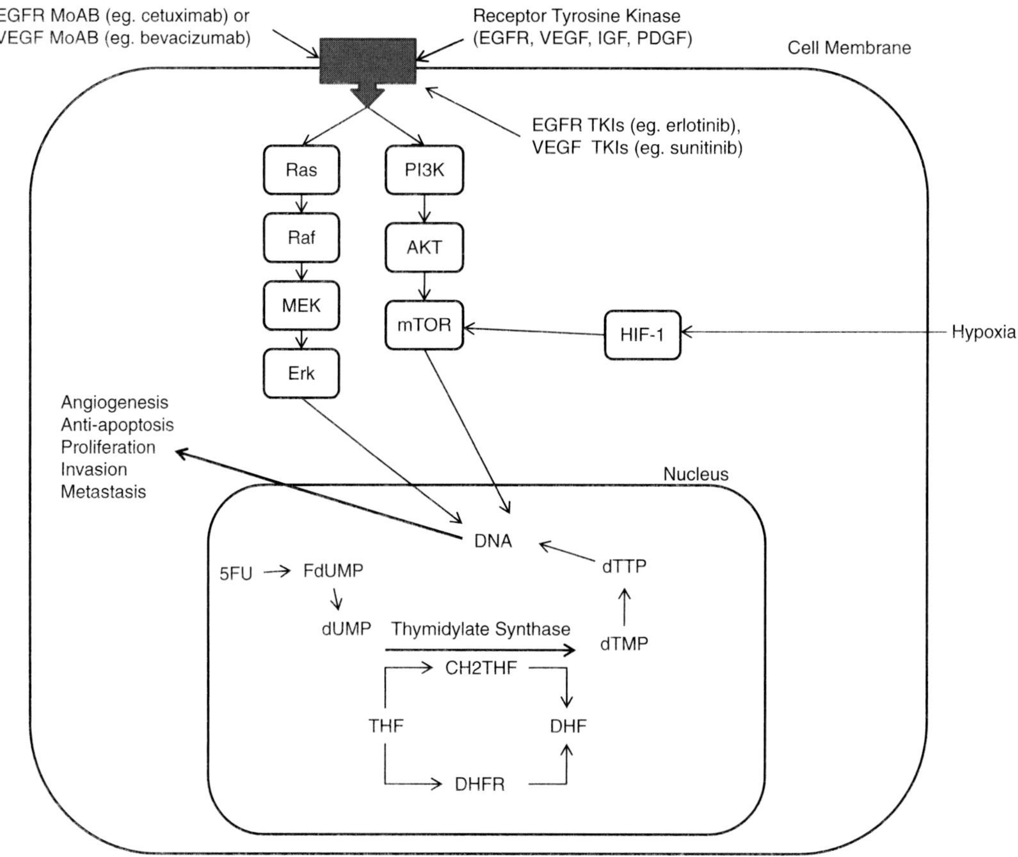

FIGURE 1 Depiction of some of the cellular signal transduction pathways targeted in the treatment of gastrointestinal malignancies.

tumor cells and are associated with dose limiting side effects. Having a better understanding of the molecular pathways involved in tumor cell growth, angiogenesis, invasion, and metastasis has resulted in the development of novel and targeted drugs. These drugs are more selective for tumor killing due to higher expression or uniqueness of the molecular target in the tumor microenvironment compared with normal cells. Some of these drugs have been shown to improve the median survival in specific malignancies. In the case of metastatic colon cancer, targeting two key pathways, the epidermal growth factor receptor (EGFR) and vascular endothelial growth factor receptor (VEGFR) signaling pathways have been especially successful and have changed the way we treat these cancers (9). The better side effects profile has emerged as a key advantage for targeted agents when compared to cytotoxic chemotherapy.

Nonetheless, these agents have relatively low activity level when used alone and are commonly incorporated with cytotoxic combinations. Numerous novel targeted and cytotoxic agents are currently under investigation and may further enhance outcomes in GI malignancies. In this review, we will discuss alternatives to traditional cytotoxic chemotherapy agents, in addition to novel molecular targeting agents and established biologic therapies.

■ ORAL 5-FU ALTERNATIVES

Infusional 5-FU requires a pump and a central venous catheter which can be cumbersome for many patients. Oral fluoropyrimidine analogs have been developed for patient convenience and have improved quality of life. Capecitabine is an oral prodrug of 5-FU that is absorbed though the GI tract and converted through multiple steps to 5-FU. Thymidine phosphorylase, an enzyme needed in the final step of capecitabine conversion to 5-FU, is present at higher concentrations in tumor tissue. This results in a degree of tumor selectivity for capecitabine (10). Two phase III studies have established equivalent efficacy of a capecitabine regimen with 5-FU/ leucovorin combination in metastatic colorectal cancer (mCRC) (11, 12). Capecitabine has a side effect profile similar to 5-FU based regimens with the exception of higher occurrence of hand-foot syndrome. Capecitabine seems to exhibit regional variation in tolerance, as grade 3/4 toxicities are reported more frequently in residents of the United States when compared to other countries (13). Currently, capecitabine can be used in first-line regimens for metastatic colon cancer (XELOX, XELIRI regimens) and the XELOX regimen is under investigation in the adjuvant setting as an alternative to FOLFOX. (14). It is also used as a replacement for infusional fluorouracil in an esophagogastric regimen that combines a fluoropyrimidine with epirubicin and a platinum agent (15).

Uftoral also known as Tegafur-uracil or UFT, is another combination that contains an oral prodrug of 5-FU. Tegafur is absorbed as an intact molecule through the GI tract and subsequently converted to 5-FU in the liver (16). Uracil is a pyrimidine derivative that competes with 5-FU for metabolism by dihydropyrimidine dehydrogenase (DPD) resulting in prolongation of 5-FU half-life (17). The efficacy of the combination of tegafur and uracil is further enhanced by adding leucovorin. Patients who received this combination had similar overall survival and time to progression in two phase III trials when compared to a standard regimen of 5-FU daily bolus with leucovorin in mCRC (18,19).

S-1 (also known as TS-1) is an oral fluoropyrimidine formulation that combines tegafur, 5-chloro-2,4-dihydroxypyridine (CDHP, which reversibly inhibits DPD), and potassium oxonate in a molar ratio of 1:0.4:1. It is approved in Japan for treating colorectal cancer and other GI malignancies including gastric cancer, pancreatic cancer, and biliary tract cancer. In a phase II study ($n = 62$) in mCRC, 35 % achieved partial response with a median survival of 12 months (20). Another phase II study ($n = 38$) showed similar 40 % response rate with a similar median survival (21). In a recent phase II study ($n = 56$) of S-1 with leucovorin in mCRC, 57 % of the patients had a partial response and the median survival was 24 months. The most common side effects were GI

in nature including diarrhea and stomatitis followed by neutropenia (22). Several phase III studies from Japan showed significant clinical activity for S-1 in gastric cancer both in the adjuvant setting (23), and advanced setting (24, 25).

<h2>■ OTHER THYMIDYLATE SYNTHASE INHIBITORS</h2>

Given the relative success of fluoropyrimidines in GI malignancies, other drugs have been sought that inhibit thymidylate synthase. Pemetrexed is a folate antagonist that inhibits several enzymes in purine and pyrimidine synthesis including thymidylate synthase, dihydrofolate reductase (DHFR) and glycinamide ribonucleotide formyltransferase (GARFT) (26). It has several indications including nonsquamous non-small cell lung cancer in first-line therapy, as well as recurrent and maintenance therapy. Pemetrexed initially gained FDA approval in 2004 for the treatment of malignant mesothelioma (27). Vitamin B12 and folate supplementation are required to reduce significant treatment related toxicities including bone marrow suppression and rash (28). Early phase studies showed promising results in pancreatic cancer when combined with gemcitabine, however, a phase III study did not show improvement in survival compared with gemcitabine alone (29). Nonetheless, a National Surgical Adjuvant Breast and Bowel Project (NSABP) phase II study ($n = 54$) has shown that combining pemetrexed with oxaliplatin in advanced colorectal cancer had a 29.6% confirmed clinical response rate with a median time to progression of 5.3 months, and median overall survival of 12.3 months (30, 31).

OSI-7904L is a novel liposomal thymidylate synthase inhibitor. A phase I study demonstrated clinical activity when combined with cisplatin in gastric adenocarcinoma (32). The drug was fairly well tolerated, with myelotoxicity, GI toxicity, and rash being the main side effects. Vitamin supplementation was not needed. In another phase I study, OSI-7904L was used in combination with oxaliplatin in advanced colorectal carcinoma. Two out of 14 patients showed partial radiological response (33).

<h2>■ TOPOISOMERASE INHIBITIORS</h2>

Type I topoisomerases are enzymes needed to relieve torsional stress in the DNA strand during replication.

Drugs that inhibit topoisomerase stabilize the normally transient bond between topoisomerase I and DNA which results in irreversible double strand breaks when a replication fork collides with the DNA-topoisomerase complex. This leads to cell cycle arrest and cell death (34, 35). Irinotecan is a camptothecin analog that is a prodrug of a topoisomerase I inhibitor. After IV administration, it is converted to its active metabolite (SN-38) by carboxylesterase enzymes which are present in the liver and other tissue. Irinotecan is approved for the treatment of metastatic colon cancer as a single agent and in combination with other cytotoxic and targeted therapies (36).

SN-38 is metabolized by the enzyme UGT1A1, which is polymorphic. Patients who are homozygous for the UGT1A1*28 (found in approximately 10% of the North American population) are thought to be at increased risk for more severe irinotecan-related toxicities including diarrhea and neutropenia (37). However, in a meta-analysis of nine studies (n = 821), the significance of toxicity was more likely related to the actual dose of irinotecan rather the genetic predisposition (38). Current manufacturer's label recommends testing for the presence of the UGT1A1*28 allele (commercial kit available, The Invader UGT1A1 molecular assay). Initial dose reduction in patients who are UGT1A1*28 homozygotes continue to be controversial.

An oral formulation of irinotecan is not currently available as the bioavailability of oral irinotecan is unpredictable (39). Liposome-entrapped SN-38 is a biologically active metabolite of irinotecan that is currently being studied. It does not need activation by carboxylesterase (40). Edotecarin is a novel more potent topoisomerase I inhibitor that is structurally different and more potent than camptothecins. Early phase studies showed the drug to be tolerable with the main side effect being hematological in nature (41). Symadex or C-1311 is a member of the imidazoacridinone family, which can bind to DNA and inhibit topoisomerase II. It is currently being tested in a phase II study in colorectal cancer (42).

CELL CYCLE AGENTS

Indisulam (E7070) is a synthetic sulfonamide that targets the G1 phase of the cell cycle and has antiproliferative activity. It has shown some activity as a single agent in colorectal cancers that have previously progressed on 5-FU (43). CF101 is a specific agonist to the A3 adenosine receptor (A3AR), that downregulates protein kinase B/Akt- and NF-kappaB–related pathways. In preclinical studies it has shown inhibition of growth of colon cancer cells. When combined with 5-FU it can potentiate its effect and prevent drug resistance (44). SB715992 is a kinesin spindle protein (KSP) inhibitor. KSP plays an important role in mitosis and cell cycle progression due to its role in formation of a bipolar mitotic spindle (45,46). It is currently being investigated in colorectal cancers.

APOPTOSIS INDUCTION

Telcyta (TLK286) is a novel glutathione S-transferase pi (GST-pi) activated prodrug that promotes stress and apoptosis. GST-pi is highly expressed in several solid malignancies including colon cancer cells as well as in drug-resistant cell populations. In a phase II study, TLK-286 was shown to have clinical activity with a favorable toxicity profile as a single agent in the salvage setting in colorectal cancers (47,48). Mapatumumab (HGS-ETR1) is a humanized monoclonal antibody that targets tumor necrosis factor-related apoptosis-inducing ligand receptor 1 (TRAIL-R1). This results in apoptosis in cancer cells that expresses this receptor. In a recent phase 1 study (n = 49) it was safely combined with gemcitabine and cisplatin. Twelve patients had partial response and 25 patients had stable disease (49).

PROTEASOME INHIBITION

Bortezomib is currently the only approved and widely used proteasome inhibitor. It binds with a high affinity to 26S proteasome and thus it affects the expression of many proapoptotic proteins (50). Currently, it is approved for multiple myeloma and mantle cell lymphoma. In a phase II study no objective response was noted to this drug as a single agent for colon cancer (51). The result of a phase II combination with irinotecan was disappointing as well (52).

MICROTUBULE STABILIZING AGENTS

Ixabepilone is an epothilone B analog that is produced by *Sorangium cellulosum*. It was approved for metastatic or locally advanced breast cancer that was resistant to treatment with an anthracycline and a taxane (53). A single agent phase II study of this drug showed no activity in advanced colorectal cancer (54). Another antimitotic agent, BT-751, that binds to the colchicine site of β-tubulin and prevents microtubule polymerization was tested in a phase II study in metastatic colorectal cancer and was found to be inactive in this setting as well (55).

■ TARGETED AGENTS

Epidermal Growth Factor Receptor

Epidermal growth factor receptor (EGFR) is thought to play an important role in the growth of cancer cells and is thought to be involved in tumor proliferation, metastasis, and induction of angiogenesis. It is expressed in about 75 % of colon cancer cells (56, 57). Targeting EGFR has proved successful in the treatment of mCRC. Two monoclonal antibodies (MoAb) are currently approved in this setting.

Cetuximab is a chimeric antibody that targets EGFR, which prevents ligand binding and induces antibody-dependent cell-mediated cytotoxicity (ADCC). It is effective both as a single agent and in combination with other drugs in mCRC. In a prospective randomized study, cetuximab was compared to best supportive care in 572 patients who have failed prior therapy and found to have a better median overall survival of 6.1 months compared to 4.6 months in the control group (58). When combined with irinotecan, cetuximab resulted in an improvement in progression-free survival from 2.4 months to 4 months in the control group. The two most common unique side effects were diarrhea and rash (59). The Bond trial confirmed the superiority of the combination of these two drugs compared to irinotecan alone (time to progression of 4.1 months compared with 1.5 months in the control arm) (60).

Panitumumab is a fully humanized monoclonal antibody that binds to the extracellular domain of EGFR. It was compared to best supportive care in a phase III trial ($n = 463$) in patients who had progressed on 5-FU, irinotecan, and oxaliplatin. Panitumumab induced an improvement in the 8-week progression-free survival from 30% to 49%. Similar to other EGFR targeted agents, panitumumab caused more diarrhea and rash (61). For both cetuximab and panitumumab, there was no correlation between response and EGFR expression. However, *K-ras* mutation, which is reported in 40% of patients with colon cancer, has been clearly linked to resistance to EGFR-targeted therapy. Analysis from several large studies, in which cetuximab was used, confirm this finding (62).

Although both cetuximab and panitumumab are monoclonal antibodies directed towards the EGFR receptor, significant differences do exist. Cetuximab is a human–mouse chimeric IgG1 monoclonal antibody, whereas panitumumab is a fully human IgG2 monoclonal antibody. Due to panitumumab's fully human structure, individuals who experience dose limiting infusion reactions to cetuximab may tolerate panitumumab (63, 64).

Cetuximab and panitumumab also do not appear to be clinically interchangeable. Despite being directed toward the same target, the agents appear to exert their effects differently. Cetuximab leads to cell-cycle arrest in the G1 phase, and induces ADCC. Panitumumab induces cell cycle arrest in the G0-G1 interphase, and does not induce antibody-dependent cellular cytotoxicity (65). When combined with cytotoxic therapies, cetuximab appears to work synergistically, whereas panitumumab has yet to demonstrate this effect clinically.

Erlotinib is an EGFR tyrosine kinase inhibitor currently approved in combination with gemcitabine for the treatment of patients with locally advanced, unresectable, or metastatic pancreatic cancer. This approval was based on a prospective placebo-controlled randomized phase III study ($n = 569$) in which the overall survival was slightly better in the erlotinib arm (6.2 vs 5.9 months, p = 0.038) (66).

Vascular Endothelial Growth Factor

Bevacizumab is a humanized monoclonal antibody that inhibits neoangiogenesis by binding vascular endothelial growth factor-A (VEGF-A) ligand. In addition to suppressing tumor neovascularization, VEGF inhibition may also normalize existing abnormal tumor vasculature and improve delivery of chemotherapy to the tumor (67). Bevacizumab is currently in wide use for multiple malignancies, but gained its initial approved indication in mCRC. A large ($n = 813$) randomized trial comparing first-line treatment of metastatic disease with irinotecan, bolus fluorouracil, and leucovorin (IFL) plus bevacizumab versus placebo showed improved response rate (34.8% vs 44.8%, p = 0.004), progression-free survival (10.6 months vs 6.2 months, $p < 0.001$), and median duration of survival (15.6 months vs 20.3, $p < 0.001$) (68). Some of the side effects that were seen more frequently in the bevacizumab arm include hypertension, proteinuria, bowel perforation, bleeding and arterial thromboembolic events, as well as delayed wound healing. Since infusional-based regimens such as FOLFOX had supplanted IFL as standard first-line treatment before the study was published, it was assumed that the benefit of adding bevacizumab would extend to FOLFOX (9). This resulted in the FOLFOX plus bevacizumab regimen becoming the standard of care. However, a subsequent phase III study showed only modest benefit in progression-free survival and no increase in response rate or overall survival when bevacizumab is combined with oxaliplatin-containing regimens in the first-line setting (69). Another large study ($n = 829$) exhibited efficacy for bevacizumab in combination with oxaliplatin-based chemotherapy in patients who have progressed on fluoropyrimidine and irinotecan. A regimen consisting of oxaliplatin, fluorouracil, and leucovorin (FOLFOX4) was compared to the same regimen with bevacizumab versus bevacizumab alone. The survival in the FOLFOX4 and bevacizumab group was 12.9 months compared with 10.8 months for the FOLFOX 4 alone group and 10.2 months for bevacizumab alone group (70). Continuation of bevacizumab beyond progression remains controversial. A large prospective observational study reported an increased overall survival rate in patients that continued to receive bevacizumab beyond initial progression versus those who did not (31.8 months vs 19.9 months, $p < 0.001$) (71). This study however was not randomized or controlled and is thus subject to bias and influence by uncontrolled variables.

The success of bevacizumab in the setting of metastatic colorectal cancer has led investigators to examine the possibility that it may reduce recurrence rates when added to adjuvant chemotherapy in stage II and III colon cancer. Unfortunately, the addition of bevacizumab to FOLFOX in the adjuvant setting did not improve disease-free survival at 3 years follow-up (72).

Bevacizumab has also been investigated in metastatic gastric and GE junction tumors. A phase II trial examined the addition of bevacizumab to cisplatin and irinotecan chemotherapy. This study demonstrated a time to progression of 8.3 months, which represents an improvement over the historical 4.2 to 5.8 month survival time for chemotherapy without

bevacizumab (73). Another study, recently presented in abstract form, examined the combination of bevacizumab with docetaxel and oxaliplatin for gastric and GE junction carcinoma. Although the combination appears to be very active, 3 of 23 patients enrolled developed fistulas (74). Phase III trials are currently underway to definitively determine whether the addition of bevacizumab to chemotherapy benefits patients with advanced gastric cancer.

Bevacizumab is generally well-tolerated but its use can result in uncommon and serious toxicities. Hemorrhage, thromboembolism, proteinuria, hypertension, wound dehiscence, and GI perforation are adverse effects associated with bevacizumab. Proteinuria should be monitored periodically to ensure the patient does not progress to nephrotic syndrome. Arterial thromboembolic events are reported in 2% to 5% of patients and may be a class effect of antiangiogenic agents. These events are more likely to occur in patients with a history of these events and are of age >65. The risk of GI perforation may be increased in patients with carcinomatosis or peptic ulcer disease. Wound-healing complications can occur if bevacizumab is administered before a wound is healed or within 28 days of major surgery. Due to bevacizumab's long half-life and concern for wound-healing effects, uncertainty exists for the amount of time that must elapse between discontinuation of the drug and when major surgery can safely be performed. A recent analysis of patients undergoing hepatic surgery of colon cancer metastases who received bevacizumab preoperatively did not identify an increase in postsurgical complication rates. The median time from bevacizumab discontinuation to surgery in this study was 58 days (31– 117 days) (75). Despite many serious potential toxicities, bevacizumab appears to be a reasonably safe drug, provided careful patient selection and monitoring is employed.

Mammalian Target Of Rapamycin

Mammalian target of rapamycin (mTOR) is a protein that plays an important role in cell growth and proliferation. Inhibitors of mTOR like temsirolimus and everolimus have been approved for the treatment of renal cell cancers. One of the ways mTOR inhibitors target cancer cells is by inhibiting the synthesis of hypoxia-inducible factor-1alpha (HIF-1alpha) which has an important role in cancer growth and angiogenesis. Topoisomerase I inhibitors, like irinotecan,

can also inhibit the synthesis of HIF-1alpha. In a preclinical study, xenografted tumors treated with combination of irinotecan and rapamycin had more potent inhibition of the mTOR/HIF-1alpha axis (76). mTOR pathways have been implicated in resistance to EGFR inhibitors. In another preclinical study, an mTOR inhibitor, everolimus was combined with anti-EGFR drugs gefitinib or cetuximab in human cancer cell lines. It was found to be active by overcoming resistance to EGFR inhibitors (77,78).

an important role in cell growth. It has been implicated in the resistance against EGFR inhibitors. A phase II of combination cetuximab, irinotecan with of MK-0646 (IGF-1 inhibitor) in colorectal patients who failed irinotecan and oxaliplatin was encouraging with 33 % response rate observed at higher dose and 14 % observed at the lower dose. The most common high grade toxicities were neutropenia, diarrhea, and hyperglycemia. A phase II/III study of this combination is currently recruiting (82).

■ MULTIKINASE INHIBITORS

Sorafenib is an oral small-molecule inhibitor of several kinases including CRAF, BRAF, KIT, FLT-3, RET, VEGFR, and PDGFR-β. Many of these pathways are activated in cancer, and inhibition of the aberrant pathway results in inhibition of tumor growth. Sorafenib also inhibits angiogenesis mainly by inhibiting VEGF receptors, particularly VEGF-R2. It is currently approved for the treatment of patients with unresectable hepatocellular carcinoma (HCC). Cellular signaling mediated by Raf kinases and VEGF have been implicated in the pathogenesis of HCC, providing a rational target for inhibition. A phase III ($n = 602$) multicenter placebo controlled randomized study was conducted with sorafenib in patients with unresectable HCC. The Sorafenib group had a better overall survival (10. 7 months vs 7.9 months, HR 0.69, $p < 0.001$) and time to progression (5.5 months vs 2.8 months). This was a breakthrough in the treatment of HCC as it is considered the first treatment ever to show a survival advantage (79).

Sunitinib is another multikinase inhibitor. Its current approved indication is in imatinib-refractory or intolerant advanced GI stromal tumor (GIST). In a phase III study ($n = 312$) of sunitinib versus placebo, the median time to tumor progression was 27.3 weeks in the sunitinib group versus 6.4 weeks in the placebo group ($p < 0.0001$) with most common adverse effects being fatigue, nausea, diarrhea, and skin changes (80). The benefit of sunitinib is more pronounced in patients with *c-kit* exon 9 mutation or a *PDGFRA* mutation. (81)

■ INSULIN-LIKE GROWTH FACTOR

Insulin-like Growth Factor 1 (IGF-1) receptor is a transmembrane tyrosine kinase receptor and plays

■ CONCLUSION

The past decade has brought forth incremental and exciting advances in the treatment of GI malignancies. Characterization of aberrant molecular pathways involved in tumorigenesis has provided rational targets for new classes of antineoplastic agents. Improvements in survival for colon cancer and HCC are largely due to the advent of molecular targeting as a cancer treatment modality. The next decade will likely advance our abilities to treat these malignancies even further. As we progress however, we must temper our expectations of these agents and proceed with caution. Despite being "targeted," these agents can exhibit significant toxicities. Some have resulted in statistically but not clinically significant benefit. For many of these agents, the rapidly rising cost has unfortunately not resulted in proportional benefit. Monthly treatments can cost thousands of dollars. In addition, many newer agents are oral medications, resulting in higher out-of-pocket expense for the patient. Clinicians must be aware of the data and have the ability to convey these factors to the patient.

■ REFERENCES

1. Sobrero AF, Aschele C, Bertino JR. Fluorouracil in colorectal cancer—a tale of two drugs: implications for biochemical modulation. *J Clin Oncol* 1997;15(1):368–381.
2. Grem JL. Systemic treatment options in advanced colorectal cancer: perspectives on combination 5-fluorouracil plus leucovorin. *Semin Oncol* 1997;24(5 Suppl 18):S18–S18.
3. Jäger E, Heike M, Bernhard H, et al. Weekly high-dose leucovorin versus low-dose leucovorin combined with fluorouracil in advanced colorectal cancer: results of a randomized multicenter trial. Study Group for Palliative Treatment of Metastatic Colorectal Cancer Study Protocol 1. *J Clin Oncol* 1996;14(8):2274–2279.

4. Buroker TR, O'Connell MJ, Wieand HS, et al. Randomized comparison of two schedules of fluorouracil and leucovorin in the treatment of advanced colorectal cancer. *J Clin Oncol* 1994;12(1):14–20.

5. de Gramont A, Bosset JF, Milan C, et al. Randomized trial comparing monthly low-dose leucovorin and fluorouracil bolus with bimonthly high-dose leucovorin and fluorouracil bolus plus continuous infusion for advanced colorectal cancer: a French intergroup study. *J Clin Oncol* 1997;15(2):808–815.

6. Wang WS, Lin JK, Chiou TJ, et al. Randomized trial comparing weekly bolus 5-fluorouracil plus leucovorin versus monthly 5-day 5-fluorouracil plus leucovorin in metastatic colorectal cancer. *Hepatogastroenterology* 2000;47(36):1599–1603.

7. Mini E, Trave F, Rustum YM, Bertino JR. Enhancement of the antitumor effects of 5-fluorouracil by folinic acid. *Pharmacol Ther* 1990;47(1):1–19.

8. Goldberg RM, Rothenberg ML, Van Cutsem E, et al. The continuum of care: a paradigm for the management of metastatic colorectal cancer. *Oncologist* 2007;12(1):38–50.

9. Segal NH, Saltz LB. Evolving treatment of advanced colon cancer. *Annu Rev Med* 2009;60:207–219.

10. Schüller J, Cassidy J, Dumont E, et al. Preferential activation of capecitabine in tumor following oral administration to colorectal cancer patients. *Cancer Chemother Pharmacol* 2000;45(4):291–297.

11. Hoff PM, Ansari R, Batist G, et al. Comparison of oral capecitabine versus intravenous fluorouracil plus leucovorin as first-line treatment in 605 patients with metastatic colorectal cancer: results of a randomized phase III study. *J Clin Oncol* 2001;19(8):2282–2292.

12. Van Cutsem E, Twelves C, Cassidy J, et al. Xeloda Colorectal Cancer Study Group. Oral capecitabine compared with intravenous fluorouracil plus leucovorin in patients with metastatic colorectal cancer: results of a large phase III study. *J Clin Oncol* 2001;19(21):4097–4106.

13. Haller DG, Cassidy J, Clarke S, et al. Tolerability of fluoropyrimidines appears to differ by region. Abstract 3514. *J Clin Oncol* 2006;24:149s.

14. Comella P, Casaretti R, Sandomenico C, Avallone A, Franco L. Capecitabine, alone and in combination, in the management of patients with colorectal cancer: a review of the evidence. *Drugs* 2008;68(7):949–961.

15. Cunningham D, Starling N, Rao S, et al.; Upper Gastrointestinal Clinical Studies Group of the National Cancer Research Institute of the United Kingdom. Capecitabine and oxaliplatin for advanced esophagogastric cancer. *N Engl J Med* 2008;358(1):36–46.

16. Hoff PM, Kopetz S, Thomas MB, et al. A phase II study of UFT with leucovorin administered as a twice daily schedule in the treatment of patients with metastatic colorectal cancer. *Br J Cancer* 2008;99(5):722–726.

17. Hoff PM, Pazdur R. UFT Plus Oral Leucovorin: A New Oral Treatment for Colorectal Cancer. *Oncologist* 1998;3(3):155–164.

18. Douillard JY, Hoff PM, Skillings JR, et al. Multicenter phase III study of uracil/tegafur and oral leucovorin versus fluorouracil and leucovorin in patients with previously untreated metastatic colorectal cancer. *J Clin Oncol* 2002;20(17):3605–3616.

19. Carmichael J, Popiela T, Radstone D, et al. Randomized comparative study of tegafur/uracil and oral leucovorin versus parenteral fluorouracil and leucovorin in patients with previously untreated metastatic colorectal cancer. *J Clin Oncol* 2002;20(17):3617–3627.

20. Ohtsu A, Baba H, Sakata Y, et al. Phase II study of S-1, a novel oral fluorophyrimidine derivative, in patients with metastatic colorectal carcinoma. S-1 Cooperative Colorectal Carcinoma Study Group. *Br J Cancer* 2000;83(2):141–145.

21. Shirao K, Ohtsu A, Takada H, et al. Phase II study of oral S-1 for treatment of metastatic colorectal carcinoma. *Cancer* 2004;100(11):2355–2361.

22. Koizumi W, Boku N, Yamaguchi K, et al. Phase II study of S-1 plus leucovorin in patients with metastatic colorectal cancer. *Ann Oncol* 2009: Oct 14. [Epub ahead of print]

23. Sakuramoto S, Sasako M, Yamaguchi T, et al.; ACTS-GC Group. Adjuvant chemotherapy for gastric cancer with S-1, an oral fluoropyrimidine. *N Engl J Med* 2007;357(18):1810–1820.

24. Boku N, Yamamoto S, Shirao K, et al. Randomized phase III study of 5-fluorouracil (5-FU) alone versus combination of irinotecan and cisplatin (CP) versus S-1 alone in advanced gastric cancer (JCOG9912). Abstract LBA 4513. *Proc Am Soc Clin Oncol* 2007:25.

25. Koizumi W, Narahara H, Hara T, et al. S-1 plus cisplatin versus S-1 alone for first-line treatment of advanced gastric cancer (SPIRITS trial): a phase III trial. *Lancet Oncol* 2008;9(3):215–221.

26. Alberts SR, Kim GP, Mahoney MR, et al. Pemetrexed and oxaliplatin for metastatic colorectal cancer: results of a phase I Mayo Cancer Center Research Consortium trial, MC0248. *Clin Colorectal Cancer* 2007;6(8):572–577.

27. Scagliotti GV, Ceppi P, Capelletto E, Novello S. Updated clinical information on multitargeted antifolates in lung cancer. *Clin Lung Cancer* 2009;10 Suppl 1:S35–S40.

28. Louvet C, de Gramont A. Pemetrexed in advanced colorectal cancer. *Oncology (Williston Park, NY)* 2004;18(13 Suppl 8):56–62.

29. Hochster HS. The role of pemetrexed in the treatment of gastrointestinal malignancy. *Clin Colorectal Cancer* 2004;4(3):190–195.

30. Atkins JN, Jacobs SA, Wieand HS, et al. Pemetrexed/oxaliplatin for first-line treatment of patients with advanced colorectal cancer: a phase II trial of the National Surgical Adjuvant Breast and Bowel Project Foundation Research Program. *Clin Colorectal Cancer* 2005;5(3):181–187.

31. Meriggi F, Di Biasi B, Caliolo C, Zaniboni A. The potential role of pemetrexed in gastrointestinal cancer. *Chemotherapy* 2008;54(1):1–8.

32. Ricart AD, Berlin JD, Papadopoulos KP, et al. Phase I, pharmacokinetic and biological correlative study of OSI-7904L, a novel liposomal thymidylate synthase inhibitor, and cisplatin in patients with solid tumors. *Clin Cancer Res* 2008;14(23):7947–7955.

33. Clamp AR, Schöffski P, Valle JW, et al.; EORTC New Drug Development Group. A phase I and pharmacokinetic study of OSI-7904L, a liposomal thymidylate synthase inhibitor in combination with oxaliplatin in patients with advanced colorectal cancer. *Cancer Chemother Pharmacol* 2008;61(4):579–585.

34. Hsiang YH, Lihou MG, Liu LF. Arrest of replication forks by drug-stabilized topoisomerase I-DNA cleavable complexes as a mechanism of cell killing by camptothecin. *Cancer Res* 1989;49(18):5077–5082.

35. Pommier Y. DNA topoisomerase I inhibitors: chemistry, biology, and interfacial inhibition. *Chem Rev* 2009;109(7):2894–2902.

36. Mitry E, Lièvre A, Bachet JB, Rougier P. Irinotecan as palliative chemotherapy for metastatic colorectal cancer: evolving tactics following initial treatment. *Int J Colorectal Dis* 2009;24(6):605–612.

37. Schulz C, Boeck S, Heinemann V, Stemmler HJ. UGT1A1 genotyping: a predictor of irinotecan-associated side effects and drug efficacy? *Anticancer Drugs* 2009;20(10):867–879.

38. Hoskins JM, Goldberg RM, Qu P, Ibrahim JG, McLeod HL. UGT1A1*28 genotype and irinotecan-induced neutropenia: dose matters. *J Natl Cancer Inst* 2007;99(17):1290–1295.

39. Kuppens IE, Beijnen J, Schellens JH. Topoisomerase I inhibitors in the treatment of gastrointestinal cancer: from intravenous to oral administration. *Clin Colorectal Cancer* 2004;4(3):163–180.

40. Pal A, Khan S, Wang YF, et al. Preclinical safety, pharmacokinetics and antitumor efficacy profile of liposome-entrapped SN-38 formulation. *Anticancer Res* 2005;25(1A):331–341.

41. Yamada Y, Tamura T, Yamamoto N, et al. Phase I and pharmacokinetic study of edotecarin, a novel topoisomerase I inhibitor, administered once every 3 weeks in patients with solid tumors. *Cancer Chemother Pharmacol* 2006;58(2):173–182.

42. Alami N, Paterson J, Belanger S, Juste S, Grieshaber CK, Leyland-Jones B. Comparative cytotoxicity of C-1311 in colon cancer in vitro and in vivo using the hollow fiber assay. *J Chemother* 2007;19(5):546–553.

43. Ryan DP, Eder J, Appleman L, et al. A phase I study of E7070, a chloroin- dolyl-sulfonamide, in combination with irinotecan in gastrointestinal and thoracic carcinomas. Abstract 2031. 2005 ASCO Annual Meeting..

44. Bar-Yehuda S, Madi L, Silberman D, Gery S, Shkapenuk M, Fishman P. CF101, an agonist to the A3 adenosine receptor, enhances the chemotherapeutic effect of 5-fluorouracil in a colon carcinoma murine model. *Neoplasia* 2005;7(1):85–90.

45. Knight SD, Parrish CA. Recent progress in the identification and clinical evaluation of inhibitors of the mitotic kinesin KSP. *Curr Top Med Chem* 2008;8(10):888–904.

46. Sakowicz R, Finer JT, Beraud C, et al. Antitumor activity of a kinesin inhibitor. *Cancer Res* 2004;64(9):3276–3280.

47. Tew KD. TLK-286: a novel glutathione S-transferase-activated prodrug. *Expert Opin Investig Drugs* 2005;14(8):1047–1054.

48. Rosen LS, Laxa B, Boulos L, et al. Phase 1 study of TLK286 (Telcyta) administered weekly in advanced malignancies. *Clin Cancer Res* 2004;10(11):3689–3698.

49. Mom CH, Verweij J, Oldenhuis CN, et al. Mapatumumab, a fully human agonistic monoclonal antibody that targets TRAIL-R1, in combination with gemcitabine and cisplatin: a phase I study. *Clin Cancer Res* 2009;15(17):5584–5590.

50. Lenz HJ. Clinical update: proteasome inhibitors in solid tumors. *Cancer Treat Rev* 2003;29 Suppl 1:41–48.

51. Mackay H, Hedley D, Major P, et al. A phase II trial with pharmacodynamic endpoints of the proteasome inhibitor bortezomib in patients with metastatic colorectal cancer. *Clin Cancer Res* 2005;11(15):5526–5533.

52. Kozuch PS, Rocha-Lima CM, Dragovich T, et al. Bortezomib with or without irinotecan in relapsed or refractory colorectal cancer: results from a randomized phase II study. *J Clin Oncol* 2008;26(14):2320–2326.

53. Higa GM, Abraham J. Ixabepilone: a new microtubule-targeting agent for breast cancer. *Expert Rev Anticancer Ther* 2008;8(5):671–681.

54. Eng C, Kindler HL, Nattam S, et al. A phase II trial of the epothilone B analog, BMS-247550, in patients with previously treated advanced colorectal cancer. *Ann Oncol* 2004;15(6):928–932.

55. Benson H, Kindler D, Jodrell, et al. 2005 ASCO Annual Meeting Proceedings. Abstract 3537A. 2005;23(16S): Part I of II (June 1 Supplement),

56. Baselga J, Arteaga CL. Critical update and emerging trends in epidermal growth factor receptor targeting in cancer. *J Clin Oncol* 2005;23(11):2445–2459.

57. Wong SF. Cetuximab: an epidermal growth factor receptor monoclonal antibody for the treatment of colorectal cancer. *Clin Ther* 2005;27(6):684–694.

58. Jonker DJ, O'Callaghan CJ, Karapetis CS, et al. Cetuximab for the treatment of colorectal cancer. *N Engl J Med* 2007;357(20):2040–2048.

59. Sobrero AF, Maurel J, Fehrenbacher L, et al. EPIC: phase III trial of cetuximab plus irinotecan after fluoropyrimidine and oxaliplatin failure in patients with metastatic colorectal cancer. *J Clin Oncol* 2008;26(14):2311–2319.

60. Cunningham D, Humblet Y, Siena S, et al. Cetuximab monotherapy and cetuximab plus irinotecan in irinotecan-refractory metastatic colorectal cancer. *N Engl J Med* 2004;351(4):337–345.

61. Van Cutsem E, Peeters M, Siena S, et al. Open-label phase III trial of panitumumab plus best supportive care compared with best supportive care alone in patients with chemotherapy-refractory metastatic colorectal cancer. *J Clin Oncol* 2007;25(13):1658–1664.

62. Allegra CJ, Jessup JM, Somerfield MR, et al. American Society of Clinical Oncology provisional clinical opinion: testing for KRAS gene mutations in patients with metastatic colorectal carcinoma to predict response to anti-epidermal growth factor receptor monoclonal antibody therapy. *J Clin Oncol* 2009;27(12):2091–2096.

63. Heun J, Holen K. Treatment with panitumumab after a severe infusion reaction to cetuximab in a patient with

metastatic colorectal cancer: a case report. *Clin Colorectal Cancer* 2007;6(7):529–531.

64. Cartwright TH, Genther R. Successful administration of panitumumab alone after severe infusion reaction to cetuximab in a patient with metastatic colorectal cancer. *Clin Colorectal Cancer* 2008;7(3):202–203.

65. Pfeiffer P, Qvortrup C, Eriksen JG. Current role of antibody therapy in patients with metastatic colorectal cancer. *Oncogene* 2007;26(25):3661–3678.

66. Moore MJ, Goldstein D, Hamm J et al. National Cancer Institute of Canada Clinical Trials Group. Erlotinib plus gemcitabine compared with gemcitabine alone in patients with advanced pancreatic cancer: a phase III trial of the National Cancer Institute of Canada Clinical Trials Group. *J Clin Oncol* 2007;25(15):1960–1966.

67. Jain RK. Normalization of tumor vasculature: an emerging concept in antiangiogenic therapy. *Science* 2005;307(5706):58–62.

68. Hurwitz H, Fehrenbacher L, Novotny W, et al. Bevacizumab plus irinotecan, fluorouracil, and leucovorin for metastatic colorectal cancer. *N Engl J Med* 2004;350(23):2335–2342.

69. Saltz LB, Clarke S, Díaz-Rubio E, et al. Bevacizumab in combination with oxaliplatin-based chemotherapy as first-line therapy in metastatic colorectal cancer: a randomized phase III study. *J Clin Oncol* 2008;26(12):2013–2019.

70. Giantonio BJ, Catalano PJ, Meropol NJ, et al.; Eastern Cooperative Oncology Group Study E3200. Bevacizumab in combination with oxaliplatin, fluorouracil, and leucovorin (FOLFOX4) for previously treated metastatic colorectal cancer: results from the Eastern Cooperative Oncology Group Study E3200. *J Clin Oncol* 2007;25(12):1539–1544.

71. Grothey A, Sugrue MM, Purdie DM, et al. Bevacizumab beyond first progression is associated with prolonged overall survival in metastatic colorectal cancer: results from a large observational cohort study (BRiTE). *J Clin Oncol* 2008;26(33):5326–5334.

72. Wolmark N, Yothers G, O'Connell MJ, et al. A phase III trial comparing mFOLFOX6 to mFOLFOX6 plus bevacizumab in stage II or III carcinoma of the colon: Results of NSABP protocol C-08. Abstract LBA4. 2009 ASCO Annual Meeting.

73. Shah MA, Ramanathan RK, Ilson DH, et al. Multicenter phase II study of irinotecan, cisplatin, and bevacizumab in patients with metastatic gastric or gastroesophageal junction adenocarcinoma. *J Clin Oncol* 2006;24(33):5201–5206.

74. El-Rayes BF, Patel B, Zalupski M. A phase II study of bevacizumab, docetaxel, and oxaliplatin in gastric and GEJ cancer. Abstract 4563. 2009 ASCO Annual Meeting.

75. Kesmodel SB, Ellis LM, Lin E, et al. Preoperative bevacizumab does not significantly increase postoperative complication rates in patients undergoing hepatic surgery for colorectal cancer liver metastases. *J Clin Oncol* 2008;26(32):5254–5260.

76. Pencreach E, Guérin E, Nicolet C, et al. Marked activity of irinotecan and rapamycin combination toward colon cancer cells in vivo and in vitro is mediated through cooperative modulation of the mammalian target of rapamycin/hypoxia-inducible factor-1alpha axis. *Clin Cancer Res* 2009;15(4):1297–1307.

77. Bianco R, Garofalo S, Rosa R, et al. Inhibition of mTOR pathway by everolimus cooperates with EGFR inhibitors in human tumours sensitive and resistant to anti-EGFR drugs. *Br J Cancer* 2008;98(5):923–930.

78. Buck E, Eyzaguirre A, Brown E, et al. Rapamycin synergizes with the epidermal growth factor receptor inhibitor erlotinib in non-small-cell lung, pancreatic, colon, and breast tumors. *Mol Cancer Ther* 2006;5(11):2676–2684.

79. Llovet JM, Ricci S, Mazzaferro V, et al.; SHARP Investigators Study Group. Sorafenib in advanced hepatocellular carcinoma. *N Engl J Med* 2008;359(4):378–390.

80. Demetri GD, van Oosterom AT, Garrett CR, et al. Efficacy and safety of sunitinib in patients with advanced gastrointestinal stromal tumour after failure of imatinib: a randomised controlled trial. *Lancet* 2006;368(9544):1329–1338.

81. Heinrich MC, Maki RG, Corless CL, et al. Primary and secondary kinase genotypes correlate with the biological and clinical activity of sunitinib in imatinib-resistant gastrointestinal stromal tumor. *J Clin Oncol* 2008;26(33):5352–5359.

82. Watkins D J, Tabernero J, Schmoll H J, et al. A phase II study of the anti-IGFR antibody MK-0646 in combination with cetuximab and irinotecan in the treatment of chemorefractory metastatic colorectal cancer. Abstract 4127. 2009 ASCO annual meeting.

Index

Note: Page numbers followed by "*f*" and "*t*" indicate figures and tables, respectively.

Abdominal dissection, for esophageal cancer, 22, 25, 27
Abdominoperineal resection (APR), for anal cancer, 167
Ablative therapy, for esophageal cancer, 29
Acute respiratory distress syndrome (ARDS)
    radiation therapy for, 64
Adenomatous polyposis coli (APC) stool test, 5–6
Adjuvant therapy
    for colorectal cancer, 118, 120–123
    for esophageal cancer, 20, 42, 47, 50, 74
    for gastric cancer, 82–85
    for gastrointestinal stromal tumors, 156, 157
    for pancreatic cancer, 140–142
    for small bowel adenocarcinoma, 176–177
Alcohol consumption
    and acute pneumonitis, 63*f*
    and gastric cancer, 81
Anal cancer, 165–171
    clinical presentation of, 166
    diagnostic workup for, 166–167
    epidemiology of, 165
    etiology of, 165
    pathology of, 166
    prognosis of, 167
    risk factors of, 165
    spread, routes of, 166
    staging of, 167, 168*t*
    treatment for, 167–171
Anal intraepithelial neoplasia, 165
Anthracycline. *See* FAM; FAMTX
Anthracycline-based regimens, for metastatic disease, 86–87
Anti epidermal growth factor receptor (anti-EGFR) therapy
    for metastatic colorectal cancer, 11
Anti vascular endothelial growth factor receptor (anti-VEGF)
        therapy
    for metastatic colorectal cancer, 11
APC stool test. *See* Adenomatous polyposis coli (APC)
        stool test
Apoptosis induction, for gastrointestinal tumors, 182
ARDS. *See* Acute respiratory distress syndrome (ARDS)

Barrett's esophagus (BE), 24–25
    long segment (LSBE), 29
Bevacizumab
    with bFOL, 128–129
    with capecitabine, 89

    with cisplatin, 75, 76, 88
    for colorectal cancer, 120–121
    with docetaxel, 76, 184
    with erlotinib, 104
    with FOLFOX4, 128, 129, 184
    with FOLFOX6, 128–129
    for GEJ adenocarcinoma, 76, 89
    for hepatocellular carcinoma, 100, 104
    with IFL, 11, 13*t*, 128, 183–184
    with irinotecan, 75, 76
    for metastatic colorectal cancer, 11, 13*t*,128–130,
        183–184
    with oxaliplatin, 184
    as second-line therapy, 130
    toxicities of, 130
    with XELOX, 128–129
bFOL with bevacizumab, 128–129
Biological therapy
    for colorectal cancer, 120–121
    for esophageal cancer, 47, 50, 53–54, 88–89
Bleomycin
    for esophageal cancer, 71
    for metastatic disease, 86
Blood-based tests, for colorectal cancer, 5
Bortezomib
    for gastrointestinal tumors, 182
    with irinotecan, 182
BRAF mutations, in metastatic colorectal cancer, 15, 16*t*
Brivanib, for hepatocellular carcinoma, 100
BT-75, for metastatic colorectal cancer, 183

Capecitabine. *See also* ECX; EOX; XELOXIRI
    with bevacizumab, 11, 14*t*
    with cetuximab, 11, 14*t*
    for colorectal cancer, 121, 124–126
    for esophageal cancer, 71
    for hepatocellular carcinoma, 93, 103, 106–109, 108*f*
    with irinotecan, 124–125, 126
    for metastatic colorectal cancer, 11, 14*t*
    with oxaliplatin, 11, 14t, 125, 126
    with PHY906, 106–109, 108*f*
    for small bowel adenocarcinoma, 177
CapeIri. *See* Capecitabine with irinotecan
CAPOX. *See* Capecitabine with oxaliplatin (CAPOX)
CCSA. *See* Colon cancer-specific antigen (CCSA)

Celecoxib-based chemoradiation regimens, for esophageal
cancer, 54
Cell cycle agents, for gastrointestinal tumors, 182
Cervical dissection, for esophageal cancer, 27
Cervical esophagogastric anastomosis, 23, 27
Cetuximab
for colorectal cancer, 120
for esophageal cancer, 88–89
with everolimus, 185
with FOLFIRI, 131
with FOLFOX4, 131
for hepatocellular carcinoma, 102, 103
with IGF-1, 185
with irinotecan, 130–131, 183
for metastatic colorectal cancer, 10, 12*t*, 130–132, 183
second-line therapy, 131
toxicities of, 131–132
Cetuximab-based chemoradiation regimens, for esophageal
cancer, 47, 48–49*t*
Chemoradiation therapy. *See also* Radiation therapy
for anal cancer, 167–170, 170*t*
with cisplatin, 167
for esophageal cancer
biological therapy, 47, 50, 53–54
celecoxib-based chemoradiation, 54
erlotinib-based chemoradiation, 50
irinotecan-based chemoradiation, 42, 45–46*t*
oxaliplatin-based chemoradiation, 42, 47, 48–49*t*
without surgery, 54–56, 55*t*
taxane-based chemoradiation, 39–42, 40–41*t*, 43–44*t*
for esophageal squamous cell carcinoma, 62–63
with 5-FU, 167–168, 170t
for gastric cancer, 82–83
with mitomycin, 167–168, 170*t*
for pancreatic cancer, 140
locally advanced, 142–144, 143*t*, 145–146*t*
for pericardial effusion, 63
versus radiation therapy alone, 169–170, 170*t*
for small bowel adenocarcinoma, 176–177
toxicity of, 168–169
Chemotherapy. *See also* Chemoradiation therapy; Cytotoxic
chemotherapy; Metronomic chemotherapy
for colorectal cancer, 118, 120–134
optimal duration of, 127–128
for gastric cancer, 83–85
for metastatic disease, 86
Chromogenic in situ hybridization (CISH)
for metastatic colorectal cancer, 10
CISH. *See* Chromogenic in situ hybridization (CISH)
Cisplatin. *See also* DCF; DMAP; ECF; ECX; FLP
with capecitabine, 87
with carboplatin, 74
with docetaxel, 76
for esophageal cancer, 32, 37, 38, 39, 47, 50, 71, 73–76
with 5-fluorouracil, 74, 76, 87
with FOLFOX, 74–75
with FOLFIRI, 74
for GEJ adenocarcinoma, 74
for hepatocellular carcinoma, 99

for metastatic disease, 86–87
with OSI-7904L, for gastric adenocarcinoma, 181
with paclitaxel, 74
with S-1, 73–74
with sorafenib, 76
Colon cancer-specific antigen (CCSA), 6
Colonoscopy, for colorectal cancer, 3
CT (virtual) colonoscopy, 3
Colorectal cancer (CRC), 1–6, 117–134
antigens mapping, 6
APC stool test for, 5–6
blood-based tests for, 5
chemotherapy for, 118, 120–134
colonoscopy for, 3
fecal occult blood test for, 2
flexible sigmoidoscopy for, 2–3
genetic model of, 5*f*
incidence of, 4
metastatic. *See* Metastatic colorectal cancer
mortality of, 4
mutant APC molecules, circulating, 6
risk factors of, 1–2, 2*f*
screening of, 2–4, 4*f*
barriers to, 4
compliance, 3–4
conduction, 3–4
early screening of, 2
single-contrast barium enema test for, 3
stages of, 118, 119*t*
stool-based DNA test for, 5
Combined-modality therapy. *See also* Trimodality therapy
for esophageal cancer, new developments in, 37–56
biological therapy, 47, 50, 53–54
celecoxib-based chemoradiation, 54
chemoradiation without surgery, 54–56, 55*t*
erlotinib-based chemoradiation, 50
irinotecan-based chemoradiation, 42, 45–46*t*
oxaliplatin-based chemoradiation, 42, 47, 48–49*t*
taxane-based chemoradiation, 39–42, 40–41*t*, 43–44*t*
Computed tomographic colonography
for colorectal cancer, 3
limitations, 3
risk of perforation with, 3
Computed tomography (CT)
in gastrointestinal stromal tumors, 155
for small bowel adenocarcinoma, 175, 176
COX-2. *See* Cyclooxygenase 2 (COX-2)
CRC. *See* Colorectal cancer (CRC)
CT. *See* Computed tomography (CT)
Cyclooxygenase 2 (COX-2)
for esophageal cancer, 54
Cytotoxic chemotherapy. *See also* Chemotherapy
for esophageal cancer, 71–74
for hepatocellular carcinoma, 97–99, 98*t*, 105*t*
with molecular targeted therapy, 104–109, 105*t*

Dacarbazine. *See* DMAP
DBE. *See* Double balloon endoscopy (DBE)
DCBE. *See* Double-contrast barium enema (DCBE)

DCF (docetaxel, cisplatin, and 5-FU). *See also individual drugs*
  for esophageal cancer, 72, 73*t*
  for gastric cancer, 83
  for metastatic disease, 86, 87–88
DDLT. *See* Deceased donor liver transplantation (DDLT)
Deceased donor liver transplantation (DDLT)
  for hepatocellular carcinoma, 96
DMAP (dacarbazine, mitomycin, doxorubicin, and cisplatin).
    See also individual drugs
  for gastrointestinal stromal tumors, 156
  for leiomyosarcomas, 156
Docetaxel. *See also* DCF
  with bevacizumab, 184
  with cisplatin, 76
  for esophageal cancer, 72
  for GEJ adenocarcinoma, 76
  with irinotecan, 76
  for metastatic disease, 86
  with sorafenib, 76
Double balloon endoscopy (DBE)
  for small bowel adenocarcinoma, 176
Double-contrast barium enema (DCBE) test. *See also* Single-
    contrast barium enema test
  for colorectal cancer, 3
Doxorubicin. *See also* DMAP
  with cisplatin, 98
  with 5 FU, 98
  for hepatocellular carcinoma, 98
  with interferon-α-PIAF, 98
  for metastatic disease, 86
  with tamoxifen, 98–99
Dual biologic therapy, for metastatic colorectal cancer, 11, 15

EBE. *See* En bloc esophagectomy (EBE)
ECF (epirubicin, cisplatin, and 5-FU). *See also individual drugs*
  for esophageal cancer, 72, 73*t*
  for gastric cancer, 83
  for metastatic disease, 86–87, 88
  for small bowel adenocarcinoma, 177
ECX (epirubicin, cisplatin, and capecitabine). *See also
    individual drugs*
  for esophageal cancer, 72
  for gastric cancer, 83
  for metastatic disease, 87
Edotecarin, for metastatic colorectal cancer, 182
EGFR. *See* Epidermal growth factor receptor (EGFR)
ELISA. *See* Enzyme-linked immunosorbent assay (ELISA)
EMR. *See* Endoscopic mucosal resection (EMR)
En bloc esophagectomy (EBE), 26–28. *See also*
    Esophageal cancer
  complications of, 27
  indications for, 27
  operative technique
    abdominal dissection, 27
    cervical dissection, 27
    right thoracotomy, 27
  outcomes of, 28
  and transhiatal esophagectomy, comparison, 28
  and vagal-sparing esophagectomy, comparison, 30

Endoscopic mucosal resection (EMR), for esophageal cancer
  with ablative therapy, 29
  indications and contraindications for, 28
  operative technique, 28
  outcomes, 28–29
Endoscopic submucosal dissection (ESD)
  for esophageal cancer, 28
Enzyme-linked immunosorbent assay (ELISA)
  for colorectal cancer, 6
EOF (epirubicin, oxaliplatin, and 5-FU). *See also individual
    drugs*
  for esophageal cancer, 72
  for metastatic disease, 87, 88
EOX (epirubicin, oxaliplatin, and capecitabine). *See also
    individual drugs*
  for esophageal cancer, 72
Epidermal growth factor receptor (EGFR), 47, 50, 53, 88, 120
  in esophageal cancer, 74–75, 75*t*
  in hepatocarcinogenesis, 100, 102–103
  mutations in metastatic colorectal cancer, 10
  -targeted therapies, for metastatic colorectal cancer, 15, 183
Epirubicin. *See* ECF; ECX; EOF; EOX; FEM
Erlotinib
  with bevacizumab, 104
  for esophageal cancer, 50, 75
  for GEJ adenocarcinoma, 75
  for hepatocellular carcinoma, 102, 103, 104
  for metastatic pancreatic cancer, 183
Erlotinib-based chemoradiation regimens, for esophageal
    cancer, 50
ESD. *See* Endoscopic submucosal dissection (ESD)
Esophageal cancer, 19–33
  chemotherapy and targeted agents, 71–76
  combined-modality therapy
    biological therapy, 47, 50, 53–54
    celecoxib-based chemoradiation, 54
    chemoradiation without surgery, 54–56, 55*t*
    erlotinib-based chemoradiation, 50
    irinotecan-based chemoradiation, 42, 45–46*t*
    oxaliplatin-based chemoradiation, 42, 47, 48–49*t*
    taxane-based chemoradiation, 39–42, 40–41*t*, 43–44*t*
  radiation therapy for, 61–68
    cardiac radiation tolerance, 62–63, 66*f*
    4D treatment planning, 67–68
    intensity-modulated radiation therapy, 67
    positron emission tomography-computed tomography,
      64–66, 66*f*
    pulmonary radiation tolerance, 63–64, 63*f*
  staging of, 20, 21*t*
  surgery for, 20*t*, 37–39, 38*t*
    ablative therapy, 29
    en bloc esophagectomy, 26–28
    endoscopic mucosal resection, 28–29
    endoscopic submucosal dissection, 28
    lymphadenectomy, extent of, 31–32
    minimally invasive esophagectomy, 30–31
    perioperative chemotherapy, 32–33
    resection for, 20
    robotic-assisted esophagectomy, 31

Esophageal cancer—*(continued)*
    transhiatal esophagectomy, 21–24, 26
    transthoracic esophagectomy, 24–26
    vagal-sparing esophagectomy, 29–30
    taxane-based chemoradiation regimens for, 39–42, 40–41*t*, 43–44*t*
    trimodality therapy for, 37–39, 38*t*
Etoposide
  for esophageal cancer, 72
  for metastatic disease, 86
Everolimus
  with cetuximab, 185
  with gefitinib, 185
  for hepatocellular carcinoma, 104

FAM (5-fluorouracil, anthracycline, and mitomycin C). *See also individual drugs*
  for metastatic disease, 87
FAMTX (5-fluorouracil, anthracycline, and methotrexate). *See also individual drugs*
  for metastatic disease, 86, 87
FDG PET. *See* Fluorodeoxyglucose positron emission tomography (FDG PET)
Fecal occult blood test (FOBT), for colorectal cancer
  guaiac based, 2
  immunologically based, 2
FEM (5-fluorouracil, epirubicin, and mitomycin C). *See also individual drugs*
  for metastatic disease, 87
FISH. *See* Fluorescence in situ hybridization (FISH)
Flexible sigmoidoscopy (FS)
  for colorectal cancer, 2–3
FLI (irinotecan, leucovorin, and 5-FU). *See also individual drugs*
  for metastatic disease, 88
FLOX (5-fluorouracil, leucovorin, and oxaliplatin). *See also individual drugs*
  for colorectal cancer, 120
  for esophageal cancer, 72–73
FLP (5-fluorouracil, leucovorin, and cisplatin). *See also individual drugs*
  for esophageal cancer, 73
Fluorescence in situ hybridization (FISH)
  for metastatic colorectal cancer, 10
Fluorodeoxyglucose positron emission tomography (FDG PET)
  for gastrointestinal stromal tumors, 155
Fluoropyrimidines
  for esophageal cancer, 47, 71, 73–74
  for gastric cancer, 82
  for gastrointestinal tumors, 179
  for hepatocellular carcinoma, 99
  for metastatic disease, 85, 87
5-Fluorouracil (5-FU). *See also* DCF; ECF; FAM; FAMTX; FEM; FLI; FLOX; FLP; FOLFIRI; FOLFOX; FOLFOXIRI; FUFOX; IFL; UFT
  for esophageal cancer, 32, 37, 39, 47, 50, 71, 73, 82, 117, 118, 123
  infusional versus bolus, 123
  for gastrointestinal tumors, 179, 180–181
  with leucovorin, 181
5-Fluorouracil-based chemoradiation regimens
  for metastatic colorectal cancer, 123
  for pancreatic cancer, 140, 141
    advanced or metastatic, 145*t*
    locally advanced, 142, 145–146*t*
FOBT. *See* Fecal occult blood test (FOBT)
FOLFIRI (5-FU, leucovorin, and irinotecan). *See also individual drugs*
  with cetuximab, 10, 12*t*, 131
  for colorectal cancer, 120, 125–126, 126*t*, 127–128, 134
  for metastatic colorectal cancer, 10, 12t, 88, 131
  with panitumumab, 131
FOLFOX (5-fluorouracil, leucovorin, and oxaliplatin). *See also individual drugs*
  with bevacizumab, 11, 13*t*, 184
  with cetuximab, 11, 12*t*
  for colorectal cancer, 118, 120, 125–128, 134
  for metastatic colorectal cancer, 11–12, 13*t*
  with panitumumab, 11, 13*t*
  for small bowel adenocarcinoma, 176, 177
FOLFOX4
  with bevacizumab, 128–129, 184
  with cetuximab, 131
  for colorectal cancer, 125, 127
  for metastatic colorectal cancer, 126, 128–129, 131
  with panitumumab, 131
FOLFOX6
  with bevacizumab, 120–121, 128–129
  for colorectal cancer, 126, 126*t*
  for metastatic colorectal cancer, 128–129
FOLFOX7, for colorectal cancer, 127
FOLFOXIRI (5-fluorouracil, leucovorin, oxaliplatin, and irinotecan). *See also individual drugs*
  for colorectal cancer, 127
FOLIRI
  with bevacizumab, 11, 13*t*
  for metastatic colorectal cancer, 11, 13*t*
  with panitumumab, 11, 13*t*
  for small bowel adenocarcinoma, 177
4D CT. *See* 4-Dimensional CT (4D CT)
4-Dimensional CT (4D CT)
  for esophageal cancer, 67, 68
FS. *See* Flexible sigmoidoscopy (FS)
5-FU. *See* 5-Fluorouracil (5-FU)
FUFOX (infusional 5-fluorouracil, leucovorin, and oxaliplatin). *See also individual drugs*
  for colorectal cancer, 126

Gastric cancer, 79–89
  diagnosis of, 81
  pathology of, 81
  prognosis of, 81–82
  risk factors of, 80–81
  screening of, 81
  signs and symptoms of, 81
  staging of, 81–82, 84*t*
  treatment for, 82–89

Gastric cancer—*(continued)*
    early stage disease, 82–85
      locally advanced disease, 85–86
      metastatic disease, 86–88
Gastroesophageal junction tumor (GEJ)
    radiation therapy for, 62*f*
    treatment for, 75, 76, 89
Gastrografin, for esophageal cancer, 23
Gastrointestinal anastomosis (GIA), 23
Gastrointestinal stromal tumors (GISTs), 151–160
    clinical presentation of, 154–155
    diagnosis of
      historical evolution, 151–152
      imaging, 155
    epidemiology of, 152
    histopathology of, 152–153, 153*f*
    molecular and genetic markers, 153–154, 154*f*
    prognostic markers
      anatomic location, 156
      histological characteristics, 156
      mutational analysis, 156
    treatment for, 156–160
      genetic predictors of efficacy in, 159–160
Gastrointestinal tumors, 179–185, 180*f*
    apoptosis induction, 182
    cell cycle agents, 182
    insulin-like growth factor receptors for, 185
    microtubule stabilizing agents, 182–183
    multikinase inhibitors for, 185
    proteasome inhibition, 182
    targeted agents for, 183–185
    thymidylate synthase inhibitors for, 181
    topoisomerase inhibitiors for, 181–182
Gefitinib
    for esophageal cancer, 50
    with everolimus, 185
    for hepatocellular carcinoma, 102
GEJ. *See* Gastroesophageal junction tumor (GEJ)
Gemcitabine
    for gastrointestinal tumors, 181
    for hepatocellular carcinoma, 99
    with mapatumumab, 182
    for pancreatic cancer, 139–140, 141
      advanced or metastatic, 144–147, 146*f*
Gemcitabine-based chemoradiation regimens
    for locally advanced pancreatic cancer, 142, 143, 143*t*
GIA. *See* Gastrointestinal anastomosis
GISTs. *See* Gastrointestinal stromal tumors
Gross tumor volume (GTV), in radiation therapy. *See also*
    Target volumes, in radiation therapy
    esophageal cancer, 64–66
GTV. *See* Gross tumor volume (GTV)
Guaiac-based FOBT test. *See also* Fecal occult blood test
    for colorectal cancer, 2

HBV. *See* Hepatitis B virus (HBV) infection
HCC. *See* Hepatocellular carcinoma (HCC)
HCV. *See* Hepatitis C virus (HCV) infection
Helicobacter pylori infection, 80

Hepatitis B virus (HBV) infection
    and hepatocellular carcinoma, 94
Hepatitis C virus (HCV) infection
    and hepatocellular carcinoma, 94
Hepatocellular carcinoma (HCC), 93–109
    epidemiology of, 93–94
    living donor liver transplantation for, 96
    Milan criteria for, 96–97, 96*t*
      in MELD allocation system, 94–95
    orthotopic liver transplantation for, 94, 97, 97*t*
    transplantation history for, 94
    treatment for, 97–109
HER2, 53, 88
HPV. *See* Human papillomavirus (HPV) infection
Human papillomavirus (HPV) infection
    and anal cancer, 165

IFL (irinotecan, 5-FU, and leucovorin). *See also individual*
    drugs
    with bevacizumab, 128, 183–184
    for colorectal cancer, 120, 123
    for metastatic colorectal cancer, 128
IGF-1R. *See* Insulin-like growth factor-1 receptor (IGF-1R)
Imatinib, for gastrointestinal stromal tumors, 156, 157–159
Immunologically-based FOBT test. *See also* Fecal occult
    blood test
    for colorectal cancer, 2
IMRT. *See* Intensity modulated radiation therapy (IMRT)
Indisulam, for colorectal cancer, 182
Insulin-like growth factor-1 receptor (IGF-1R)
    with cetuximab, 185
    for gastrointestinal tumors, 185
    with irinotecan, 185
    role in metastatic colorectal cancer, 15
    with oxaliplatin, 185
Intensity modulated radiation therapy (IMRT). *See also*
    Radiation therapy
    for anal cancer, 169, 169*f*
    for esophageal cancer, 67
    for gastric cancer, 86
    for locally advanced pancreatic cancer, 143–144
Intraoperative endoscopy, for small bowel adenocarcinoma, 175
Irinotecan, 184–185. *See also* FLI; FOLFIRI; FOLFOXIRI;
    IFL; XELOXIRI
    with bortezomib, 182
    with cetuximab, 130–131, 183
    for colorectal cancer, 120*t*, 124
    for esophageal cancer, 72, 73
    with fluorouracil and leucovorin, 11, 13*t*
    with IGF-1, 185
    for metastatic colorectal cancer, 10, 11, 13*t*, 86,
      130–131, 182
    with mTOR, for xenografted tumors, 185
Irinotecan-based chemoradiation regimens, for esophageal
    cancer, 42, 45–46*t*
Irinotecan-based chemotherapy regimens, for metastatic
    disease, 88
Ivor Lewis esophagectomy. *See* Transthoracic esophagectomy
Ixabepilone, for gastrointestinal tumors, 182–183

KIT mutations, in gastrointestinal stromal tumors, 153, 156
KRAF mutations, in metastatic colorectal cancer, 10
    response to anticancer drugs, 10–15, 12–14*t*
KRAS mutations
    for gastrointestinal tumors, 182–183
    in hepatocellular carcinoma, 103

Lapatinib
    for hepatocellular carcinoma, 102, 103
    for HER2-positive gastric cancer, 88
    with paclitaxel, 88
LDLT. *See* Living donor liver transplantation (LDLT)
Leiomyosarcomas, DMAP for, 156
Leucovorin. *See also* FLI; FLOX; FLP: FOLFIRI; FOLFOX;
        FOLFOXIRI; FUFOX; IFL
    with 5-fluorouracil, 181
    for gastric cancer, 82, 83
Living donor liver transplantation (LDLT)
    for hepatocellular carcinoma, 96
        survival rate after, 96*t*
Lymphadenectomy extent, during esophageal cancer surgery,
        31–32

Magnetic resonance imaging (MRI)
    in gastrointestinal stromal tumors, 155
    for small bowel adenocarcinoma, 175
Mammalian target of rapamycin (mTOR) inhibitors
    for gastrointestinal tumors, 184–185
    for hepatocellular carcinoma, 104
    with irinotecan, for xenografted tumors, 185
    role in metastatic colorectal cancer, 15
Mapatumumab
    for gastrointestinal tumors, 182
    with gemcitabine, 182
Masitinib mesylate, for gastrointestinal stromal
        tumors, 158
mCRC. *See* Metastatic colorectal cancer (mCRC)
Mediastinal dissection, for esophageal cancer, 22–23
Metastatic colorectal cancer (mCRC), 9–16
    BRAF mutations in, 15
    chemotherapy for, 86, 123, 126, 128–131
    dual biologic therapy for, 11, 15
    EFGR mutations in, 10
    EFGR-targeted therapies for, 15
    KRAF mutations in, 10–15, 12–14*t*
Metastesectomy, for colorectal cancer, 133–134
Methotrexate, for metastatic disease, 86
Metronomic chemotherapy. *See also* Chemotherapy
    for hepatocellular carcinoma, 104
Microtubule stabilizing agents, for gastrointestinal tumors,
        182–183
MIE. *See* Minimally invasive esophagectomy (MIE)
Minimally invasive esophagectomy (MIE). *See also* Esophageal
        cancer
    comparison with OE, 31
    indications and contraindications for, 30
    operative technique, 30
    outcomes of, 30–31
Mitomycin. *See* DMAP

Mitomycin C. *See also* FAM; FEM
    for esophageal cancer, 71
    for metastatic disease, 86
MoAb. *See* Monoclonal antibodies
Molecular targeted therapy (MTT)
    with cytotoxic therapy, 104–109, 105*t*
    for esophageal cancer, 74–76, 75*t*
    for hepatocellular carcinoma, 99–109, 101–102*t*
Monoclonal antibodies (MoAb)
    for metastatic colorectal cancer, 183
MRI. *See* Magnetic resonance imaging (MRI)
mTOR. *See* Mammalian target of rapamycin inhibitors
        (mTOR)
MTT. *See* Molecular targeted therapy (MTT)
Multikinase inhibitors, for hepatocellular carcinoma, 185

NASH. *See* Nonalcoholic steatohepatitis (NASH)
Neoadjuvant therapy
    for colorectal cancer, 134
    for esophageal cancer, 20, 32, 39, 42, 47, 50, 64, 74
    for gastrointestinal stromal tumors, 155, 157–158
    for small bowel adenocarcinoma, 176–177
NGR-hTNF, for hepatocellular carcinoma, 100
Nirlotinib, for gastrointestinal stromal tumors, 159
Nolatrexed, for hepatocellular carcinoma, 97
Nonalcoholic steatohepatitis (NASH)
    and hepatocellular carcinoma, 94

OLT. *See* Orthotopic liver transplantation (OLT)
Oncogel, for esophageal cancer, 47
Orthotopic liver transplantation (OLT)
    for hepatocellular carcinoma, 94
        outcomes of, 97*t*
        survival rate after, 97
OSI-7904L
    with cisplatin, for gastric adenocarcinoma, 181
    with oxaliplatin, for colorectal cancer, 181
Oxaliplatin. *See also* EOF; EOX; FLOX; FOLFOX;
        FOLFOXIRI; FUFOX; XELOXIRI
    with bevacizumab, 184
    for colorectal cancer, 125
    for esophageal cancer, 71
    for hepatocellular carcinoma, 99
    with IGF-1, 185
    with irinotecan, 88
    for metastatic colorectal cancer, 10–11, 88
    with OSI-7904L, 181
    with pemetrexed, 181
Oxaliplatin-based chemoradiation regimens, for esophageal
        cancer, 42, 47, 48–49*t*

Paclitaxel
    for esophageal cancer, 47, 50, 72
    for metastatic disease, 86
Paclitaxel-based neoadjuvant chemoradiation regimens, for
        esophageal cancer, 39–42, 40–41*t*, 43–44*t*
Paclitaxel poliglumex (PPX)
    for esophageal cancer, 47
Palliative therapy, for esophageal cancer, 89

Pancreatic cancer, 139–147
adjuvant therapy for, 140–142
advanced or metastatic, 144–147, 146f
locally advanced, 142–144, 143t, 145–146t
Pancreaticoduodenectomy (Whipple procedure), 176
Panitumumab
for esophageal cancer, 53
for metastatic colorectal cancer, 11, 13t, 131–132, 183
Particle beam therapy, for locally advanced pancreatic cancer,
143–144
Pazopanib, for hepatocellular carcinoma, 100
PCR. See Polymerase chain reaction (PCR)
PDGFR. See Platelet-derived growth factor
receptor (PDGFR)
Pemetrexed
for gastrointestinal tumors, 181
with oxaliplatin, for colorectal cancer, 181
Perioperative chemotherapy. See also Chemotherapy
for esophageal cancer, 32–33
PET-CT. See Positron emission tomography-computed
tomography (PET-CT)
PGE2. See Prostaglandin E2 (PGE2)
PHY906, for hepatocellular carcinoma, 106–109
with capecitabine, 106–109, 108f
Planning target volume (PTV), in radiation therapy. See also
Target volumes, in radiation therapy
esophageal cancer, 65
Platelet-derived growth factor receptor (PDGFR)
in gastrointestinal stromal tumors, 153, 154
Platinum, for hepatocellular carcinoma, 99
Pneumonia, radiation therapy for, 64
Polymerase chain reaction (PCR)
for metastatic colorectal cancer, 10
Positron emission tomography-computed tomography
(PET-CT)
for esophageal cancer, 64–66, 66f
Postoperative chemoradiotherapy. See also Chemoradiation
therapy
for gastric cancer, 82–83
Postoperative chemotherapy. See also Chemotherapy
for gastric cancer, 85
PPX. See Paclitaxel poliglumex (PPX)
Pre-operative chemotherapy. See also Chemotherapy
for gastric cancer, 83–85
Prostaglandin E2 (PGE2), for esophageal cancer, 54
Proteasome inhibitors, for gastrointestinal tumors, 182
PTV. See Planning target volume (PTV)
Push enteroscope, for small bowel adenocarcinoma, 175
Pyloromyotomy, for esophageal cancer, 25
Pyloroplasty, for esophageal cancer, 25

Radiation therapy
for esophageal cancer, 61–68
for pancreatic cancer, 141–142
advanced or metastatic, 147
locally advanced, 142–144, 143t, 145–146t
Radiosensitizing drugs, for esophageal cancer, 47
Ras/Raf pathway, in esophageal cancer, 76
Robotic-assisted esophagectomy, 31

S-1
with cisplatin, 73–74, 87
for esophageal cancer, 47, 71, 73–74
with 5-flurouracil, 85
for gastric cancer, 82, 85
for gastrointestinal tumors, 181
with gimeracil, 85
for metastatic disease, 86, 87
with oteracil, 85
SB715992, for metastatic colorectal cancer, 182
SBA. See Small bowel adenocarcinoma (SBA)
SBFT. See Small bowel follow-through (SBFT)
SCBE test. See Single-contrast barium enema (SCBE) test
Single-contrast barium enema (SCBE) test. See also Double-
contrast barium enema test
for colorectal cancer, 3
Sirolimus, for hepatocellular carcinoma, 104
Small bowel adenocarcinoma (SBA), 173–178
clinical presentation of, 174
diagnosis of, 175–176
etiology of, 174
histology of, 173–174
prognosis of, 174–175
staging of, 174, 175t
treatment for, 176–177
Small bowel follow-through (SBFT)
for small bowel adenocarcinoma, 175
Sorafenib
with cisplatin, 76
with docetaxel, 76
for esophageal cancer, 76
for hepatocellular carcinoma, 100, 185
Split-course hypofractionated radiation, for esophageal
cancer, 38
Stereotactic radiation therapy. See also Radiation therapy
for locally advanced pancreatic cancer, 143, 144
Stool-based DNA test, for colorectal cancer, 5
Sunitinib
for gastrointestinal stromal tumors, 159
GI stromal tumors, 185
for hepatocellular carcinoma, 100
Surgery
for advanced or metastatic gastrointestinal stromal tumors, 156
for early gastrointestinal stromal tumors, 156
for small bowel adenocarcinoma, 176

Tamoxifen plus doxorubicin, for hepatocellular carcinoma,
98–99
Target volumes, in radiation therapy
esophageal cancer, 64–66
Taxane-based chemoradiation regimens, for esophageal cancer,
39–42, 40–41t, 43–44t
Taxane-based chemotherapy regimens, for metastatic disease,
87–88
TCM. See Traditional Chinese medicine (TCM)
Tegafur. See UFT
Telcyta, for gastrointestinal tumors, 182
Thalidomide, for hepatocellular carcinoma, 104
THE. See Transhiatal esophagectomy (THE)

3D conformal radiation therapy (3DCRT)
    for esophageal cancer, 67
3DCRT. *See* 3D conformal radiation therapy (3DCRT)
Three-field lymph node dissection, for esophageal cancer, 26
Thymidylate synthase inhibitors, for gastrointestinal
        tumors, 181
Topoisomerase inhibitiors, for gastrointestinal tumors, 181–182
Traditional Chinese medicine (TCM)
    for hepatocellular carcinoma, 104–109
Transhiatal esophagectomy (THE), 22–24. *See also* Esophageal
        cancer
    complications of, 23–24
    and en bloc esophagectomy, comparison, 28
    indications and contraindications for, 22
    operative technique
        abdominal phase, 22
        cervical esophagogastric anastomosis, 23
        cervical phase, 22
        mediastinal dissection, 22–23
    and transthoracic esophagectomy, comparison, 26
    and vagal-sparing esophagectomy, comparison, 30
Transthoracic esophagectomy, 24–26. *See also* Esophageal
        cancer
    complications of, 26
    indications and contraindications for, 24–25
    operative technique
        abdominal portion, 25
        right thoracotomy, 25–26
    and transhiatal esophagectomy, comparison, 26
Trastuzumab, for HER2-positive gastric cancer, 88
Trimodality therapy. *See also* Combined-modality therapy
    versus definitive chemoradiation, for esophageal cancer,
        54–56, 55*t*
    versus surgery, for esophageal cancer, 37–39, 38*t*

UFT (5-fluorouracil, tegafur, and uracil). *See also individual*
        drugs
    for esophageal cancer, 71
    for hepatocellular carcinoma, 99
    for metastatic colorectal cancer, 181
Uracil. *See* UFT

Vagal-sparing esophagectomy (VSE). *See also* Esophageal cancer
    and en bloc esophagectomy, comparison, 30
    operative technique, 29–30
    outcomes of, 30
    and transhiatal esophagectomy, comparison, 30
Vascular endothelial growth factor (VEGF) inhibitors, 53–54,
        89, 120
    in esophageal cancer, 75–76
    -targeted therapy, for gastrointestinal tumors, 183–184
VCE. *See* Video capsule endoscopy (VCE)
VEGF. *See* Vascular endothelial growth factor (VEGF)
    inhibitors
Video capsule endoscopy (VCE)
    for small bowel adenocarcinoma, 175, 176
Vindesine, for esophageal cancer, 71–72
Vinorelbine
    for esophageal cancer, 71–72
    for metastatic disease, 86
VSE. *See* Vagal-sparing esophagectomy (VSE)

XELIRI, for metastatic colorectal cancer, 181
Xeloda. *See* Capecitabine
XELOX, for colorectal cancer, 121–123, 125
    metastatic, 123, 181
    stage I, 122
    stage II, 122
    stage III, 122–123
XELOXIRI (irinotecan, oxaliplatin, and capecitabine). *See also*
        individual drugs
    with cisplatin, 62–63, 74, 76
    for colorectal cancer, 118, 123
    for hepatocellular carcinoma, 99
    for HER2-positive gastric cancer, 88
    with leucovorin, 118, 121–123, 124, 140,
        141, 144
    with levamisole, 118, 123
    for metastatic colorectal cancer, 62–63, 74, 76, 118,
        121–123, 124, 127
    for pancreatic cancer, 140, 141, 144
    for small bowel adenocarcinoma, 176
    with trastuzumab, 88